ADVANCES IN CANCER RESEARCH

VOLUME 26

Contributors to This Volume

P. Bentvelzen   Luka Milas

Pelayo Correa   Martin T. Scott

William Haenszel   Jack G. Stevens

J. Hilgers   Lee W. Wattenberg

ADVANCES IN
CANCER RESEARCH

Edited by

GEORGE KLEIN

Department of Tumor Biology
Karolinska Institutet
Stockholm, Sweden

SIDNEY WEINHOUSE

Fels Research Institute
Temple University Medical School
Philadelphia, Pennsylvania

Volume 26—1978

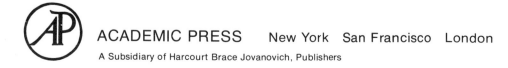

ACADEMIC PRESS   New York   San Francisco   London
A Subsidiary of Harcourt Brace Jovanovich, Publishers

ACADEMIC PRESS, INC.
111 Fifth Avenue, New York, New York 10003

United Kingdom Edition published by
ACADEMIC PRESS, INC. (LONDON) LTD.
24/28 Oval Road, London NW1

LIBRARY OF CONGRESS CATALOG CARD NUMBER: 52–13360

ISBN 0–12–006626–2

PRINTED IN THE UNITED STATES OF AMERICA

CONTENTS

The Epidemiology of Large-Bowel Cancer

PELAYO CORREA AND WILLIAM HAENSZEL

Interaction between Viral and Genetic Factors in Murine Mammary Cancer

J. HILGERS AND P. BENTVELZEN

Inhibitors of Chemical Carcinogenesis

LEE W. WATTENBERG

Latent Characteristics of Selected Herpesviruses

JACK G. STEVENS

Antitumor Activity of *Corynebacterium parvum*

LUKA MILAS AND MARTIN T. SCOTT

CONTRIBUTORS TO VOLUME 26

Numbers in parentheses indicate the pages on which the authors' contributions begin.

P. BENTVELZEN, *Radiobiological Institute TNO, Rijswijk, The Netherlands* (143)

PELAYO CORREA, *Louisiana State University Medical Center, New Orleans, Louisiana* (1)

WILLIAM HAENSZEL,* *National Cancer Institute, Bethesda, Maryland* (1)

J. HILGERS, *The Netherlands Cancer Institute, Amsterdam, The Netherlands* (143)

LUKA MILAS, *Central Institute for Tumors and Allied Diseases, Zagreb, Croatia, Yugoslavia* (257)

MARTIN T. SCOTT, *Department of Experimental Immunobiology, Wellcome Research Laboratories, Beckenham, England* (257)

JACK G. STEVENS, *Reed Neurological Research Center and Department of Microbiology and Immunology, School of Medicine, University of California, Los Angeles, California* (227)

LEE W. WATTENBERG, *Department of Laboratory Medicine and Pathology, University of Minnesota, Minneapolis, Minnesota* (197)

* Present address: Illinois Cancer Council, Chicago, Illinois.

THE EPIDEMIOLOGY OF LARGE-BOWEL CANCER

Pelayo Correa and William Haenszel[1]

Louisiana State University Medical Center, New Orleans, Louisiana,
and National Cancer Institute, Bethesda, Maryland

[1] Present address: Illinois Cancer Council, Chicago, Illinois.

1

I. Introduction

Prior to the 1960 decade, large-bowel cancer received only cursory attention from epidemiologists. For many years virtually all the epidemiological data for this site had been assembled as a by-product of periodic multipurpose analyses of death certificates and of reports of newly diagnosed cancer cases sent to tumor registries. Within the digestive tract, stomach attracted more attention and the systematic assembly of descriptive data to develop or test etiological hypotheses for cancer of the colon and rectum remained a neglected field.

Why did this condition prevail? While there is no certain answer, one probable reason was that epidemiologists in North America and western Europe were bemused by the impression of little variation in risk for large-bowel cancer within their respective countries. This, coupled with the fact that clinical investigators had assembled substantial amounts of data on genetically determined diseases (familial polyposis, Gardner's syndrome, Crohn's disease, etc.) associated with high risks for large-bowel cancer that emphasized the role of host characteristics, tended to direct interest away from the study of possible environmental factors. The outcome was that epidemiologists in North America and western Europe ignored large bowel because they viewed the local experience as "normal," while investigators working in low-risk countries had little incentive to study these neoplasms, which were unimportant sources of morbidity in their populations.

The turning point in the epidemiology of large-bowel cancer came with the systematic compilation of incidence data from cancer registries throughout the world. While these efforts were antedated by Segi's compilations of cancer mortality statistics beginning with 1950 (Segi, 1960), which described sizable gradients in large-bowel cancer death rates—the differences being on the order of 6 to 1 between countries at the two extremes of the risk spectrum—the mortality data had been discounted on the grounds that the contrasts were inflated by intercountry differences in diagnostic and treatment facilities and death certification practices. This attitude began to change when the data in the first edition of "Cancer Incidence in Five Continents" (Doll *et al.*, 1966) proved to be consistent with and reinforced the mortality findings. Within a short time span, the concept of substantial intercountry variation in large-bowel cancer risk gained wide acceptance as a prime epidemiologic characteristic of this disease. This feature was stressed at the meeting of the International Working Party of the World Organization of Gastroenterology in 1963, which also noted differences in the presentation of tumors by anatomical segment in high- and low-risk populations (Boyd *et al.*, 1964). Interpopulation differences were the source and inspiration for Burkitt's hypothesis on the causal role of a low-bulk, high-starch diet in large-bowel cancer (Burkitt, 1971a; Burkitt *et al.*, 1972). Burkitt's conjectures have been followed by more systematic correlations of global data on food consumption and incidence and/or mortality from large-bowel cancer (Howell, 1974, 1975; Armstrong and Doll, 1975), which have generated other dietary hypotheses.

The international comparisons pointing to environmental factors as important risk determinants have been reinforced by observations that showed migrants coming to the United States from low-risk European countries and Japan to acquire within their lifetime the high risks characteristic of the host population of U.S. whites (Haenszel, 1961; Haenszel and Kurihara, 1968). The latter in turn stimulated studies of diet and related factors among migrants and control populations in the countries of origin and destination (Haenszel *et al.*, 1973; Bjelke, 1974).

The contrasts of high- and low-risk populations revived some earlier work on associated pathologies. Helwig's autopsy studies in St. Louis on the distribution of adenomatous polyps, published in 1947, had described a congruence in the anatomical distribution of adenomatous polyps and intestinal carcinomas and identified adenomatous polyps as a possible precursor lesion (Helwig, 1947). Helwig's findings stimulated other work in the United States (Blatt, 1961; Chapman, 1963; Arminski and McLean, 1964; Spratt *et al.*, 1958), but the issue of presence or absence of congruence in the distribution of polyps and tumors remained unresolved, not because of lack of diligence or ingenuity on the part of the investigators, but primarily from the inability of observational settings within a single country to distinguish and choose among the alternatives. Correa *et al.* (1972) in their work stressed the need for comparative autopsy studies in populations at high risk and low risk to large-bowel cancer. This approach established striking differences in prevalence and anatomic distribution in the two types of populations and strengthened the case for intestinal polyps (or certain subtypes of polyps) as precursors of large-bowel carcinomas. The polyp findings raise the possibility of transforming the epidemiology of large-bowel cancer into the epidemiology of intestinal polyps and other suspect antecedent conditions, a step that would facilitate investigations of dietary factors. Diet histories are notoriously difficult to collect and the problems of response are magnified when the data sought relate to practices in the distant past. Case-control studies that focus on a condition presenting early in the sequence of events culminating in large-bowel cancer should afford better opportunities of uncovering dietary associations.

Wynder and Shigematsu (1967) reviewed the literature up to 1966. Haenszel and Correa (1971) later considered the epidemiological findings on magnitude of incidence rates, the sex–age patterns of incidence, and the anatomic localization of tumors in relation to the findings from autopsy studies on the distribution of intestinal polyps. Undoubtedly the most comprehensive review of the epidemiological literature bearing on large-bowel cancer has been carried out by Bjelke as part of his studies of digestive tract cancers among Norwegian "sedentes" and migrants. Bjelke's complete dissertation (1973) is available only as a microfilm reproduction, but a summary of the dissertation highlights has been published (Bjelke, 1974). The present review touches on many of the topics covered in earlier reviews, and when possible the findings have been updated. We have made extensive reference to the most recent cancer registry data published in the third edition of "Cancer Incidence in Five Continents" (Waterhouse *et al.*, 1976) and have considered information from comparative studies of intestinal polyps in high- and low-risk populations that has become available since 1970. An assessment of animal studies and the development of animal models to test and elaborate mechanisms for the production of large-bowel tumors, which have been stimulated by the epidemiological findings, is outside the scope of this review. We do attempt to identify profitable areas for epidemiological studies that are suggested by findings from animal work, since a review of the rapidly expanding field presented by research on large-bowel cancer requires one to place past and current events in context of their implications for future work.

II. Demographic Factors

A. INTERCOUNTRY VARIATION

"Cancer Incidence in Five Continents," third edition (Waterhouse *et al.*, 1976), is the primary source of information on interpopulation variation in risk of large-bowel cancer. Figure 1 summarizes the inci-

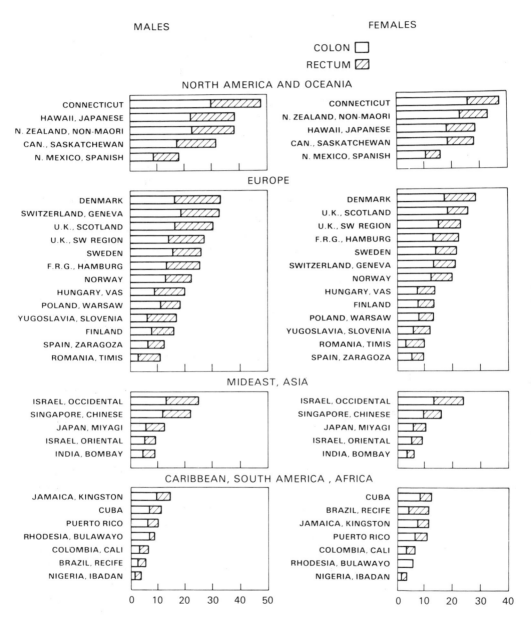

FIG. 1. Age-adjusted incidence rates for cancer of the large bowel (colon and rectum), by sex. Selected registries, variable periods close to 1970. Source: Waterhouse *et al.* (1976).

dence rates, age-adjusted to the world population standard, for selected registries contributing to that publication. The conventional subdivision of large bowel into colon and rectum is somewhat arbitrary and differences in classification and reporting practices may have introduced incomparabilities into the results for the two anatomical segments. For this reason the initial presentation represented by Fig. 1 emphasizes the incidence rates for total large bowel, although the separate contributions for colon and rectum are indicated. The presentation has been organized by regions of the world to highlight the interregional variation which has been and remains a distinctive epidemiological characteristic of this cancer site. Two criteria were followed for the inclusion of registries in Fig. 1. Registries with representative experience for each region were chosen, supplemented by countries deviating from regional norms to underscore the presence of variations in risks within individual regions. The inclusion of the Spanish-surname population of New Mexico (of predominantly Mexican origin) documents the presence within the United States of groups at relatively low risk to bowel cancer. To condense the presentation, data available from several cancer registries in the United States, Canada, England, and Japan reporting comparable experience were omitted. For example, the Connecticut and Saskatchewan registries were selected to describe the rates typical of registries in the Northern United States and Canada.

For males the ratios in risk between populations at the two extremes of the disease spectrum are on the order of 6–8 to 1; a similar, but slightly weaker, relationship prevails for females. Both sexes yield essentially similar rankings of countries by order of large-bowel cancer risk. The highest incidence is reported by registries in North America and Oceania (United States, Canada, New Zealand). The European registries assume an intermediate position and can be further subdivided into western Europe and Scandinavia and eastern Europe and the Balkans, the first group of countries having generally higher rates. The lowest rates are found in Asia, Africa, and Latin America.

Not all populations are covered by cancer registries, and we have consulted the mortality data assembled by Segi for countries with adequate diagnostic and medical care facilities (Segi and Kurihara, 1972) and the relative frequency information from hospital and necropsy sources compiled by Dunham and Bailar (1968) for supplementary information to round out the global description of large-bowel cancer risk. The essential findings of Dunham and Bailar on the geographical distribution of large-bowel cancer are contained in the map for males reproduced from their publication (Fig. 2). Their infor-

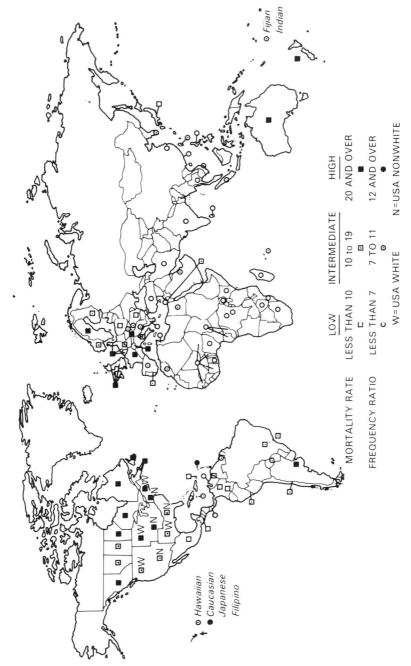

FIG. 2. World map of risks for cancer of the colon and rectum among males. Source: Dunham and Bailar (1968).

mation based on sources available as of 1967 agrees in most respects with the picture portrayed by the incidence data.

The mortality data for most of the west European countries (Austria, Denmark, England and Wales, France, Germany, Switzerland) appear to be consistent with the general characterization of this part of the world by the incidence data as a high-to-intermediate risk zone. However, it should be noted that the mortality data collected by Segi have consistently described Scotland to be a high-risk population. Doll (1969) considered Scotland to have the world's highest bowel cancer rate, certainly much higher than that of England, and Berg (1972) after review of the distribution of bowel cancer deaths within Scotland commented that, unlike in the United States, Denmark, and Norway, bowel cancer did not appear to be a predominantly urban disease in Scotland. The highest rates were in predominantly rural counties, 7 of which formed a contiguous band across north-central Scotland.

Dunham and Bailar were unable to secure much detail on the status of the Balkan and east European countries, but the information at their disposal placed these populations in the low-to-intermediate range. The establishment of more registries in these countries and the steady accumulation of new incidence data now confirm the presence there of relatively low risks, although for the most part the incidence rates tend to be higher than in Asian, African, and Latin American populations. The low incidence reported by the recently established registry in Zaragoza, Spain is consistent with the scanty relative frequency data for the Iberian peninsula assembled by Dunham and Bailar, and the collective information strongly suggests that bowel cancer risk in Spain more closely resembles the experience of eastern than western Europe.

All the tumor registries in Asia have consistently described low incidence rates for large-bowel carcinoma, and the results for selected registries from these continents in Fig. 1 can be viewed as typical. No populations with rates approaching those attained in North America or western Europe have been pinpointed, and the evidence from relative frequency data based on necropsy and hospital admission data coincide closely with the registry findings. The two population outliers with risks approaching the European intermediate level are Israeli Jews born in Europe or North America and the Singapore Chinese. The environmental exposures and food habits of the Israeli probably reflect their earlier experience abroad more closely than their current life-style in Israel. The contrast between Israelis born in North Africa or Asia and those born in Europe or North America is substantial, the bowel cancer risks for the latter being roughly 2.5 times greater.

The two African registries included in Fig. 1 rank close to the bottom of the list in magnitude of bowel cancer rates. These findings are consistent with those reported for the South African Bantu by Higginson and Oettlé (1960). The relative frequency data of Dunham and Bailar uniformly describe very low risks for Africa south of the Sahara and suggest no more than low-to-intermediate risks for African countries bordering on the Mediterranean.

Latin America presents a more heterogeneous pattern of bowel cancer risks than Africa or Asia. While many Latin American populations (Cali, Colombia; Recife, Brazil) display low rates comparable to those encountered in Africa and Asia, other populations appear to be at higher risk. The inter-American study of mortality (Puffer and Griffith, 1967) reported bowel cancer mortality in La Plata, Argentina to be only slightly less than that in San Francisco, California and Bristol, England, and the same source described intermediate rates for São Paulo and Ribeirão Prêto in Brazil (see Table I). The relative frequency data of Dunham and Bailar depict intermediate risks for Paraguay, and the collective information suggests a zone of intermediate to high bowel cancer risk extending from southern Brazil to Uruguay, Paraguay, and Argentina. The risk in the São Paulo area may be even higher than indicated by the reported data. There has been substantial migration from poverty-stricken, northeast Brazil (which the Recife data suggest to be a low-risk area) to the São Paulo

TABLE I

AGE-ADJUSTED MORTALITY RATES PER 100,000 POPULATION
FOR CANCER OF THE LARGE BOWEL IN 12 CITIES[a]

City (country)	Bowel cancer (ICD 153–154)
San Francisco (United States)	13.0
Bristol (England)	12.9
La Plata (Argentina)	12.6
São Paulo (Brazil)	7.1
Santiago (Chile)	6.8
Ribeirão Prêto (Brazil)	6.4
Lima (Peru)	6.0
Caracas (Venezuela)	5.6
Mexico City (Mexico)	4.0
Guatemala City (Guatemala)	3.6
Bogotá (Colombia)	3.4
Cali (Colombia)	3.3

[a] Source: Puffer and Griffith (1967).

region, and the presence of a low-risk migrant population may have depressed the rates reported for São Paulo. Future studies should determine whether the São Paulo rate represents an average of a high risk among natives and a low rate for recent migrants.

The available information on operations and completeness of case coverage of the several registries would contraindicate interpretation of the findings as due solely to differences in diagnostic and medical care facilities. While the adequacy of diagnostic and medical care facilities vary, they seem unlikely to account for differences of the magnitude observed. The more recent incidence data collected by newly established tumor registries are important in elaborating and confirming earlier impressions from relative frequency presentations of necropsy and hospital admission data on striking geographical differences in bowel cancer risks.

B. COLON–RECTUM RATIOS

Inspection of Fig. 1 suggests a rough parallelism in the separate population rankings by order of risk for cancer of the colon and rectum, although the ranking for rectum deviates in some respects from the pattern presented for colon. The variation in rectal cancer incidence among the high-risk populations of North America and western Europe falls into a narrower range than does that for colon. While the lower colon cancer incidences in eastern Europe, Asia, Africa, and Latin America have their counterparts in lower rectal cancer rates, the internal relationships between colon and rectal cancer incidence rates become more variable in the latter populations. Despite obvious exceptions for individual registries the graph of the joint distribution of rates for colon and rectum for 28 registries in 26 countries (Fig. 3) reveals a strong correlation in the incidence rates for the two conventional subdivisions of the large bowel. A significant feature of Fig. 3 is the sex difference in the relationship between the incidence rates for colon and rectum. Females show a steeper rise in colon incidence for each unit increase in rectum incidence, the slope of the female regression curve being estimated as 1.72, substantially in excess of the slope estimate of 1.26 for males.

Discordances or systematic differences in the relationships of incidence for the two localizations can be simply expressed as colon–rectum ratios. The colon–rectum ratios of age-adjusted incidence for selected registries are given in Fig. 4. The greater female slope values for the regression of colon against rectal cancer incidence implies the presence of higher colon–rectum ratios for females in populations at

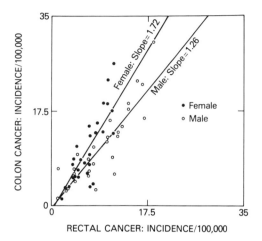

FIG. 3. Joint distribution of age-adjusted incidence rates for cancer of the colon and rectum, by sex. Selected registries, variable periods close to 1970. Source: Waterhouse *et al.* (1976).

high-risk to bowel cancer, and this feature is well expressed in Fig. 4. The Connecticut and the Hawaiian Japanese results are typical of those for North America. The registries in western Europe present more variable colon–rectum ratios. The results for Sweden, which are

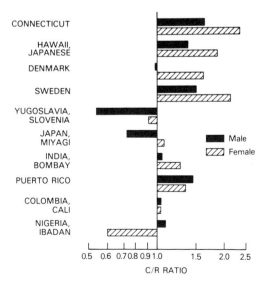

FIG. 4. Colon–rectum (C/R) ratios of age-adjusted incidence rates, by sex. Selected registries, variable periods close to 1970. Source: Waterhouse *et al.* (1976).

similar to those for Switzerland and Norway, resemble those reported from North American registries. The Danish data describe a distinctive and atypical low colon–rectum ratio of 0.93 for males which is primarily attributable to the high male incidence of rectal cancer in that country; this feature is not shared by Danish females who have a colon–rectum ratio of 1.61 that typifies western European populations. The eastern European registries on the other hand report distinctly lower colon–rectum ratios that are often below unity. The results for Yugoslavia (Slovenia) are characteristic of the ratios obtained in Hungary and Romania. The registry for the city of Warsaw, Poland is exceptional in describing colon–rectum values of 1.42 and 1.59 for males and females, respectively. The registries in Finland and Spain also exhibit colon–rectum ratios intermediate to those reported from eastern and western Europe.

Generally lower colon–rectum ratios prevail in Asian and African populations and the results for Japan (Miyagi), India (Bombay), and Nigeria (Ibadan) appear representative of the prevailing pattern in that part of the world. The findings for Caribbean and South American countries are more variable. The results for Puerto Rico in Fig. 4 are representative of the more elevated colon–rectum ratios reported from Cuba and Kingston, Jamaica. They deviate markedly from the colon–rectum ratio close to unity reported by the registry in Cali, Colombia. The data from Recife, Brazil coincide with the Cali experience of a colon–rectum ratio close to unity for males, but Recife is exceptional in exhibiting a female deficit in colon cancer (colon–rectum ratio of 0.53), which runs contrary to the normal rule of higher colon–rectum ratios for females. This same feature of a female deficit in colon cancer also appears in the data from Ibadan, Nigeria.

Part of the population variation in colon–rectum ratios presumably arises from different practices in classifying tumors presenting near the rectosigmoid flexure. Registries do not follow completely uniform practices in assignment of these tumors to sigmoid colon or rectum, which introduces an extraneous source of variation into the calculation of colon–rectum ratios. For example, the colon–rectum ratios in Norway have been inflated in the past by assignment of rectosigmoid tumors to sigmoid colon rather than to rectum (Eisenberg et al., 1964), the latter being the usual practice and one followed in Connecticut and the U.S. cancer morbidity surveys. Data from the latter two sources suggest that rectosigmoid lesions may account for 15–25% of the rectal cancers in high-risk populations, which probably represents a maximum estimate for the concentration of rectosigmoid tumors. This figure does not appear to be large enough to make classification artifacts an attractive explanation of the pattern of results described in Figs. 3 and 4. The most extreme assumptions would not reduce the colon–rectum ratios for North America and western Europe to the values close to or below unity described for Asian and African registries. The sex differences in the behavior of the colon–rectum ratios also argue against an explanation based on classification artifacts, since this would imply sex differences in criteria for tumor localizations in some populations.

C. ANATOMIC LOCALIZATION

The variable colon–rectum ratios suggest that colon and rectum may have related, but not identical, etiologies. The somewhat greater interpopulation variation in colon cancer risks raises the possibility that the variation may be concentrated in certain segments proximal to the rectosigmoid flexure, an idea supported by earlier reviews of the localization of colon tumors that had described low-risk communities to present an excess of right-sided cancers and high-risk communities to have an excess of left-sided cancers (Boyd *et al.*, 1964; Correa and Llanos, 1966; Payne, 1963). Haenszel and Correa (1971) collected more detailed data from cancer registries covering high- and low-risk populations and calculated the ratio of sigmoid tumors to those located in the cecum–ascending colon and in the rectum. Their results in the form of sigmoid–ascending and sigmoid–rectum ratios for 7 tumor registries arranged in ascending order of total colon cancer incidence are reproduced in Table II. Although interpretation was complicated by the substantial number of tumors of unspecified location, they concluded that the sigmoid–ascending and sigmoid–rectum ratios increased with overall level of colon cancer risk and that this particular feature was more pronounced among males. This pattern pointed to greater interpopulation variability in the sigmoid segment than in either the cecum-ascending or rectum segments. de Jong *et al.* (1972) investigated this subject in greater detail with similar results. For populations at widely different levels of colon cancer risk, they found differences in the segmental ratios of tumors similar to that described by Haenszel and Correa, but in the intermediate range they found no regular progression in ratios with increasing colon cancer risks.

The studies of Haenszel and Correa and de Jong *et al.* shared the defect that the basic tumor registry data relied on subjective criteria for tumor location, which vary from country to country and among physicians. J. W. Berg and W. Haenszel (personal communication, 1976) attempted to replace the subjective observations with objective mea-

TABLE II

RATIOS OF AGE-ADJUSTED INCIDENCE RATES OF SIGMOID
COLON/CECUM-ASCENDING COLON AND SIGMOID COLON/RECTUM
FOR CANCER REGISTRIES LISTED IN ASCENDING ORDER
OF TOTAL COLON CANCER INCIDENCE RATES[a]

Registry	Males		Females	
	Sigmoid/ cecum ascending	Sigmoid/ rectum	Sigmoid/ cecum ascending	Sigmoid/ rectum
India (Bombay), 1964–1967	0.20	0.04	0.33	0.04
Colombia (Cali), 1962–1968	0.20	0.10	0.42	0.12
Japan (Miyagi), 1959–1961	0.41	0.10	0.48	0.14
Puerto Rico, 1950–1968	0.71	0.16	0.89	0.28
Finland, 1964–1965	0.60	0.16	0.86	0.27
Norway, 1965–1966	1.17	0.55	0.92	0.76
Connecticut, 1960–1962	1.56	0.68	1.04	0.83

[a] Source: Haenszel and Correa (1971).

surements based on distance of the lower margin of the tumor from the pectinate line in six populations drawn from the extremes of bowel cancer incidence. In four populations covered by population-based tumor registries, incidence data were available, thus the observations could be converted into estimates of segment-specific incidence assuming that the sample of cases studied were representative of all cases diagnosed and reported to the tumor registries. The nature of the findings is illustrated in Table III contrasting a high-incidence population (Iowa) with a low-incidence population (Cali, Colombia). The segment-specific incidence rates to the sigmoid at least 16 cm distant from the anus are based on direct measurements; for the more proximal colon segments above the reach of a sigmoidoscope, the data still depend on subjective, nonquantitative criteria. The Iowa and Cali comparisons permit some tentative conclusions:

1. In the low-risk population (Cali) the cancer incidence for men and women was distributed much more uniformly by segments of the bowel. In the high-incidence population (Iowa), women presented the higher incidence in the segments proximal to the descending colon, whereas men presented the higher incidence not only in the sigmoid, but in the region 2–16 cm from the anus.

2. The Iowa–Cali ratios of incidence emphasized the great disparity in risk for the upper sigmoid (≥16 cm from the anus) and for the descending colon in both sexes. Cancer was extremely uncommon in these two segments in Cali (and the other low-risk populations studied); in Iowa more cancers were found there than in other colon segments. Proceeding proximally and distally from this region the ratios become progressively smaller for both sexes, and within 2–4 cm of the anus the differences between Cali and Iowa become minimal whether measured in absolute or relative terms.

3. While the incidence ratios emphasized the great disparity between Iowa and Cali in the upper sigmoid experience for men, the absolute differences in risk pinpoint the nearly equal importance of cancers in the 6–15-cm segment for both sexes. When the Iowa–Cali differences are examined on a per centimeter of length basis, the increments of risk in the 8–15-cm and 6–7-cm segments appear to be equal or greater than those for the upper sigmoid. (Although reference books disagree on the length of the sigmoid, none suggest that the length of the sigmoid above 15 cm is less than 10 cm) This 6–15-cm segment, then, encompassing what has traditionally been considered the upper rectum as well as the rectosigmoid, appears to be the locus of the greatest carcinogenic activity in populations at high bowel cancer risk.

TABLE III

ESTIMATED SEGMENT-SPECIFIC INCIDENCE RATES PER 100,000 POPULATION FOR BOWEL CANCER IN IOWA (HIGH RISK) AND CALI, COLOMBIA (LOW RISK), BY SEX

Segment	Estimated incidence				Difference: Iowa − Cali		Ratio: Iowa/Cali	
	Male		Female					
	Iowa	Cali	Iowa	Cali	Male	Female	Male	Female
Cecum	2.7	0.93	4.7	1.1	1.7	3.6	2.9	4.2
Ascending colon	2.9	0.78	3.8	0.61	2.1	3.2	3.7	6.3
Transverse colon	3.4	0.75	3.9	0.58	2.6	3.4	4.5	6.8
Descending colon	2.4	0.20	1.9	0.22	2.2	1.6	12.	8.5
Sigmoid colon								
≥16 cm	9.5	0.58	7.3	0.89	8.9	6.4	16.	8.4
8–15 cm	9.2	1.5	6.6	1.3	7.7	5.4	6.1	5.2
6–7 cm	2.7	0.80	2.0	0.48	1.8	1.5	3.3	4.2
4–5 cm	1.9	0.99	1.1	0.70	0.9	0.4	1.9	1.6
2–3 cm	1.3	0.66	0.67	0.64	0.7	0.03	2.0	1.0
0–1 cm	0.39	0.37	0.36	0.47	0.02	−0.1	1.1	0.8

[a] Source: J. W. Berg and W. Haenszel, personal communication (1976).

With only qualitative data on the segmental distribution of tumors available, Haenszel and Correa had no choice but to describe differences in sigmoid cancer incidence as the most characteristic separators of low- and high-incidence populations. Looking at quantitative changes, the most recent data suggest that in Iowa (and by inference the United States) the hypothesized bowel cancer factor may be exerting its greatest effect distal to the upper sigmoid colon, in the segment 6–15 cm above the anus. On a per unit length basis the sigmoid would be a region of somewhat less carcinogenic activity. In men the most distal 2 cm and in women the most distal 4 cm seem essentially to be unaffected by any bowel cancer factor peculiar to the United States. These anatomic differences in response could be due to differential sensitivity of the bowel to a carcinogen, but the contrasting locations of cancer in low- and high-risk populations exemplified by Iowa and Cali favor instead different levels of concentration of the responsible factor. Epidemiologically, many questions raised by the data on tumor location remain to be answered. However, the recent results derived from more precise measurements of tumor location appear to have important epidemiological implications. This information can be considered in the design of case-control studies of diet, for example. In the search for case-control differences bowel location may permit separations analogous to those achieved for stomach cancer by the intestinal-diffuse histologic separation made by Järvi (1962) and Lauren (1965). These separations, however, require that one abandon the old descriptive terms—rectum, rectosigmoid, etc.—and describe the location of distal large-bowel cancer more precisely.

D. MALE–FEMALE RATIOS

Figure 5 describes for colon and rectum the deviations from unity of the male–female ratios of age-adjusted incidence for representative registries covering high-, intermediate-, and low-risk populations. Little change has occurred in recent years as can be established by review of data from the three successive editions of "Cancer Incidence in Five Continents." The results suggest colon and rectum to have distinctive, rather than common, profiles of variation. Male–female ratios of less than unity are more frequently observed for colon, but each site is characterized by population differences in sex ratios. The sex ratios are more variable for rectum, with extreme values ranging from 1.7 to 0.6, as opposed to the narrower limits of 1.3 to 0.7 for colon. A more pronounced male excess for rectum is not an invariable rule. Several registries, including Puerto Rico; Kingston, Jamaica; Recife, Brazil; and Ibadan, Nigeria have reported lower sex ratios for colon.

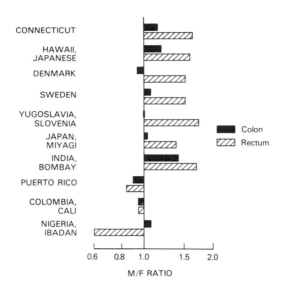

FIG. 5. Male-female (M/F) ratios of age-adjusted incidence rates for cancer of the large bowel (colon and rectum). Selected registries, variable periods close to 1970. Source: Waterhouse *et al.* (1976).

For the higher-risk populations of North America and western Europe the male–female ratios for colon tend to fall within a narrow band of deviations from unity. The most recent finding for the Hawaiian Japanese is close to normal limits and no longer exhibits the substantial and anomalous male excess reported in earlier years. An assessment for low-risk populations is more difficult, because the smaller number of colon cases observed led to wide confidence limits on the ratio estimates. Nevertheless, enough registries report a female predominance of colon cancer to support the belief of a true difference rather than a sampling variation artifact.

The higher male–female ratios of age-adjusted incidence for rectum than colon combined with the suggestion of a female excess of colon cancers in low-risk populations raises the possibility of segmental differences in sex ratios for the proximal bowel above the rectosigmoid flexure. The best and most extensive data on incidence specific for tumor location were collected in the U.S. Cancer Morbidity Survey of 1969–1971 (Cutler and Young, 1975). The results summarized in Table IV show the characteristic male excess for rectum to persist in the rectosigmoid and to be present in somewhat attenuated form in the sigmoid colon. A smaller male excess remains for descending and transverse colon, but the sex ratios for ascending colon and cecum are

TABLE IV

MALE–FEMALE (M/F) RATIOS OF AGE-ADJUSTED INCIDENCE RATES FOR CANCER
OF THE LARGE BOWEL BY ANATOMIC SEGMENT. UNITED STATES, 1969–1971[a]

| Segment | Incidence | | M/F ratio |
	Male	Female	
Cecum	5.7	5.5	1.04
Ascending colon	4.0	4.1	0.98
Transverse colon	5.2	4.7	1.11
Descending colon	2.9	2.6	1.12
Sigmoid colon	11.8	9.6	1.23
Rectosigmoid junction	4.8	3.1	1.55
Rectum	12.8	7.5	1.71

[a] Source: Cutler and Young (1975).

close to unity. Documentation of segmental differences in sex ratios from other sources is more difficult, because tumor location has not always been precisely specified and recorded by registries. Inspection of data from the Connecticut tumor registry appear to be consistent with the U.S. survey finding of a progressive dimunition in sex ratio as one traverses the large bowel from rectum to cecum.

Within the United States and other high-risk populations, the presence of higher male–female ratios for rectum can be traced to the earlier age at which the male excess risks become manifest. The data from the several U.S., Canadian, and western European sources indicate that the male incidence for rectum becomes clearly differentiated from the female risk by no later than age 55 or 60, a distinction that then persists to the end of the life-span. This contrasts sharply with colon cancer, for which the crossover from female to male dominance is delayed until age 65 or later, so that the smaller male–female ratios for colon reflect primarily a balance between the higher female risks at younger ages, and the higher male risks at older ages. Such findings suggest that the epidemiologic picture based on comparisons of age-adjusted rates alone may be obscured by sex–age interactions in the schedule of incidence rates and that examination of sex- and age-specific incidence is required.

E. SEX- AND AGE-SPECIFIC INCIDENCE

While the incidence of both colon and rectal cancers increases with age, the progression with age varies by anatomic site, population, and sex. Cook et al. (1969) computed the slopes of log incidence plotted against log age for 11 cancer registries with the following results: (a) the slopes of the male curves were consistently higher for both colon and rectum in all populations studied by them except Finland; (b) the variation in male–female differences for slope values was greater for colon than for rectum.

Although the slope values summarize the gross features of the incidence curves, they share with age-adjusted rates the inability to reveal the finer details of age–sex interactions. Haenszel and Correa (1971) inspected the sex- and age-specific incidence for several registries as of 1963–1965 from this point of view and believed that for colon cancer they could identify six rather distinct rate configurations. In developing their typology they first took note of the absolute magnitude of the incidence rates for the age group 65–74 years and grouped the registries into four categories as follows: A (150–300 new cases per 100,000 population per year); A_1 (80–<200); B (50–<150); C (10–40). Within each risk category the curves were then characterized with respect to slope, degree of curvature at older ages, and the relative positions of the male and female incidence curves. However, examination of the incidence data as of 1972–1974 did not reproduce the distinction drawn earlier between type A and A_1 registries. All the registries with age-specific incidence at 65–74 years of >100 exhibited similar slopes, and the presence or absence of a downturn in rates after age 75 was no longer correlated with the magnitude of incidence rates. The only feature continuing to differentiate the type A registries was the degree of male dominance in incidence after age 60 or 65. The Connecticut (United States), 1968–1972 excess in male risks after age 60 was more pronounced than in previous years, and the results for that registry shown in Fig. 6 are representative of those for Saskatchewan (Canada), 1969–1972; New Zealand, 1968–1971; Birmingham (England), 1968–1972, which we label type A_1. There is another subset of registries with a similar level of incidence for which the sex differential in risk at the older ages remains minimal, which we assign to the category A_2. The Southwest Region (England and Wales), 1966–1970 typifies the latter group, which includes Denmark, 1963–1967; Sweden, 1966–1970; Iowa (United States), 1969–1971.

Examination of the rates for low-risk, type C communities reveals several examples of higher female rates past age 60. This category, labeled C_1, includes Cali (Colombia), 1962–1971; Cuba, 1968–1972; Timis (Romania), 1970–1972; Oriental Jews (Israel), 1967–1971; Slovenia (Yugoslavia), 1968–1972. Other populations present several crossover points in the male and female incidence curves, giving the impression of a pattern changing from female to male predominance;

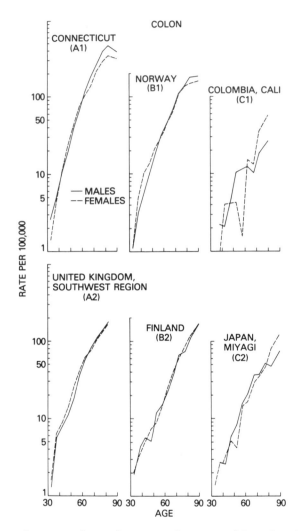

FIG. 6. Sex- and age-specific incidence rates for cancer of the colon. Selected registries, variable periods close to 1970. Source: Waterhouse *et al.* (1976).

Miyagi (Japan), 1968–1971 and Puerto Rico, 1968–1972 can be placed
in category C_2, retaining the same status held early in the 1960 decade.
The low-risk group also has clear examples of populations with dominant male risks after age 60; Kingston (Jamaica), 1967–1972 and Bombay (India), 1968–1972 can be placed in this group.

Review of the intermediate B-level registries discloses a similar
dichotomy. A majority exhibit modest male excesses at the older ages.

The results for Norway, 1968–1972 are representative of those for Hamburg (German Federal Republic), 1969–1972 and Vas (Hungary), 1968–1972, placed in category B_1. Registries that early in the 1960 decade displayed patterns suggesting a transition from female to male dominance subsequent to age 60 (Warsaw City, Poland; Slovenia, Yugoslavia) now appear to have emerged from the transitional phase to exhibit male dominance after age 65. The sex-specific incidence rates for Singapore, 1968–1972 and Zaragoza (Spain) 1968–1972, showed several crossover points, and these populations may be in a transitional phase leading to higher rates for older males at a future date. Finland, 1966–1970, still presents dominant female rates after age 60, type B_2. This feature was also exhibited by the New Mexico (United States) Spanish-surname population, 1969–1972.

The incidence patterns for rectal carcinoma can be related to the colon cancer typology by superimposing on the latter a stronger displacement to higher rectal cancer risks among older males. In the type A registries the male dominance at older ages for rectal cancer is universally accentuated, as illustrated by the results for Connecticut (United States) and the Southwestern Region (England and Wales) in Fig. 7. The same effect can be discerned for Norway (B_1), and this displacement suffices to transform the female colon cancer excess in Finland (B_2) to a male excess for rectal cancer. The shift to higher male rates also narrows the gap between male and female rates for several C-type registries. The results for Cali (Colombia) describe the situation for Cuba, Puerto Rico, Timis (Romania), and Oriental Jews (Israel). The dominant male risk in Miyagi (Japan) prevails also for Bombay (India).

The more detailed configurations of sex- and age-specific incidence may help elaborate some of the differences in sex ratios by anatomic segment described by the age-adjusted incidence rates, and to illustrate this point we refer again to the data for whites collected by the U.S. cancer morbidity survey for 1969–1971. Figure 8 shows the sex relationship of the incidence curves for cecum to diverge markedly from the pattern for ascending and sigmoid colon. In the high-risk United States white population the ascending and sigmoid segments are the major contributors to male predominance in colon cancer incidence after age 60. It is worth remarking that this particular feature of sex differentiation for ascending colon was lost in the presentation of age-adjusted rates in Table IV. The results for Connecticut, 1970–1972 are in substantial agreement with the picture portrayed by the United States survey data.

Differences in the anatomical distribution of colon tumors may be

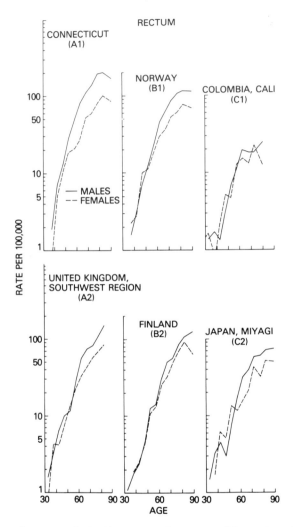

FIG. 7. Sex- and age-specific incidence rates for cancer of the rectum. Selected registries, variable periods close to 1970. Source: Waterhouse *et al.* (1976).

linked to the different configurations of male and female dominance for colon cancer portrayed by Fig. 9. For selected low- and intermediate-risk populations typed as B_1, B_2, C_1, and C_2, it would be desirable to conduct special studies of anatomic localization to ascertain whether the patterns of male and female dominance are correlated with different distributions of tumor localization.

F. INTRACOUNTRY (REGIONAL) VARIATION

The magnitude of the intercountry differences suggests the probable presence of intracountry differences as well, at least for countries with large land masses, since political boundaries are often artificial and unrelated to climate, terrain, and other environmental factors that control agricultural and food distribution practices that may influence the level of bowel cancer risk. Data from registry and vital statistics offices on this point are not routinely available for many countries, so that this topic cannot be treated in a systematic manner. Most of the information comes from developed countries at high- or intermediate-risk to the disease and the fortuitous presence of local registries in several countries (Brazil, Canada, England and Wales, United States) has provided additional data on regional variation.

This subject has been more intensively pursued in the United States than elsewhere, and elevated risks for both colon and rectum in the Northeast and in North Central regions and a below-average risk in the South have been demonstrated using a variety of source materials and study techniques. The National Cancer Institute morbidity surveys conducted in 1947–1948 and 1969–1971 (Dorn and Cutler, 1959; Cutler and Young, 1975) showed both white and black residents of the northern cities surveyed to have higher incidence than in the South (Table V). San Francisco–Oakland metropolitan area on the West

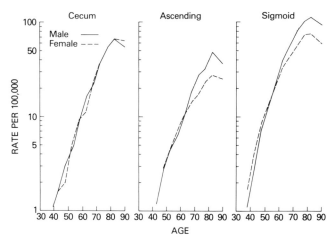

FIG. 8. Sex- and age-specific incidence rates for cancer of the cecum, ascending colon, and sigmoid colon. United States whites, 1969–1971. Source: Cutler and Young (1975).

TABLE V

NORTH–SOUTH RATIO OF AGE-ADJUSTED INCIDENCE RATES FOR CANCER OF THE COLON AND RECTUM, BY SEX. UNITED STATES, WHITES AND BLACKS, 1947–1948 AND 1969–1971[a]

| | 1947–1948 | | | | 1969–1971 | | | |
| | White | | Black | | White | | Black | |
Segment and survey area	Male	Female	Male	Female	Male	Female	Male	Female
Colon								
North								
Detroit	23.3	25.4	9.6	10.4	30.0	24.9	27.9	25.7
Pittsburgh	28.9	31.0	28.5	19.8	31.3	25.2	22.6	32.2
Iowa[b]	21.0	25.9	—	—	28.1	28.2	34.6	33.9
South								
Atlanta	19.2	12.0	6.8	4.8	26.7	24.1	21.3	24.0
Birmingham	17.4	24.9	14.4	6.8	21.1	22.7	18.0	20.8
Dallas–Forth Worth[c]	22.7	21.4	24.1	21.7	23.2	22.1	24.1	25.3
Ratio: North/South[d]	1.23	1.41	1.26	1.36	1.26	1.14	1.34	1.31
Rectum								
North								
Detroit	20.2	11.4	14.1	12.2	18.0	9.4	14.9	8.6
Pittsburgh	21.8	14.2	13.8	21.8	17.6	10.9	17.7	12.5
Iowa[b]	14.2	10.5	—	—	14.7	9.4	20.4	6.6
South								
Atlanta	8.8	10.4	7.1	9.0	11.3	6.8	10.2	6.9
Birmingham	13.9	7.2	13.4	8.8	9.5	7.9	6.8	4.7
Dallas–Forth Worth[c]	15.5	12.6	7.5	19.3	13.3	9.1	13.3	6.9
Ratio: North/South[d]	1.47	1.20	1.49	1.37	1.48	1.25	1.75	1.50

[a] Source: Dorn and Cutler (1959).

[b] Iowa data from 1950 instead of 1947–1948; 1950 black population too small for calculation of rates.

[c] Dallas only in 1947–1948.

[d] Ratio based on unweighted average of rates.

Coast displayed the incidence rates typical of northern cities. The same regional gradients have been reproduced in death certificate studies. Burbank (1971) in his review of the mortality data for 1950–1967 commented on the cluster of Northeast and Great Lake states with high death rates for colon and rectum among whites and the generally lower rates elsewhere, particularly in the South. His data for blacks also depicted lower risks in a tier of southern states extending from North Carolina to Texas. More detailed county maps based on data for 1950–1969 (Mason *et al.*, 1975) reinforced Burbank's presentation by states and showed the deficits in risk to be almost universal and widely dispersed in the area south of the Ohio River. This characteristic was displayed most prominently by white males.

The higher risks in the North can be attributed in part to elevated rates for residents of metropolitan areas, which tend to be concentrated in that part of the United States, but this factor alone cannot account for the regional gradient. Haenszel and Dawson (1965) studied a sample of deaths from bowel cancer with control for residence and found the deficit in the South to persist in urban and rural areas and metropolitan and nonmetropolitan counties. Nor was the North–South gradient related to the greater number of foreign-born in the Northeast and North Central regions, since the regional gradients in risk for large bowel remained unaltered when the contrasts were limited to native-born whites (Haenszel, 1961). In the latter respect large bowel differed from stomach, the concentration of foreign-born in the North being responsible for the higher stomach cancer risks there.

The third U.S. National Cancer Survey for 1969–1971 secured data on tumor localization for over 90% of bowel cancers. Analysis of the summary, age-adjusted rates did not demonstrate any differences in the proportion of tumors localized in the sigmoid and rectosigmoid segments among the areas surveyed, which would suggest that the North–South gradient in incidence was not confined to specific portions of the intestinal tract. Similar findings had been based on death certificate studies reported earlier by Haenszel and Dawson (1965).

Although the age-adjusted comparisons of the United States incidence and mortality data failed to uncover regional differences in tumor localization, the presence of interactions by age, sex, and anatomic segment noted earlier suggested that the more detailed information contained in the incidence curves by sex and age be explored. For total colon, the 3 northern areas combined (Detroit, Pittsburgh, State of Iowa) exhibit a more pronounced male excess risk at the older ages than the 3 southern communities (Atlanta, Birmingham, Dallas–Ft. Worth). The segment-specific data shown in Fig. 9 suggest this feature of regional difference to be concentrated in the sigmoid colon. For this segment the white male predominance appears well established by age 60 and sharply defined in the North in contrast to the South, where the male predominance in incidence appears to be delayed until after age 70. For both cecum and ascending colon, there is little sex difference in incidence at older ages in the North. In the South, the data at older ages show a female excess incidence for ascending colon, but a slight male excess in the cecum. The nature of the

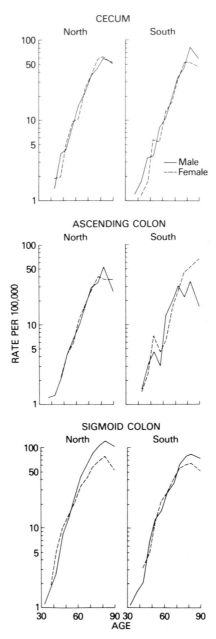

FIG. 9. Sex- and age-specific incidence rates for cancer of the cecum, ascending colon, and sigmoid colon. United States whites, 3 northern and 3 southern areas, 1969–1971. Source: Cutler and Young (1975).

United States findings are sufficiently promising and provocative to warrant pursuit in other study settings as the requisite information becomes available.

The Canadian provinces, in contrast to the United States, exhibit a more restricted range of variation in bowel cancer incidence, the peak rates, 25–30% above those for other provinces, being reported from Newfoundland at one end and British Columbia at the other end of the country (Table VI) (Waterhouse *et al.*, 1976). The results for British Columbia resemble those reported from the San Francisco Bay area of California. The more homogeneous data for the inland provinces may be related to the fact that the population of Canada is concentrated in a relatively narrow strip of land about 50–100 miles wide running from East to West.

The Scandinavian countries present a pattern of gradients in risk with latitude that resembles in certain respects the United States situation. Denmark presents higher bowel cancer risks than the other Scandinavian countries, and it has been observed that the highest rates in Sweden occur in the southwestern part of the country immediately adjacent to Denmark and that the risks diminish as one proceeds northward (National Board of Health and Welfare, 1971). Figure 10 describes the situation for colon cancer in Sweden as of 1959–1965. Data from Finland (Teppo *et al.*, 1975) present a similar geographic configuration. The lowest colon cancer incidence occurs in the northern and eastern regions of the country, and the rates in districts adjacent to the capital city of Helsinki in the south of Finland are more than 50% above those in the most northern districts; somewhat smaller

TABLE VI

AGE-ADJUSTED INCIDENCE RATES PER 100,000 POPULATION FOR CANCER
OF THE COLON AND RECTUM FOR 7 CANADIAN PROVINCES, BY SEX, 1969–1972[a]

Province	Colon		Rectum	
	Male	Female	Male	Female
Alberta	17.1	18.5	10.6	6.9
British Columbia	23.5	24.1	15.9	10.5
Manitoba	20.7	20.4	13.7	9.0
Maritime Provinces	19.3	23.4	13.5	9.9
Newfoundland	24.7	24.2	13.1	6.0
Quebec	16.2	18.1	12.7	8.5
Saskatchewan	17.8	18.9	13.8	9.4

[a] Source: Waterhouse *et al.* (1976).

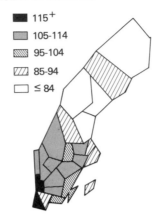

PERCENT OF AVERAGE

FIG. 10. Geographic variation in age-adjusted incidence of cancer of the colon, both sexes, in Sweden, 1959–1965. Source: National Board of Health and Welfare (1971).

differentials paralleling those for colon are also present for rectum. Figure 11 shows the variation in male colon cancer incidence within Finland. The results for Norway follow closely the pattern described for Sweden and Finland. The highest incidence of large-bowel cancer occurs in Oslo and adjacent counties in south Norway, and the lowest rates are found in the northern counties (Bjelke, 1973). The metropolitan conurbations in Scandinavia are located in the more southerly

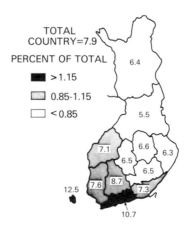

FIG. 11. Geographic variation in age-adjusted incidence of cancer of the colon, males, in Finland, 1966–1970. Source: Teppo et al. (1975).

latitudes, and the risk gradients are diminished, but do not disappear, with control for urbanization.

Clinicians in Brazil have felt large-bowel cancer to be a more serious problem in the south of Brazil than in the poverty-stricken northeast. These impressions have recently been reinforced by incidence data collected by tumor registries in Recife and São Paulo. The Recife registry covering the State of Pernambuco in the northeast has reported an age-adjusted bowel cancer incidence rate about half of that for São Paulo; 5.5 per 100,000 for males and 11.8 for females in Recife, compared to 15.6 for males and 17.8 for females in São Paulo (Waterhouse et al., 1976).

A systematic pattern of regional variation is not demonstrable everywhere. In England and Wales the several regional registries reveal a rather compressed range of incidence rates for large-bowel cancer, the difference between the extremes being on the order of 25% (Waterhouse et al., 1976). No obvious geographic configuration is suggested, although somewhat higher risks prevail in the Birmingham and Liverpool regions. Differences of this magnitude might arise from local differences in reporting and completeness of coverage of cases. The variation in mortality from large-bowel cancer in Japan has been studied by Segi et al. (1965), who found no regular pattern of changes in risk with latitude. The prefectures at higher risk tended to be located in the central part of the main island of Honshu bordering on the Japan Sea. Review of the published and unpublished data from prefectural tumor registries in Japan coincide with the mortality studies in suggesting regional variation not to be a prominent epidemiological feature of bowel cancer in Japan.

The status of within-country variation in bowel cancer risk might be summarized as follows. In large countries or in those extending over a wide range of latitudes, regional differences that mimic the international variations in total bowel cancer incidence have been observed. In small, geographically compact countries even if regional differences did exist, the observational situation would not favor their detection. The use of summary, age-adjusted data has not described important regional differences in risk associated with specific tumor localizations for countries where the requisite data are available. This failure may be consistent with the inability of de Jong et al. (1972) to find differences in the proportion of sigmoid tumors in comparisons of populations with relatively minor differences in incidence of bowel cancer.

Information on the variation in bowel cancer risk by counties or small geographical units had been lacking until the publication of U.S.

county maps by Mason *et al.* (1975). Since bowel cancer had not been intensively investigated from this point of view, it is not surprising that studies of soil and drinking water content in relation to small area variation for this disease have not been pursued with the same diligence as for stomach cancer and cardiovascular disease. The observations on the role of selenium in inhibiting tumorigenesis (Schwartz, 1975), coupled with the inverse relationship between selenium occurrence in the soil and forage crops and the death rates for cancer of all sites and of the large bowel in the United States and Canada (Shamberger and Frost, 1969), ensure that environmental geochemistry and the distribution of trace metals in relation to bowel cancer will receive greater attention in the future.

G. MIGRANT POPULATIONS

The intercountry comparisons of cancer risks confound the effects of diagnostic practices, environmental factors, and host characteristics. With respect to diagnostic artifacts the presumption of true intercountry differences in large-bowel cancer is strengthened by observations on migrant populations. For example, Jews coming to Israel from Yemen and North Africa have experienced in the years immediately after arrival lower bowel cancer incidence than Jews from western Europe and North America (Doll *et al.*, 1966), a result consistent with global population contrasts for this disease.

A more fundamental application of these data comes from recognition that population migration represents an unplanned experiment of nature. Several investigators have recognized the importance of comparing the experience of natives and migrants residing in the same areas to elicit information on the potential role of environmental and endogenous factors in specific diseases (Steiner, 1954) as well as to elaborate the interpretation of intercountry differences in risk. Migration to the United States in the late 19th and early 20th centuries was a major contribution to its population growth, and the presence of a substantial foreign-born population stimulated comparative studies of cancer mortality in the foreign- and native-born. The initial efforts reporting data on cancer deaths by country of birth of decedent for selected states and cities in a few years prior to 1920 did not consider individual cancer sites (Dublin and Baker, 1920; Dublin, 1922). Lombard and Doering (1929) were the first to report systematically on site-specific mortality in their Boston study. Comprehensive coverage of ethnic group variation in large-bowel cancer was provided by Haenszel (1961) in his study of 34,000 deaths of foreign-born whites in

35 states as of 1950. The results from that source for intestines (colon) and rectum in the form of standardized mortality ratios (SMRs) are summarized in Fig. 12. The companion data for stomach are shown to emphasize the site-specific nature of the nativity-group findings. As of 1950, cancer of the colon and rectum was characterized by a limited range of variation among ethnic groups compared to that presented by stomach and esophagus. Similar conclusions were reached by Lilienfeld *et al.* (1972) in their study covering the 3 years 1959–1961. A precise reconciliation of the two sets of results is not possible because Haenszel's analysis adjusted for region of residence in calculating the base-line experience of the U.S. native-born, while Lilienfeld *et al.* used the rates for total U.S. native whites as their standard of reference. Since bowel cancer mortality was higher in the North where most of the foreign-born resided, the rates for the foreign-born in the presentation by Lilienfeld *et al.* tended to exceed the base-line native-white level.

The compressed range of SMRs by ethnic group for colon and rectum in Fig. 12 stands in sharp contrast to the magnitude of the international variation in mortality for these same sites. Few of the foreign-born groups had SMRs substantially in excess of that for the U.S. native-born. The higher SMRs for Irish males for intestine and rectum forms part of a larger pattern of excess mortality for all digestive tract sites except stomach in this ethnic group. The group of U.S.S.R.-born contained a high concentration of Jews, for whom excess risks of large bowel cancer have been reported by other studies (Greenwald *et al.*, 1975).

When the U.S. foreign-born rates as of 1950 and 1959–1961 were positioned against those in the countries of origin, the mortality from large-bowel cancer among migrants from the low-risk European countries proved to be more closely aligned with the host population of U.S. whites and suggested the following generalization for large bowel (and for breast, corpus uteri, ovary, and prostate as well): rates for migrants from low-risk areas converge during their lifetime to the higher risks of the host population. The rule for stomach is quite different: migrants from high-risk areas experience some reduction in rates, but still display the risks characteristic of the country of origin. A similar upward displacement of large bowel cancer mortality in Australia among Poles who migrated there after World War II has also been observed (Staszewski *et al.*, 1971). The U.S. and Australian data suggest that events in adult life associated with migration can visibly affect the level of bowel cancer risk within 2–3 decades.

Tabulations of U.S. mortality data have routinely included race as a

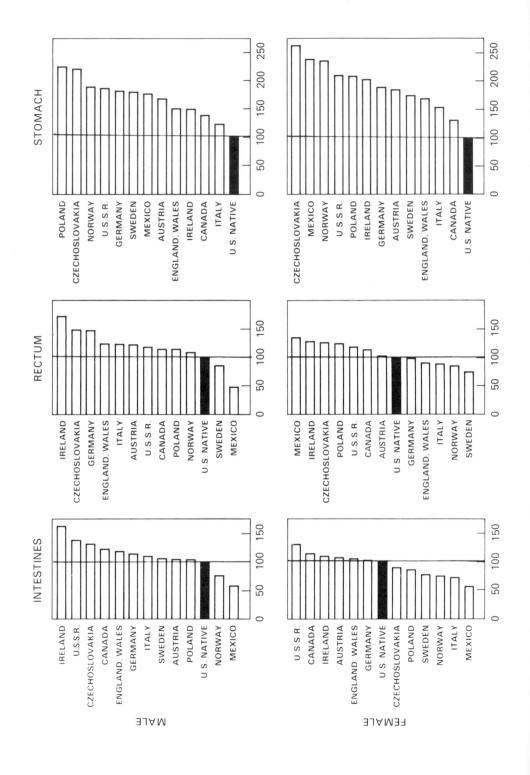

TABLE VII

STANDARDIZED RATIOS[a] FOR CANCER OF THE COLON AND RECTUM, U.S.
JAPANESE: MORTALITY 1949–1952, 1959–1962, 1969–1971; INCIDENCE, 1968–1972

Parameter	Year	Intestines (colon)		Rectum	
		Male	Female	Male	Female
Mortality	1949–1952	65	34	78	66
	1959–1962	69	47	94	63
	1969–1971	61	60	115	86
Incidence	1968–1972	95	86	126	121

[a] Standardized ratios for U.S. whites, each sex = 100.

study variable, a practice that has made it relatively easy to document
the changing large bowel mortality among Japanese in Hawaii and the
continental United States. When Smith (1956a) reviewed the cancer
mortality among Japanese in the United States as of 1949–1952, he
reported lower death rates from cancer of the colon among U.S.
Japanese than for U.S. whites, with a tendency, more pronounced
among males, for the U.S.-Japanese rates to be higher than rates for the
Japanese in Japan. Haenszel and Kurihara (1968) updated the results
as of 1959–1962. At that time the colon cancer rates for Issei (the
original migrants) and Nisei (their U.S.-born offspring) males had risen
to closely approximate those for white males; a similar, but smaller,
translation had occurred among females. This process of accommoda-
tion has continued into the 1960 decade (Table VII). The incidence
rates for Miyagi and for Hawaii Japanese and Caucasians show that, for
colon, Miyagi rates are lower than rates for Hawaii, where the
Caucasians and Japanese have similar rates up to age 70 (probably
mostly Nisei) but the rates for ages over 70 are higher for Caucasians
than for Japanese (mostly Issei). For rectum, Hawaii Caucasians and
Japanese rates are similar, both higher than for Miyagi, but the differences are smaller than for colon (Fig. 13).

The Japanese experience for colon seems quite consistent with that
presented by European migrants although the Issei did not make as
complete a transition within one generation as did migrants from Poland (Staszewski and Haenszel, 1965). The shift to higher U.S. risks

FIG. 12. Standardized mortality ratios by country of birth and by sex for cancer of the
intestines, rectum, and stomach, United States (35 states), 1950. Source: Haenszel
(1961).

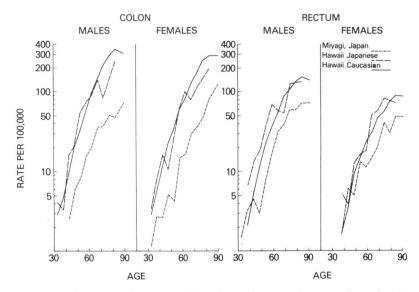

FIG. 13. Incidence rates for cancer of the colon and rectum, by sex and age, for Miyagi, Japan 1968–1971 and for Japanese and Caucasians in Hawaii 1968–1972. Source: Waterhouse *et al.* (1976).

continued in the second-generation Nisei. The mortality and incidence data as of circa 1950 probably understated the rising risk among the U.S. Japanese. In 379 autopsies of Japanese patients over 70 in a Honolulu hospital, Stemmermann (1966) discovered clinically unsuspected cancer of the large intestine in 13, or 3.4%, and suggested that " . . . careful autopsy study of the large intestine in all Japanese dying after 70 might double the yield of new tumors in this age group." In the light of later events his finding suggests that the migrant effect for this site was first expressed in older persons as small, asymptomatic tumors.

One distinction between Japanese and Polish migrants should be noted. The Polish migrants experienced a substantial rise in risk for both colon and rectum, while the Japanese data emphasized selective effects within the intestinal tract. The U.S.–Japan differential in mortality from rectal cancer has never been marked, so that little change in the risk for rectum among Japanese migrants might have been anticipated and the facts conformed to expectation. However, the relative stability in overall rates for cancer of the rectum may have concealed a shift in the anatomic localization of these tumors among the migrants. As discussed in the section on anatomic localization, it was possible from measurements of tumor location for samples of cases in conjunction with tumor registry data to estimate segment-specific incidence for Japanese in Japan and Hawaii (J. W. Berg and W. Haenszel, personal communication, 1976). The age-adjusted incidence per 100,000 males for specific segments tabulated here show that the overall contrast for rectum has partially concealed a rising incidence among the Hawaii Japanese concentrated in tumors in the upper rectum and rectosigmoid region.

Distance from pectinate line (cm)	Japan (Miyagi prefecture)	Hawaii Japanese
0– 1.9	0.4	0.2
2.0– 3.9	0.7	1.5
4.0– 5.9	1.1	1.9
6.0– 7.9	0.7	3.5
8.0–15.9	2.3	8.7

The magnitude and anatomical specificity of the effects make the Hawaiian Japanese an attractive population in the search for more sophisticated parameters (intestinal flora, fecal chemistry, mutagenic activity of stools) that may differentiate them from the low-risk populations in Japan. Exploratory studies along these lines are underway.

Apart from the Japanese, the possibilities for new descriptive and analytic epidemiologic studies in the United States on migrants who have come from low-risk areas may be about exhausted. The U.S.-born offspring of the migrants now present the same large bowel cancer risks as the native born, and continued observation of these groups is unlikely to reveal new information. Further work along these lines might be initiated in other countries, such as Canada and Australia, where substantial numbers of migrants arrived after World War II. Another interesting observational situation is presented in Brazil, where there has been recent extensive migration from the poverty-stricken northeast part of the country (where large-bowel cancer is rare) to São Paulo and the south of Brazil, where large-bowel cancer is more frequently seen. The reverse phenomenon—migration from high- to low-risk areas—is not generally available for exploitation, the best possibility from this point of view being Israel.

H. Time Trends

The status of intercountry variation in risks of large-bowel cancer has not been completely static, and the differences among countries may be diminishing with the passage of time. For a comprehensive overview of time trends one must rely on mortality data. The establishment of tumor registries is a recent phenomenon, and only a handful of registries have been reporting incidence data for as long as 15 years. Table VIII gives the slopes of straight-line regressions fitted to the log mortality rates for colon and rectum cancer in 17 countries since 1950 (Segi and Kurihara, 1972; World Health Organization, 1972–1975). The countries have been arranged in descending order of male colon cancer death rates to make the point that the most pro-

TABLE VIII
SLOPES OF LINEAR REGRESSIONS FITTED TO LOGARITHMS OF AGE-ADJUSTED
MORTALITY RATES FOR CANCER OF THE COLON AND RECTUM;
17 COUNTRIES, 1950–1971[a]

| | Slope, per year | | | |
| | Colon | | Rectum | |
Country[a]	Male	Female	Male	Female
Scotland	-0.006^b	-0.006^b	-0.005^b	-0.001
England, Wales	-0.005^b	-0.005^b	-0.007^b	-0.004^b
Canada	$+0.002$	-0.003^b	-0.001	-0.003^b
Australia	-0.001	-0.002^b	-0.003^b	-0.003
United States, white	$+0.002^b$	-0.004^b	-0.009^b	-0.012^b
Denmark	-0.001	-0.001	-0.006^b	-0.003
New Zealand	$+0.004$	-0.002	$+0.002$	-0.002
Switzerland	$+0.002$	-0.002	-0.003	-0.005^b
France	$+0.004^b$	-0.003^b	$+0.001$	$+0.001^b$
Austria	$+0.004$	$+0.001$	$+0.002$	$+0.003$
Sweden	$+0.003$	$+0.001$	-0.001	(<0.0005)
Netherlands	$+0.006^b$	$+0.002^b$	-0.003^b	-0.005^b
United States, nonwhite	$+0.008^b$	$+0.004^b$	-0.005	-0.010^b
Norway	$+0.005^b$	$+0.005^b$	$+0.005$	$+0.006^b$
Germany, Federal Republic	$+0.016^b$	$+0.016^b$	$+0.003$	$+0.006^b$
Italy	$+0.015^b$	$+0.009^b$	$+0.012^b$	$+0.007^b$
Finland	$+0.005^b$	$+0.002$	$+0.005$	$+0.003$
Japan	$+0.013^b$	$+0.009^b$	$+0.006^b$	$+0.005^b$

[a] Countries arranged in descending order of male colon cancer mortality rates at beginning of time period.

[b] Denotes slopes significantly different from zero at 1% level.

nounced rise in recorded mortality has occurred in those countries where the risks have been historically low. In certain high-risk populations, such as Scotland and England, the colon cancer rates have declined and there is a group of intermediate-risk countries for which the changes in mortality have been minimal. The differences in time trends between the two extremes of the spectrum of risk are clearly evident.

There is a perceptible tendency for the higher colon cancer slope values (or smaller negative values) to occur among males. Countries in the intermediate- and low-risk category for bowel cancer also tend to exhibit smaller displacements in mortality over time for rectum than for colon.

To illustrate the nature of the changes that have been summarized in the form of estimated slope values, Fig. 14 plots curves of age-adjusted mortality for selected populations. Mortality in Japan and Norway has risen almost continuously with few interruptions, while the tendency

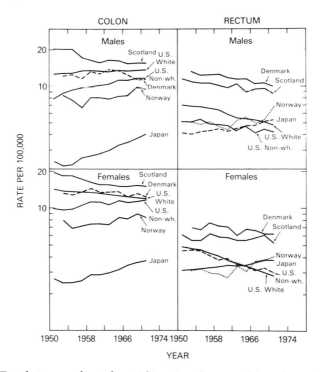

FIG. 14. Trends in age-adjusted mortality rates of cancer of the colon and rectum, by sex. Selected countries, 1950–1971. Source: World Health Organization (1972–1975).

to lower rates in Scotland, particularly for females, was concentrated in the interval between 1950 and 1965.

In interpreting mortality trends it should be remembered that this source will tend to understate rises in risk because advancements in treatment methods since World War II have improved the survival experience of bowel cancer patients (Cutler and Lourie, 1963). The improvement in survival among patients with rectal cancer has been particularly impressive, and this feature may account in part for the generally smaller slope values in log mortality for cancer of the rectum. The companion text figure for cancer of the rectum for the same populations presents a more consistent pattern of declining mortality than the results for colon cancer. The tendency for a rise in rectum cancer in Norway and Japan is overshadowed by the impression of declining mortality in the other countries. For both colon and rectum, the graphic presentations appear consistent with the summary information contained in the slope estimates of mortality.

Figure 15 presents information on the changes in age-adjusted incidence for cancer of the colon and rectum occurring in 4 areas for which data have been assembled over a substantial time interval either by cancer registries or morbidity surveys. The incidence data for U.S. whites (supplemented by data for Connecticut), U.S. nonwhites, Denmark, and Norway for colon cancer among males show a more pronounced upward trend than that revealed by the corresponding mortality data. The steeper slopes in colon cancer rates for U.S. blacks is a highlight of Fig. 15. The rise in incidence among blacks since 1947 has substantially outpaced that for whites. The incidence data also reinforce the impression of different time trends for colon and rectum. The composite incidence curves for cancer of the rectum display a pattern of declining incidence, particularly among females, as opposed to a pattern of stationary or rising incidence for colon. Even in Norway, which represents a possible counterexample to the pattern of declining incidence for rectum, the rise for rectum has not been as regular and persistent as for colon.

The different behavior in incidence trends for colon and rectum raises the more general question about the behavior of the several segments of the large bowel in this respect. Data on this point are available from Connecticut, and age-adjusted rates by segments from that source for 1940–1971 are plotted in Fig. 16. There is a slight upward bias in the segmental curves due to greater specificity in anatomic localization of bowel tumors reported to the tumor registry over time (incidence for colon, site not specified, declined from about 5/100,000 to 1.5 between 1940 and 1971 in Connecticut), but this

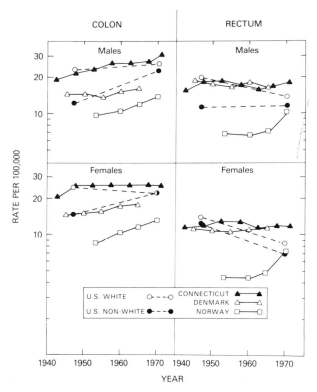

FIG. 15. Trends in age-adjusted incidence rates of cancer of the colon and rectum, by sex. Selected countries, variable time periods, 1940–1972. Sources: Dorn and Cutler (1959), Cutler and Young (1975), Norwegian Cancer Society (1959, 1964, 1973), Clemmesen (1965b, 1969, 1974), Connecticut State Dept. of Health (1966, 1969, 1973).

factor can account for only a small fraction of the rise in segment-specific incidence. The upward trend has been most pronounced for both sexes in the proximal colon, with cecum and ascending colon showing the steepest rise. Unfortunately, the Connecticut registry did not segregate the data for cecum and ascending colon. The rise for descending colon was somewhat greater than that for sigmoid colon. The slopes of the regression lines fitted to log incidence summarized in Table IX reveal a pattern of diminishing change over time as one goes from cecum and ascending colon to rectum. Since comparable information is not available from other registries, it is not possible to state whether the results are specific for Connecticut or whether similar tendencies are present in the data from other cancer registries covering high-, intermediate-, and low-risk populations for bowel

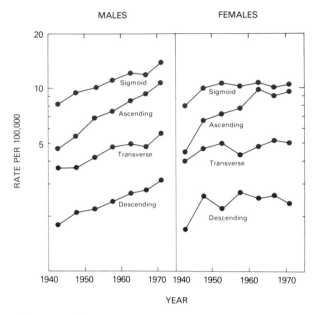

FIG. 16. Trends in age-adjusted incidence rates of cancer of the colon, by anatomic segment, by sex. Connecticut, 1940–1971. Source: Cutler (1975).

cancer. Fragmentary data from Denmark suggest that the results for Connecticut may not be universal. The publications of the Danish Cancer Registry distinguished sigmoid from the remainder of the colon, and Figure 17 shows a steeper rise in incidence for sigmoid

TABLE IX

SLOPES OF LINEAR REGRESSIONS FITTED TO LOGARITHMS OF AGE-ADJUSTED INCIDENCE RATES FOR CANCER OF THE LARGE BOWEL, BY ANATOMIC SEGMENT, BY SEX. CONNECTICUT, 1940–1971

Anatomic segment	Male		Female	
	Slope, per 5 years	±2 SE	Slope, per 5 years	±2 SE
Cecum, ascending colon	0.064	0.007	0.054	0.021
Transverse colon	0.033	0.010	0.014	0.013
Descending colon	0.042	0.006	0.020	0.025
Sigmoid colon	0.037	0.008	0.014	0.015
Rectum	0.002	0.012	−0.007	0.012

colon, which implies a smaller slope value for at least one segment proximal to the sigmoid.

The presentation to this point has dealt with age-adjusted mortality or incidence. The age-specific incidence rates for Connecticut and Denmark have also been examined for time trends, and the results for Connecticut are shown in Fig. 18. In Connecticut the rise in colon incidence has been most evident among males over age 65. The upward tendency is less pronounced among younger males, and it is difficult to judge whether there has been in fact a sustained rise in colon incidence among males under 55 years. The rise in colon cancer incidence for Connecticut women over 65 years has been more gradual than for men. The age differentials in time trends that characterize the Connecticut results are also apparent in Denmark, and the major feature that distinguishes the two areas is the less pronounced sex differences in time trends in Denmark.

An upward displacement in rectal cancer incidence for Connecticut males over age 65, while present, did not match the magnitude of the

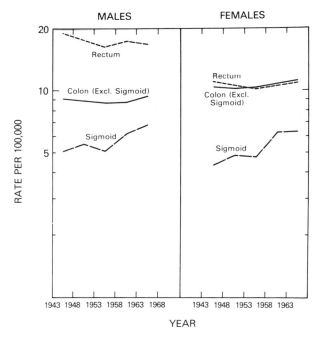

FIG. 17. Trends in age-adjusted incidence rates for cancer of the large bowel, by anatomic segment, by sex. Denmark, 1943–1967. Source: Clemmesen (1965b, 1969, 1974).

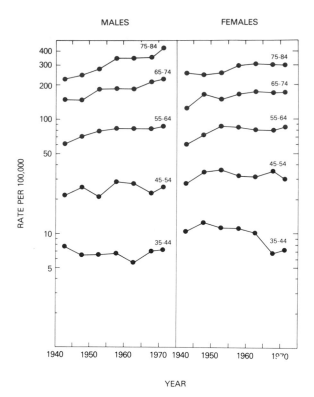

FIG. 18. Trends in age-specific incidence rates for cancer of the colon, by sex. Connecticut, 1940–1972. Source: Connecticut State Dept. of Health (1966).

colon finding, and for males under 65 the dominant impression was one of decreases (Fig. 19). The female incidence for rectum remained relatively stable for each age group in Connecticut except for 35–44 age group, in which a decline was noted. Similar tendencies were evident in Denmark, where a rise in incidence for rectum was limited to ages over 75; at younger ages in both sexes declines were the rule.

Figures 20 and 21 examine the trends in age-specific incidence by individual segments. Cecum and ascending colon were the primary contributors to the Connecticut rise in colon cancer in the older age groups, and for that bowel segment the rise in incidence over time is well expressed for both sexes. Under age 55 the time trends for ascending colon showed no strong pattern of increase or decrease. The Connecticut data for sigmoid colon present a different pattern for each sex; the rise in incidence for males over 55 sets them apart from younger males and also from females of all ages, who showed pronounced trends. The situation in Connecticut is summarized in Table X presenting the regression slopes of log incidence by age and anatomic localization. For cecum and ascending colon a consistent progression in slope values with age can be discerned, and this feature is better expressed by males. The smaller slope values for females do not form as regular a pattern with age. The results for both ascending and sigmoid colon contrast sharply with the slope values for rectum, where negative values predominate at ages under 65 years and do not significantly differ from zero at ages over 65.

The Danish data on age- and segment-specific incidence reinforce the impression gained from the age-adjusted incidence. Contrary to the experience in Connecticut, the rise in incidence for males and females over 65 years appears attributable primarily to sigmoid colon, although this was accompanied by a rise in incidence for "other colon" at ages over 75. Male and female incidence for "other colon" showed little change with time in the younger age groups.

The possibility that the increase in colon cancer incidence among older persons reflects improved diagnosis of tumors located in the

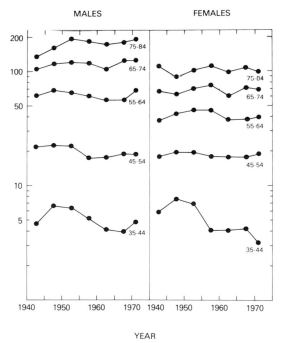

FIG. 19. Trends in age-specific incidence rates for cancer of the rectum, by sex. Connecticut, 1940–1972. Source: Connecticut State Dept. of Health (1966), Connecticut Tumor Registry, personal communication.

TABLE X

SLOPES OF LINEAR REGRESSIONS FITTED TO LOGARITHMS OF AGE-SPECIFIC
INCIDENCE RATES FOR SELECTED ANATOMIC SEGMENTS OF THE
LARGE BOWEL BY SEX. CONNECTICUT, 1940–1972

Anatomic segment	Age	Males Slope, per 5 years	±2 SE	Females Slope, per 5 years	±2 SE
Cecum and ascending	35–44	+0.003	0.033	+0.024	0.064
	45–54	+0.020	0.042	+0.008	0.020
	55–64	+0.057	0.028	+0.046	0.028
	65–74	+0.065	0.018	+0.053	0.026
	75–84	+0.101	0.021	+0.090	0.026
Sigmoid colon	35–44	+0.021	0.044	−0.004	0.079
	45–54	+0.025	0.018	+0.042	0.044
	55–64	+0.040	0.019	+0.024	0.019
	65–74	+0.034	0.005	+0.018	0.041
	75–84	+0.062	0.006	−0.006	0.027
Rectum	35–44	−0.027	0.016	−0.057	0.016
	45–54	−0.018	0.007	−0.004	0.005
	55–64	−0.005	0.008	−0.004	0.008
	65–74	+0.008	0.006	+0.003	0.007
	75–84	+0.020	0.008	+0.001	0.008

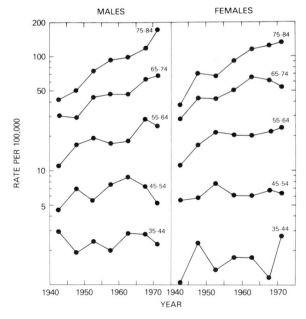

FIG. 20. Trends in age-specific incidence rates for cancer of the cecum and ascending colon, by sex. Connecticut, 1940–1972. Sources: Connecticut State Dept. of Health (1966), Connecticut Tumor Registry, personal communication.

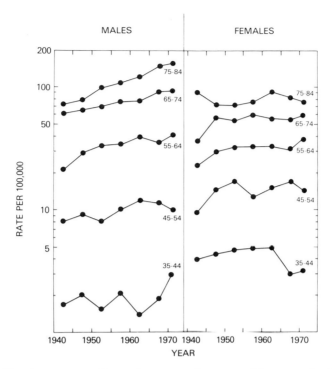

FIG. 21. Trends in age-specific incidence rates for cancer of the sigmoid colon, by sex. Connecticut, 1940–1972. Sources: Connecticut State Dept. of Health (1966), Connecticut Tumor Registry, personal communication.

right bowel must be considered, but part of the change presumably represents a true increase in risk, at least in Connecticut. There can scarcely be any question that the characteristic segmental time trends in incidence distinguish rectum from the large bowel proximal to the rectosigmoid flexure. The End Results Group in the United States had noted a consistent increase in the colon–rectum ratio between 1940 and 1962, and after review of the detailed data on assignments to subsites, it concluded that the changing colon–rectum ratio arose from an increased incidence in colon cancer, not from changing criteria in the assignment of bowel cancers (Axtell and Chiazze, 1966).

I. URBAN–RURAL DIFFERENCES

A high risk in urban populations is a well-defined, prominent feature of esophageal cancer, a characteristic shared to a lesser, but still pronounced degree, by large bowel, but not by stomach. There is abundant documentation from countries at high-, intermediate-, and low-risk to bowel cancer of the presence of higher risks among urban residents (Levin *et al.*, 1960; Clemmesen, 1974; Doll *et al.*, 1970; Teppo *et al.*, 1975; Registrar General of England and Wales, 1971). The urban-rural gradients in the U.S. incidence data have their counterparts in Denmark, Finland, Norway, and to a lesser degree, England so that this phenomenon appears to be universal and not limited to a few populations.

Figure 22 summarizes the evidence from several sources and indicates a generally more pronounced urban excess for colon than rectum that is better expressed by males. The stability in the urban–rural ratios seems surprisingly good when one considers the variation in definitions and data collection procedures in the source materials. The outliers for colon cancer in Fig. 22 are England and Wales and Finland; the experience for Scotland parallels that for England and Wales (Curwen, 1954), and a recent review of incidence and mortality data from Poland reports urban–rural ratios of risk commensurate with those described for Finland (Staszewski, 1976). The mortality data compiled by the Registrar General of England and Wales (1971) has consistently described a small rural deficit in risk of large-bowel

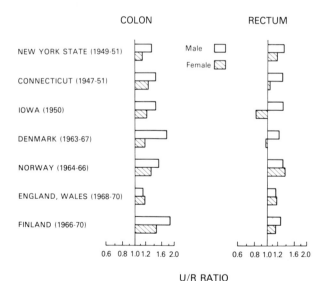

FIG. 22. Urban–rural (U/R) ratios of age-adjusted incidence rates for cancer of the colon and rectum. Selected registries, variable time periods. Sources: Levin *et al.* (1960), Clemmesen (1974), Waterhouse *et al.* (1976), Teppo *et al.* (1975), Registrar General of England and Wales (1971).

cancer in England that has persisted for over 30 years. The densely populated "rural" areas of England and Scotland may be more subject to exposures characteristic of urban areas and in this respect may be further removed in terms of potential exposures from the rural environments of Finland, Norway, and Poland. The very sizable urban excess of colon cancer in Finland and Poland may represent in part the presence of superior diagnostic and treatment facilities in the large cities; however, the possibility that the data also relate to a transitional period, during which exposures conducive to higher risks were introduced at an earlier date into the urban environment, should not be dismissed. Changes occurring later in the rural areas may eventually lead to a delayed rise in rural incidence and thus depress the urban–rural risk ratio.

There is evidence that the urban-rural risk relationships are not constant and Table XI reports on changes that have occurred in three areas where data on this point have been accumulated over at least a 15-year time span. In the United States (Iowa) and Norway diminishing urban–rural ratios for colon cancer have been observed for both sexes, attributable to a more rapid rise in rural incidence rates. A similar tendency was present for rectal cancer, except for Iowa females. The pattern of results for Denmark was quite different. No significant change was observed in the urban–rural ratios for colon; there was a decline in the urban–rural ratios for cancer of the rectum, but the latter was due primarily to a decline in incidence among urban residents.

The urban–rural ratios based on age-adjusted rates provide a reasonably representative picture of the comparative risks. The more detailed age-specific data, not shown, portray a rather consistent urban excess at all ages in three countries at two different points in time, and much of the variation by age could be attributed to small numbers and attendant sampling variation.

The nature of the urban–rural gradients in risk have been more extensively investigated in the United States than elsewhere. Mortality tabulations for 1949–1951 (Haenszel and Dawson, 1965) comparing metropolitan and nonmetropolitan counties (a classification yielding results almost identical with those based on urban–rural contrasts) showed the U.S. urban excess for large-bowel cancer to persist within each major region of the country (Table XII). The same pervasive pattern of an urban excess risk has also been described in Norway (Bjelke, 1973). Detailed residence histories collected for a 10% sample of deaths from cancer of the colon and rectum in the United States for 1958 rule out the attribution of the excess urban risk to the migration of

TABLE XI

TRENDS IN URBAN–RURAL (UR) RATIOS OF AGE-ADJUSTED[a] INCIDENCE RATES FOR CANCER OF THE COLON AND RECTUM. SELECTED REGISTRIES, VARIABLE TIME PERIODS[b]

Registry	Year	Colon						Rectum					
		Male			Female			Male			Female		
		Urban	Rural	U/R	Urban	Rural	U/R	Urban	Rural	U/R	Urban	Rural	U/R
Iowa	1950	22.1	15.5	1.43	25.0	20.6	1.21	14.6	11.0	1.33	8.7	9.7	0.90
	1969–1971	26.0	23.7	1.10	26.2	23.6	1.11	14.0	12.2	1.15	8.4	8.1	1.04
Norway	1953–1954	14.2	8.8	1.61	12.1	8.2	1.48	9.4	5.9	1.59	6.0	3.7	1.62
	1968–1972	15.0	11.2	1.34	14.6	11.6	1.26	11.2	9.4	1.19	8.0	6.2	1.29
Denmark	1943–1947	19.2	11.3	1.70	16.0	13.5	1.19	23.5	15.9	1.48	13.2	10.2	1.29
	1963–1967	21.7	12.6	1.72	19.2	16.1	1.19	18.8	15.4	1.22	10.8	11.0	0.98

[a] Adjusted to world standard population (Doll et al., 1970).
[b] Sources: Haenszel et al. (1955), Clemmesen (1974), Doll et al. (1970), Waterhouse et al. (1976).

TABLE XII

STANDARDIZED MORTALITY RATIOS[a] FOR CANCER OF THE COLON AND RECTUM, BY
REGION, AND METROPOLITAN (M) AND NONMETROPOLITAN (N) COUNTIES.
U.S. WHITES, 1959–1951[b]

Survey area	White males			White females		
	Metro- politan counties	Nonmetro- politan counties	Ratio: M/N	Metro- politan counties	Nonmetro- politan counties	Ratio: M/N
Northeast	147	115	1.28	131	115	1.14
North Central	123	90	1.37	107	94	1.14
South	85	57	1.49	87	68	1.28
West	98	73	1.34	89	77	1.16

[a] Standardized mortality ratios for U.S. whites, both sexes combined = 100.
[b] Source: Haenszel and Dawson (1965).

ill persons to urban centers for medical care (Haenszel and Dawson, 1965). In fact, the urban excess risk based on the conventional concept of "usual residence" was somewhat enhanced when the contrast was restricted to "long-term" residents—persons who have resided in the same community for more than 40 years. The same study found the metropolitan–nonmetropolitan county (and urban–rural) gradient in risk to be displayed at all localizations within the intestinal tract. This suggests that the urban–rural contrasts within the United States or similar high-risk areas to not reproduce the anatomical site specificity elicited in the more extreme international comparisons of risk.

The urban–rural ratios should not be interpreted as a measure of the difference in risks between farm and urban populations. Within the United States farmers account for only a small proportion of the rural population, and the data for rural Iowa are a better reflection of the farm experience than those for "rural" Connecticut or upstate New York, where suburban areas and small towns of less than 2500 population are heavily represented. Despite the differences in composition of rural populations, the respective urban–rural ratios for colon cancer are quite similar. This point is reinforced by the observation that the urban–rural ratios for metropolitan counties in upstate New York as of 1949–1951 (Levin et al., 1960) were only slightly smaller than those for nonmetropolitan counties (see tabulation on page 50).

Such results suggest that modest, ill-defined contrasts in life style and/or work and environmental exposures can evoke substantial differences in large-bowel cancer risk.

Population	Colon	Rectum
Metropolitan countries		
Male	1.30	1.24
Female	1.13	1.16
Nonmetropolitan countries		
Male	1.35	1.27
Female	1.23	1.25

J. RACE

The international comparisons have described low risks for large-bowel cancer in Africa, Asia, and Latin America, and the presence of low risks among black and Oriental populations on those continents is beyond dispute. These results, however, confound the effects of race and allied genetic characteristics with those attributable to environmental exposures and different standards of diagnosis and medical care. More precise comparisons of racial differences in risk require that they be made within circumscribed geographic areas, and the available U.S. data can be used for this purpose to good advantage.

The national cancer morbidity surveys in 1947–1948 (Dorn and Cutler, 1959) and 1969–1971 (Cutler and Young, 1975) collected incidence data for both white and black populations. Table XIII gives the age-adjusted rates for cancer of the colon and rectum for the areas surveyed in 1969–1971. Both blacks and whites still exhibited as of 1969–1971 the North–South gradient in risk for all segments of the large bowel, although the difference has narrowed since 1947–1948. Within each community and region of the country the white-black differentials are now minimal, a situation that contrasts sharply with the status as of 1947–1948 (Dorn and Cutler, 1959). At that time the incidence of colon cancer among whites in the North and West was almost double that for blacks, and for rectum the white excess was of the order of 50%; the same white–black ratio for colon cancer prevailed in the South as in the North, but the racial difference in rectal cancer incidence was even then almost negligible in the South. The changed racial relationship for colon is due primarily to the rise in incidence among blacks (see Fig. 15); for rectum the narrowing race differential appears traceable to a recorded drop in incidence among whites. Figure 15 depicts little change in risk since 1947 among black males and females. The reduced rectal cancer incidence among both U.S. blacks and whites may reflect in part recent changes in describing and classifying tumors located close to the rectosigmoid flexure. With due allowance for the latter factor one may still state that the rise in colon cancer incidence for blacks in the short time span of less than 25 years constitutes one of the strongest pieces of evidence for downplaying the effect of race and allied host factors for this site and for upgrading the role of environmental etiologies.

The black–white contrast of age-adjusted rates conceals no anomalous relationships in the age-specific incidence for colon and rectum. The age-specific incidence curves are essentially the same for both races and the lower rates for blacks after age 60 is due in part to the greater concentration of older blacks in the lower-risk areas of the

TABLE XIII

AGE-ADJUSTED INCIDENCE RATES PER 100,000 POPULATION FOR CANCER OF THE COLON AND RECTUM, BY SEX, FOR WHITES AND BLACKS U.S. CANCER MORBIDITY SURVEY AREAS, 1969–1971[a]

Survey area	Sex	Colon		Rectum	
		White	Black	White	Black
Northern and western					
Detroit	Male	30.0	27.9	18.0	14.9
	Female	24.9	25.7	9.4	8.6
Pittsburgh	Male	31.3	22.6	17.6	17.7
	Female	25.2	32.2	10.9	12.5
Iowa	Male	28.1	34.6	14.7	20.4
	Female	28.2	33.9	9.4	6.6
Minneapolis–St. Paul	Male	33.2	36.1	17.7	17.5
	Female	27.5	16.9	9.7	3.2
Colorado	Male	22.6	22.3	11.1	10.2
	Female	21.9	24.9	6.5	10.8
San Francisco–Oakland	Male	31.7	27.7	16.9	14.4
	Female	26.6	22.3	11.2	7.2
Total,[b] 6 areas	Male	29.5	28.5	16.0	15.8
	Female	25.7	26.0	9.5	8.1
Southern					
Atlanta	Male	26.7	21.3	11.3	10.2
	Female	24.1	24.0	6.8	6.9
Birmingham	Male	21.1	18.0	9.5	6.8
	Female	22.7	20.8	7.9	4.7
Dallas–Ft. Worth	Male	23.2	24.1	13.3	13.3
	Female	22.1	25.3	9.1	6.9
Total,[b] 3 areas	Male	23.7	21.1	11.4	10.1
	Female	23.0	23.4	7.9	6.2

[a] Source: Cutler and Young (1975).
[b] Total = unweighted arithmetic average.

South. [Older blacks did not participate to the same degree as younger blacks in migration from the South to northern cities (Young *et al.*, 1975).]

The best evidence on possible racial differences in risk among the Japanese, Chinese, Filipinos, and Polynesians (Hawaiians) come from the Hawaii Tumor Registry, and Table XIV summarizes the findings from that source. Some of the apparent racial differences in age-adjusted incidence for colon and rectum are probably due to the small numbers of cases observed, particularly for the Chinese, Filipinos, and Hawaiians, and the pertinent point is rather how small the differences are in that locale when measured on the scale of intercountry variation. The Filipinos are the most recent arrivals in Hawaii, and part of their low risk should still reflect exposures prior to migration; with continued residence in Hawaii, the present risk differential may be diminished.

The current convergence of Hawaiian Japanese and white incidence for large-bowel cancer represents the culmination of a long-term rise in risk among Japanese migrants and their descendants. The incidence and mortality data for 1959–1962 and earlier periods (Haenszel and Kurihara, 1968; Quisenberry *et al.*, 1966; Smith, 1956a) portrayed a deficit in risk for the Japanese vis-à-vis whites in Hawaii and the U.S.

TABLE XIV

AGE-ADJUSTED INCIDENCE RATES PER 100,000 POPULATION FOR CANCER OF THE COLON AND RECTUM, BY RACE AND SEX. HAWAII, 1960–1964, 1968–1972[a]

Race	Colon		Rectum	
	Male	Female	Male	Female
1960–1964				
Caucasian	19.3	27.5	12.6	9.8
Chinese	35.9	23.5	15.8	9.4
Filipino	12.6	14.8	12.4	13.4
Hawaiian	20.2	12.1	6.8	6.9
Japanese	20.7	15.3	11.7	9.8
1968–1972				
Caucasian	23.9	22.9	13.4	12.0
Chinese	28.7	20.9	20.4	5.9
Filipino	16.8	15.3	14.5	0.0
Hawaiian	14.0	16.9	9.4	2.9
Japanese	22.4	18.8	16.3	10.1

[a] Source: Doll *et al.* (1970), Waterhouse *et al.* (1976).

mainland, more pronounced for colon than rectum and concentrated among females. Given the earlier parallels between the Hawaii and mainland experience, one can with confidence extrapolate the most recent Hawaiian findings of minimal Japanese–white differences in risk to the continental United States.

The mortality data for the U.S. Chinese as of 1949–1952 (Smith, 1956b) and 1959–1962 (King and Haenszel, 1973) reinforce the Hawaii incidence data that describe minimal Chinese–white differences for large bowel and leave open the possibility of slightly elevated colon cancer rates among the U.S. Chinese. Recent data from Hongkong (1961–1964) and Singapore (1959–1962) (King and Haenszel, 1973) indicate that large-bowel cancer, particularly in the colon, is seen about half as often among the Chinese in these communities as in the United States.

Smith (1957) in his review of the American Indian cancer experience as of 1949–1952 reported their risk of large-bowel cancer to be less than half that of U.S. whites and to be materially lower than that for U.S. blacks as well. Part of the apparent risk deficit for the American Indian may be attributable to poor access to medical care and diagnostic facilities due to low economic status and the isolation of several tribes on remote Indian reservations, but this appears unlikely to be the complete explanation. As of 1950, the Mexican-born in the United States (who are of predominantly Indian blood) were also reported to experience lower large-bowel cancer risks (Haenszel, 1961), and the more recent 1959–1961 results of Lilienfeld et al. (1972) showed deficits for colon and rectum commensurate with those described for 1950.

The low risks among American Indians still persist (Creagan and Fraumeni, 1972). The New Mexico Tumor Registry covering the State of New Mexico and the Navajo Indian Reservation in Arizona reports substantially lower incidence rates for Indians than whites (New Mexico Tumor Registry, 1975).

K. SOCIAL CLASS

Most of the information on social-class gradients in cancer risk has come from data collected in England and Wales, Denmark, and the United States. The decennial supplements on occupational mortality published by the Registrar General of England and Wales (1962) have provided the most systematic and extensive series of data on this point. This office has grouped individual occupations for males into five broad social classes ranging from "professional" to "unskilled" on the assumption that mortality is influenced by life-styles associated with different occupational levels as well as by specific occupational hazards and has extended this approach to women by classifying female deaths by occupation of the husband. This source of information was exploited once in the United States, when Guralnick (1963a,b) reported on occupational mortality among males as of 1950. By relating death certificate statements on occupation to the corresponding census data on population at risk age-adjusted mortality rates, usually presented as standardized mortality ratios (SMRs), can be calculated for individual occupations and combinations thereof. The data from mortality sources have two defects that complicate interpretation: (a) a tendency to upgrade occupation of the decedent on the death certificate relative to statements made on census returns, which imparts an upward bias to risks calculated for the upper socioeconomic classes, and (b) possible socioeconomic differentials in patient survival. Improved survival due to better medical care for upper-income groups would tend to neutralize higher risks and exaggerate lower risks for the upper socioeconomic classes. To mitigate the problem of incomparable census and death certificate statements of occupation, another measure, age-standardized proportionate mortality ratios (PMRs) that depend solely on internal variation in the distribution of occupations by specific causes, is often used.

In Denmark the Cancer Registry employed a different criterion for determining social class. All cancer cases reported in Copenhagen during 1943–1947 were classified by district of residence at time of diagnosis and the districts were grouped according to average rental, which Clemmesen (Clemmesen and Nielsen, 1951; Clemmesen, 1965a) stated to be a better indicator of social status than income in the immediate postwar period. A variation of this technique was adopted for the U.S. cancer morbidity survey of 10 metropolitan areas in 1947–1948 (Dorn and Cutler, 1959). All the areas surveyed had been divided into census tracts (areas homogeneous in population characteristics) that were assigned to one of five classes according to median family income. The same relative population distribution by income class was maintained in each area to minimize the confounding of income–class effects with those attributable to other intercity differences.

The findings from the four sources cited are summarized in Table XV. The value of the data for England and Wales is enhanced by the continuity of observations made in a consistent manner over an extended time period. The composite data for colon in that country displayed a tendency for the highest SMRs among males to occur in the upper social classes (classes 4 and 5); a risk rising with social class is

TABLE XV

STANDARDIZED INCIDENCE AND MORTALITY RATIOS FOR CANCER OF THE COLON AND RECTUM, BY SOCIAL CLASS AND SEX. SELECTED COUNTRIES, VARIABLE TIME PERIODS[a]

Segment and survey area and time	Male					Female				
	Class 1 (low)	Class 2	Class 3	Class 4	Class 5 (high)	Class 1 (low)	Class 2	Class 3	Class 4	Class 5 (high)
A. Intestines (colon)										
Denmark—incidence: 1943–1947										
Total	93	116	88	99	101	126	115	87	79	100
Sigmoid colon only	88	105	109	97	135	100	71	75	117	160
England and Wales—mortality										
1921–1923 Total	97	87	100	112	132	—	—	—	—	—
Sigmoid only	95	82	100	114	155	—	—	—	—	—
1930–1932 Total	94	99	102	104	110	102	89	102	99	119
1950–1953 Total	99	92	102	101	121	95	101	99	106	115
1959–1963 Total	109	92	105	99	120	121	95	106	94	90
United States—Total										
Incidence: 1947–1948	100	94	102	102	101	105	105	97	97	99
Mortality: 1950	98	92	103	99	116	—	—	—	—	—
B. Rectum										
Denmark—incidence: 1942–1947	100	103	106	100	85	106	100	93	109	70
England and Wales—mortality										
1921–1923	98	96	102	102	93	—	—	—	—	—
1930–1932	98	97	103	103	89	106	86	105	97	100
1950–1953	104	94	108	86	86	93	105	104	93	107
1959–1963	120	98	106	89	79	132	106	107	81	69
United States										
Incidence: 1947–1948	104	97	99	108	92	108	103	99	93	100
Mortality: 1950	102	99	104	90	86	—	—	—	—	—

[a] Sources: Registrar General of England and Wales (1962), Guralnick (1963b), Clemmesen (1965a), Clemmesen and Nielsen (1951), Dorn and Cutler (1959).

suggested even though irregularities in the gradient of risk are present. The female results for colon were more erratic and inconsistent, and a relationship with social class is not easy to discern for that sex. The findings on rectum from England and Wales portray an inverse social-class gradient, particularly for the two most recent time periods—1950–1953, 1959–1963. The same feature was exhibited in the 1959–1963 results for females, but the latter is of doubtful significance since this characteristic was weakly present, if at all, in earlier time periods. Supplemental contrasts for 1959–1963 based on PMRs covering the age group 65–74 years lead to the same general conclusions gained by inspection of the SMRs, and tend to reinforce the impression of a small colon cancer excess and rectal cancer deficit in the highest social class.

The U.S. occupational mortality data for 1950 (Guralnick, 1963a,b) described an excess colon cancer risk for professional workers (class 5), but apart from this little variation was observed among the other social classes. A small deficit in rectal cancer among the same group of professional workers was accompanied by slightly elevated risks for that localization among the lower social classes. Agricultural workers were not included in the comparison presented in Table XV. The low SMRs for agricultural workers (colon, 76; rectum, 58) reflect in another guise the rural deficit in risk of large-bowel cancer. The U.S. cancer morbidity survey for 1947–1948 (Dorn and Cutler, 1959) agreed with the mortality data in describing minimal income class variation in risk for both colon and rectum. Smaller-scale studies in New Haven (Cohart and Muller, 1955) and Buffalo (Graham et al., 1960) also reached the same conclusions. The U.S. information can be updated when the findings from the 1969–1971 morbidity survey become available. This source will also be useful for investigating social-class differences in large-bowel cancer risk by individual anatomic segments. The 1969–1971 data may also provide clues on possible changes in risk gradients in the interval since 1947–1948, although the experience in England might suggest that dramatic changes in this characteristic over time are unlikely to be uncovered.

The Copenhagen incidence data did not depict a consistent, well-defined social class gradient for total colon among males; the female data suggested a possible elevated risk in the upper classes. A lower risk for cancer of the rectum in the uppermost class was reported for both sexes, a feature reminiscent of the English male experience. Clemmesen distinguished sigmoid from the remainder of the colon, and it is worth noting that the Copenhagen data pinpointed an elevated sigmoid colon risk in the highest social classes for both sexes. On the one occasion, the 1921–1923 supplement, when the data for sigmoid colon were examined separately, the Registrar General of England and Wales described a risk gradient rising with social class. However, an excess risk in the higher social classes concentrated in the descending, sigmoid, and rectosigmoid segments was not demonstrable for cases reported in Oslo, Norway during 1961–1965 (Bjelke, 1973).

The composite evidence from populations at relatively high risk to large-bowel cancer leaves some uncertainty as to presence and/or magnitudes of the social class differences in risk. The absence of clear-cut, consistently observed gradients in the United States and western Europe, coupled with methodological uncertainties in the analysis of the mortality data, suggest that social class differences in risk are not a prime epidemiological characteristic of the disease in economically developed countries. In any event the lower digestive tract does not share the classical inverse relationship with social class revealed for cancer of the esophagus and stomach by the identical sources cited for large bowel. The fact that the slope values are numerically small should be emphasized and less attention paid to whether the data support hypotheses of positive or negative associations with social class. The suggestion of different slopes for colon and rectum (positive for colon, negative for rectum) does raise the possibility that individual anatomical segments may possess their own characteristic social class gradient and that the relatively flat gradient for colon is a composite of variable segmental relationships. The latter point should be pursued and elaborated by the collection of more precise data on tumor location.

The findings reviewed to this point relating the experience in economically developed countries supply no evidence on the situation in low-risk populations. The recent findings from Cali (Colombia) where the overall incidence of large-bowel cancer is one-fifth that reported by U.S. registries, stand in sharp contrast to those from developed countries (Haenszel et al., 1975). The census tract approach, employed in the analysis of data from Denmark and the United States, revealed a marked excess of newly diagnosed cases from the upper socioeconomic classes reported to the cancer registry in Cali during 1962–1971 (Table XVI). These data tend to overstate the social class gradient because of underreporting in low-income groups, but the difference is undoubtedly real, and collateral evidence from autopsy studies of adenomatous polyps supports the impression of a minimal risk of large-bowel cancer in the poorest socioeconomic class (Haenszel et al., 1975).

TABLE XVI

STANDARDIZED INCIDENCE RATES FOR CANCER OF THE LARGE BOWEL, BY
SOCIOECONOMIC CLASS AND SEX. CALI (COLOMBIA), 1962–1971[a]

Socioeconomic class	Both sexes	Males	Females
All classes	100	100	100
1 (very low)	29	19	38
2	92	97	88
3	147	142	150
4 (high)	140	157	123

[a] Source: Haenszel et al. (1975).

What is even more interesting is that the Cali results depict the social class differences to be concentrated in the segments between the ascending and rectosigmoid colon, a feature that corresponds well with the anatomical specificity in risk gradients noted in international comparisons of populations at the extreme ends of the spectrum of risk for this disease (J. W. Berg and W. Haenszel, personal communication, 1976). Nutritional studies have shown a marked deficit in Cali and throughout Colombia in protein intake, mainly animal protein (Interdepartmental Committee on Nutrition for National Defense, 1961), and a very large socioeconomic difference in meat consumption has been reported in Cali (Aragon, 1964).

L. OCCUPATION

The bulk of the evidence on variation in risks by occupation comes from mortality data. The brief statements of cause of death given on death certificates limit use of this source to delineate occupation-specific rates for cancer of the colon and of the rectum without extension to more-detailed anatomical localization. Utilization of cancer registry and survey data for more elaborate studies of anatomical localization effects is conceptually feasible, but their exploitation will require special queries of patients to obtain detailed histories of occupational exposures.

The Registrar General of England and Wales (1962) presented the SMRs for cancer of the colon and rectum for only 27 broad occupational categories in contrast to stomach, lung, and other selected sites, for which data were supplied for over 200 occupations. The failure to prepare a more comprehensive review reflects in part the past disinterest in large bowel as a candidate for serious epidemiological study, although it must be admitted that the results for occupational groups provided no powerful incentive to pursue this topic in depth. Apart from professional and administrative workers, already identified by the social-class data as groups at above-average risk for colon cancer, the 1959–1963 supplement uncovered no consistent patterns of occupational risk. Findings of a somewhat elevated colon cancer risk among clothing and textile workers and an excess mortality for rectal cancer among textile workers appear almost anecdotal in nature, and the justification for mentioning them here is that the periodic reports on cancer incidence issued by the same office (Registrar General of England and Wales, 1971) suggested an excess number of cases registered for male textile workers in 1966–1967 and for male clothing workers in 1968–1970.

The U.S. 1950 results in the form of SMRs for males 20–64 years of age (Guralnick, 1963b) agreed with the English data in singling out professional and white-collar occupations (clergymen, lawyers, managers, accountants, salesmen, etc.) as at high risk to colon cancer. Excess risks for large-bowel cancer (colon and rectum combined) were also suggested for craftsmen and laborers in metal manufacturing, machinists, firemen, and operatives and kindred workers in the leather products industry (Guralnick, 1963a).

Both the English and U.S. materials described deficits in risk among farmers roughly commensurate with the urban–rural gradients for this disease prevailing in the two countries.

Milham (1976) reviewed occupational statements on all death certificates for white males filed in the state of Washington for the years 1950–1971. Since census data on the corresponding populations at risk were unavailable, his analysis relied on the calculation of age-standardized proportionate mortality ratios (PMRs). While the PMRs provide no information on absolute cause-specific mortality for a given occupation, the author pointed to the good correspondence between findings based on PMRs and the conventional SMR approach in other materials to support his contention that a PMR analysis can yield useful leads. The suggestive associations of occupation with large-bowel cancer in this set of data are few in number and small in magnitude when compared to cancer of the lung and bladder (for which a substantial body of collateral evidence on occupational effects exists). The modestly elevated PMRs for colon cancer among physicians, lawyers, and engineers reflect the general colon cancer experience of the higher social classes and conversely, the few occupations, such as janitors and garbage collectors, displaying excess risks for rectum come from the lower classes, a pattern that fits other suggestive findings on opposite socioeconomic gradients in risk for colon and rectum. A few specific occupations (railroad engineers, plasterers, pressmen, policemen, gardeners, workers in fruit orchards) displayed above-average colon cancer risks, but in view of the large number of occupations examined the results are better interpreted as reflecting the influence of sampling variation rather than specific occupational exposures.

The collective information reinforces impressions of a diffuse, ill-defined excess colon cancer risk among persons in professional and related occupations that may be attributable to general, nonoccupational environmental factors. The failure of the several sources to consistently reproduce findings on individual occupations suggests that any single result for colon cancer be viewed with reserve. The same situation holds for cancer of the rectum in that it does not seem possible to use these data to incriminate specific occupations as major, consistent contributors to the inverse social-class gradient that probably characterizes the lower bowel. Identification of specific occupational factors for colon and rectum will require long-term prospective observations of employee groups with well-defined exposures along the lines of the follow-up studies of men occupationally exposed to asbestos that have indicated an increased incidence of large-bowel cancer in that group (Selikoff *et al.*, 1973; McDonald *et al.*, 1971).

M. Religion

Comparative studies of religious groups have been motivated by the search for leads on factors linked to the life-style of individual groups that might influence directly or indirectly their site-specific cancer risks. In the United States, MacMahon (1960) and later Newill (1961) investigated cancer mortality among Catholics, Protestants, and Jews in New York City during the 1950 decade and found the variation in total death rate from neoplastic diseases among the three religious groups to be minimal but detected some site-specific differences including an excess of large-bowel cancer, confined to the colon, among Jews. The relevant data from Newill's report are summarized in Table XVII. Subsequent studies of cancer mortality among Jews were undertaken in New York City (Seidman, 1970, 1971), upstate New York (Greenwald *et al.*, 1975), and the United States (Haenszel, 1971) utilizing information on religious affiliation of the funeral home and cemetery of burial and taking advantage of the fact that Jews comprise a high proportion of the Russian-born in the United States. The later findings consistently described U.S. Jews to be at higher risk of large-bowel cancer and coincided with Newill's report in revealing the ex-

TABLE XVII

AGE-ADJUSTED MORTALITY RATES PER 100,000 FOR CANCER OF THE COLON AND RECTUM, FOR WHITES AGE 45 AND OVER, BY RELIGION. NEW YORK CITY 1953–1958[a]

Religion	Colon		Rectum	
	Male	Female	Male	Female
Jewish	81.4	74.5	39.8	26.3
Protestant	59.8	60.2	40.5	25.0
Catholic	59.1	59.9	43.2	27.2

[a] Source: Newill (1961).

cess risk to be concentrated in the segments above the rectosigmoid flexure (Table XVIII).

While the observations on Jews are confounded with other factors, notably ethnicity and country of birth, social class, and residence, it seems unlikely that the latter factors can account completely for the excess colon cancer risk among Jews. Seidman (1970, 1971) examined his New York City data by socioeconomic class and discovered the effect to be present at all levels with the largest excess risks for Jews appearing in the upper classes. The demonstration of this effect within a single conurbation, New York City, also suggests that control for urban residence is unlikely to account for the observed association. Similarly, the composite U.S. data indicated the excess cancer mortality among the Russian-born (Jews) to be a broadly-based

TABLE XVIII

STANDARDIZED MORTALITY RATIOS[a] FOR CANCER OF THE COLON AND RECTUM AMONG THE RUSSIAN BORN, BY RESIDENCE AND SEX[b]

Survey area	Colon		Rectum	
	Male	Female	Male	Female
United States (1950)	137	128	119	120
New York City (1949–1951)	120	117	90	102
New York State (1969–1971) (excluding N.Y.C.)	142	130	106	126
Jewish	156	110	93	101

[a] Standardized mortality ratios for total population in each area = 100.

[b] Sources: Haenszel (1961), Seidman (1970), Greenwald et al. (1975).

phenomenon, which persisted in metropolitan and nonmetropolitan counties and within the several regions of the country.

The U.S. observations do not mean that elevated colon risks prevail in Jewish populations everywhere. The incidence of large-bowel cancer in Israel is aligned with that for intermediate-risk populations in western Europe (Waterhouse *et al.*, 1976). Within Israel there is substantial heterogeneity in risk for both colon and rectal cancer, the incidence among Oriental Jews from Asia and Africa being less than half that for persons migrating from Europe and America (Table XIX).

Burbank's review of U.S. mortality data for 1950–1967 identified Utah as the state with the lowest overall cancer death rates for white males and females (Burbank, 1971). Since members of the Church of Jesus Christ of Latter-Day Saints (Mormons), a religious group which advocates abstention from the use of tobacco, alcohol, tea, and coffee, comprise slightly more than 70% of the Utah population, the reasonable inference was that Mormons have lower cancer risks than other U.S. white populations. Enstrom (1975b) extended the U.S.–Utah contrast of site-specific mortality to encompass Utah County (approximately 85% Mormon) and demonstrated pronounced deficits in both Utah County and Utah State for cancer of the large bowel (Table XX) and for other sites including buccal cavity, esophagus, lung, and bladder. He also reported that mortality surveillance of a study population of Mormons in California for the years 1970–1972 depicted a deficit in deaths from cancer of the colon and rectum.

The information from vital statistics sources has recently been elaborated by incidence data from the Utah Cancer Registry (Lyon *et al.*, 1976). The incidence and mortality sources are in close agreement as to the magnitude of the deficit in cancer risk in Utah and the sites contributing to the deficit. Since Lyon *et al.* had access to church

TABLE XIX

Age-Adjusted Mortality Rates per 100,000 for Cancer of the Colon and Rectum among Israeli Jews, by Place of Birth and Sex. Israel, 1967–1971[a]

	Colon		Rectum	
Place of birth	Male	Female	Male	Female
Israel	8.7	5.4	5.1	8.3
Africa or Asia	5.1	5.3	4.2	4.1
Europe or America	12.9	13.4	11.9	11.2

[a] Source: Waterhouse *et al.* (1976).

TABLE XX
AGE-ADJUSTED MORTALITY RATES PER 100,000 FOR CANCER OF THE COLON
AND RECTUM, BY SEX. UTAH COUNTY, UTAH STATE, AND UNITED
STATES WHITE POPULATION, 1950–1969[a]

	Colon		Rectum	
Survey Area	Male	Female	Male	Female
Utah County (85% Mormon)	9.7	10.2	4.5	2.6
Utah State (70% Mormon)	10.9	10.8	4.3	3.0
United States (0.5% Mormon)	16.5	16.3	7.7	4.8

[a] Source: Enstrom (1975b).

membership records, they were able to present cancer incidence rates for the Mormon and non-Mormon populations. Their results in the form of standardized incidence ratios depict not only below-average risks for cancer of the colon and rectum among Mormons but among non-Mormons as well, and for males they found no significant difference between the Mormon and non-Mormon experience (Table XXI). Furthermore, the anatomic distribution of colon cancer did not differ significantly between Mormons and non-Mormons. This outcome can be reconciled with the evidence from mortality data. Burbank's (1971) geographical comparisons for large-bowel cancer had not indicated exceptionally low rates for Utah, particularly for males; 9 states, mostly in the South but including some in close proximity to Utah, had lower colon cancer rates for white males. The same tendency was also apparent for rectum. While the favorable Mormon experience for large-bowel cancer seems to be firmly established, in the present state of knowledge the presence of local environmental factors in Utah and

Table XXI
STANDARDIZED INCIDENCE RATIOS[a] FOR CANCER OF THE COLON AND RECTUM
AMONG WHITE MORMONS AND NON-MORMONS. UTAH, 1966–1970[b]

	Colon		Rectum	
Group	Male	Female	Male	Female
Mormon	61.7	64.0	31.5	37.7
Non-Mormon	71.5	92.3	39.3	41.7

[a] Standardized incidence ratios for whites in the Third National Cancer Survey = 100.
[b] Source: Lyon et al. (1976).

adjacent states that may depress the rates for both Mormons and non-Mormons cannot be ruled out.

Attention was initially directed to the Seventh-Day Adventists because church doctrine proscribes the use of tobacco and alcohol. To utilize this observational situation the cancer mortality experience of a cohort of 35,000 Seventh-Day Adventists in California was monitored for 8 years (1958–1965) with special attention to sites thought to be related etiologically to tobacco use (Lemon and Walden, 1966; Lemon *et al.*, 1964). The results indicated the total cancer mortality of the cohort, adjusted for age and sex, to be about 60% of the comparable California rate. Since the Seventh-Day Adventists also possess a distinctive pattern of dietary habits, approximately half adhering to a milk–egg–vegetarian diet, Lemon *et al.* also investigated colon cancer mortality and reported it to be 60–70% of the rate for total California. Information on the anatomic distribution of tumors also supports the presumption of lower risks for large-bowel cancer among Adventists. In series from two California hospitals the site of colon–rectal cancers among Adventists were displaced to the right side when compared to non-Adventist controls, the deficit in Adventist patients being concentrated in the descending, sigmoid, and rectosigmoid segments (Phillips, 1975).

Other opportunities to observe the experience of religious groups with special characteristics are presented from time to time. For example, the Bombay Cancer Registry has contrasted the site-specific cancer incidence of the local Parsi community (a highly inbred group of about 80,000 survivors of Zoroastrians who left Persia in the seventh century A.D.) with that of the predominantly Hindu population of Bombay and found the Parsis to exhibit a higher incidence of bowel cancer than is typical of Bombay and of many Asian communities (Table XXII) (Jussawalla and Jain, 1976). The elevated risk for large-

TABLE XXII

AGE-ADJUSTED INCIDENCE RATES PER 100,000 FOR CANCER OF THE COLON AND RECTUM AMONG PARSI. BOMBAY, INDIA, 1970–1972[a]

Bombay	Colon		Rectum	
	Male	Female	Male	Female
Parsi	7.9	12.6	3.8	2.6
All others	3.7	2.7	4.7	2.5

[a] Source: Jussawalla and Jain (1976).

bowel cancer among the Parsis is of interest, since this population is known to have a high female breast cancer rate by Asian standards. The Parsis thus are consistent with the general tendency for breast and large-bowel cancer rates to be closely correlated in interpopulation comparisons.

III. Environmental and Host Factors

A. TOBACCO USE

No important new information on tobacco smoking and large-bowel cancer has been accumulated since this topic was reviewed by Wynder and Shigematsu (1967). The findings from three well-known prospective studies on smoking and health conducted by Doll and Hill (1964), Kahn (1966), and Hammond (1966) and from a recent study in Sweden (Cederlöf et al., 1975) are summarized in Table XXIII. All sources agree that the association of colon cancer with tobacco use is weak. The numerically small excess mortality among smokers compared to nonsmokers is insignificant when compared to that observed for other digestive organs—esophagus, pancreas, and stomach. The data from England and Sweden suggest a somewhat stronger relationship between rectal cancer and smoking, but this feature does not appear in the U.S. Veterans Administration study. The collective evidence does not demonstrate a regular, consistent gradient in risk by amount smoked for either colon or rectum.

All four studies described a slightly more elevated mortality for pipe and/or cigar smokers than for cigarette smokers, a feature also found in case-control studies by Stocks (1957) (an excess of pipe smokers among rectal cancer deaths) and by Pernu (1960) (an excess of male pipe smokers among colon cancer patients). Other case-control studies, however, have not reported effects linked with specific forms of tobacco use (Schwartz et al., 1961; Higginson, 1966).

Wynder et al. (1967) in their case-control study pursued smoking history in relation to tumor localization in detail and described an apparent excess of heavy cigar smokers among patients presenting sigmoid and rectosigmoid lesions. However, there was a concentration of Jews and obese persons among cigar smokers in their series which suggests that cigar use may have been confounded with other potential etiological factors, and the authors concluded that no inferences of a direct association between cigar smoking and large-bowel cancer could be drawn.

TABLE XXIII
STANDARDIZED MORTALITY RATIOS (SMR)[a] FOR CANCER OF THE COLON
AND RECTUM, BY SMOKING HISTORY, MALES. FOUR STUDIES[b]

	SMR	
Study	Colon	Rectum
1. U.S. veterans study (Kahn, 1954–1962)		
Current smokers	1.18	0.95
Cigarettes only	1.27	0.98
>39 per day	1.43	0.84
Pipe and/or cigars only	1.20	1.07
Ex-smokers	1.21	1.02
2. American Cancer Society Study (Hammond, 1959–1963)		
History of regular use		
Cigarettes	1.09	
Pipe and/or cigars	1.31	
3. British physicians study (Doll et al., 1951–1961)		
History of regular use		
All smokers	0.97	2.2
Cigarettes only	0.84	2.4
Cigarettes with pipe and/or cigar)	1.03	2.4
Pipe and/or cigar	1.26	1.6
Current smokers	1.03	2.2
>25 gm/day	1.42	4.4
Ex-smokers	0.74	2.4
4. Sweden, 10-year follow-up (Cederlof et al., 1963–1972)		
Current smokers	1.02	1.72
Cigarettes	0.90	1.64
>15 per day	1.64	—
Pipe only	1.17	2.08
>5 gm per day	1.39	2.42

[a] Standardized mortality ratio for males who never smoked regularly = 100.
[b] Sources: Kahn, (1966), Hammond (1966), Doll and Hill (1964), Cederlöf et al. (1975).

Drexler (1967, 1968, 1971) has reported that by proctosigmoidoscopy he detected a higher prevalence of polyps, a suspect precursor of large bowel carcinoma, among cigarette, cigar, and pipe smokers. He also noted a greater tendency for smokers to present multiple polyps. Only a fraction of the polpys in the study series were biopsied and studied microscopically, and their histologic characteristics are not well defined. It is not clear how Drexler's data may be reconciled with the other predominantly negative comparisons that have relied on mortality from large-bowel cancer as the observational end point and further efforts to reproduce and assess Drexler's results are needed. At this stage in development of the evidence the conservative conclusion would be that no convincing case for a causal relationship between tobacco smoking and large-bowel cancer has been demonstrated.

B. Diet

The international variations in risk of large-bowel cancer closely parallel the ranking of countries by stage of economic development (Higginson, 1967). Burkitt (1971a,b) felt that no other site was so closely linked to changes in dietary habits that usually accompany economic development. Burkitt recognized the rarity of bowel cancer in most African populations and relied heavily on these observations in formulating his ideas on the etiology of bowel cancer. He was cognizant of the general findings on intercountry variations in risk summarized earlier in this review, but he did not rely on systematic correlations between indices of large-bowel cancer risk and per capita consumption of various foodstuffs. Burkitt was impressed by the high fiber and low carbohydrate content of the diet in Africa and other less developed areas of the world in contradistinction to Western countries, an observation made by Cleave et al. (1969). In formulating his ideas on the cause of bowel cancer, Burkitt concentrated his attention on key facts regarded by him to be of critical importance: (1) the relationship between diet and bowel behavior and content; (2) the epidemiologic association between noninfective bowel diseases and low-residue diet; (3) the parallel geographic distributions of bowel cancer and noninfective bowel diseases and their tendency to present jointly in individual patients; (4) the geographical association between noninfective bowel diseases and other conditions, such as diabetes, atherosclerosis, and obesity; (5) the role played by bacteria in producing bowel cancer in experimental models.

He reasoned as follows: reduction in fiber content and bulk favors increased consumption of refined carbohydrates; a cellulose-depleted diet can produce diverticular disease (Painter and Burkitt, 1971); changes in cellulose content of food alter colonic activity and bowel transit time; excess carbohydrates alter the bacterial composition of feces. Differences in intestinal transit time and stool weight between African villagers, boys in an African boarding school on a semi-European-type diet, and boys in an English boarding school have been demonstrated (D. P. Burkitt, personal communication, 1976), and other studies have shown the major differences in intestinal flora between English as compared to Ugandan stools to be an increase in bacteroids and bifidobacteria and a decrease in streptococci and lactobacilli (Aries et al., 1969). The association between noninfective

bowel diseases and conditions linked to excess consumption of refined carbohydrate, such as diabetes, atherosclerosis, and obesity,
could be accounted for by the fact that lack of unabsorbable fiber
results in increased consumption of refined products to satisfy appetite
(Burkitt, 1970). Carcinogens produced by bacterial action on bile salts
or other bile constituents are the probable cause of bowel tumors. Any
carcinogen ingested or formed in the gut of refined carbohydrate
eaters would be present in a more concentrated form and would be
held in contact with the mucosa for a more prolonged period in the
constipated colon. Bacterial activity and colonic stasis could account
for the anatomical distribution of tumors found maximally in the area
where fecal retention is most prolonged and bacterial action most pronounced. The chain of reasoning is summarized in a diagrammatic
representation (Fig. 23).

Although Burkitt exercised great ingenuity in combining a series of
observations into a coherent chain of evidence to support his hypothe-

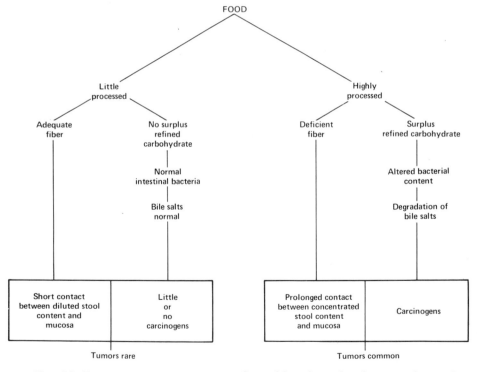

FIG. 23. Diagrammatic representation of possible relationship between diet and
cancer of the bowel. Source: Burkitt (1971a).

sis, there is a weakness. It stems from singling out low-residue diets and refined carbohydrates as the critical differences distinguishing food consumption patterns in high-risk populations from those in populations at low risk to bowel cancer. Food patterns in individual countries tend to present distinctive patterns of use and nonuse resulting in strong positive or negative correlations between specific food items. Under these circumstances international comparisons of per capita food consumption can and do reveal foods or combinations of foods that appear to discriminate among high- and low-risk populations. For example, Gregor *et al.* (1969) have remarked on the close correlation between national dietary levels of animal protein and mortality from intestinal cancer.

Despite the analytical difficulties, several authors have examined systematically and reported on the correlations between per capita consumption of food items (based on data collected by the Food and Agricultural Organization) and the incidence and/or mortality of large-bowel cancer (Bjelke, 1973; Armstrong and Doll, 1975; Howell, 1974, 1975). The findings of the several authors are in good agreement, which is not surprising since they all relied on the same primary data sources. Generally speaking, the pattern of relationships was the same for men and women and for colon and rectum, so that for present purposes the discussion can be restricted to the results for colon cancer among males. The strongest negative correlations were observed for cereals and pulses and nuts, and the strongest positive correlations were with meat, animal protein, and total fat.

Bjelke limited himself to computation of a descriptive set of correlation coefficients for individual food items and did not attempt in his analysis to compute partial correlation coefficients or use other devices to control specifically for effects attributable to other foods. Armstrong and Doll (1975) from their use of partial correlation coefficients concluded that the environmental variables most highly correlated with colon cancer rates were meat and animal protein consumption. They noted that control for either of these two variables substantially reduced the correlations with colon cancer for all other food variables (for example, the partial correlation coefficient for total fats was reduced to values between 0.11 and 0.24); conversely, control for other foods did not reduce the correlation between meat consumption and large-bowel cancer incidence to less than 0.70. Total fat consumption appeared more highly correlated with rectal cancer mortality, but even this correlation was substantially reduced by control for animal protein consumption. The authors also examined their data bearing on the highly publicized negative association of colon cancer with fiber consumption (cereals being considered to be the major source of dietary fiber) and found that in their material much of the negative correlation with cereals could be accounted for by control for meat consumption, the latter reducing the partial correlation coefficient for cereals to rather negligible dimensions, -0.10 to -0.20.

Howell (1975) pointed out that the vegetable sources of food were independent of or tended to be negatively related to colon cancer and that the associations with the disease were concentrated in the animal sources of food. Total meat protein tended to yield somewhat higher correlations with incidence than did total meat fat, but this relationship was not reproduced in her analysis using mortality data. Howell felt that there was little basis for preferring dietary protein or dietary fat as the more suspect or more significant association. The problem is that total fat and meat consumption are so highly correlated that it is difficult by use of statistical techniques to estimate separate effects attributable to each factor. Rice, cattle meat, eggs, and milk were the individual items most strongly associated, positively or negatively, with cancer of the colon and rectum. Of the meat items, beef was the most strongly associated. The results for pork and poultry were less suggestive, and fish appeared to be an unrelated factor. Howell concluded that the weight of the evidence indicates that the immediate study focus for future work should be directed to meat, specifically beef, as the dietary component most likely to be a causative factor in the development of colorectal cancer.

In principle, the approach based on population aggregate data for food consumption and large-bowel cancer used to study international variations could be extended to within-country differences. Bjelke (1973) reviewed the data for Norway and the United States in this connection and concluded that this would be an unproductive exercise requiring probably unwarranted statistical manipulation; the difficulties in interpretation of the international comparisons would be compounded by the limited range in variation in food consumption and disease risk in the more homogeneous setting presented by a single country. For within-country investigations only case-control or cohort studies would have any promise of producing reasonably accurate clues on dietary factors.

A limited number of studies have searched for case-control differences in the use of foods. One of the earliest of these was carried out by Stocks (1957). The major findings from a series of subsequent investigations are summarized in Table XXIV. The results from case-control studies up to 1970 were essentially negative, although Wynder's work in Japan (Wynder *et al.*, 1969) did suggest that bowel cancer patients

TABLE XXIV

SUMMARY OF FINDINGS FROM CASE-CONTROL STUDIES OF DIET AND BOWEL CANCER

Reference	Study locale	Findings
Stocks (1957)	North Wales and Liverpool	Beer drinking positively associated with large bowel cancer for males. Very weak suggestion of deficit in green vegetable intake by colorectal cancer patients
Pernu (1960)	Finland	No case-control differences found
Higginson (1966)	Kansas City, U.S.	No case-control differences found
Wynder and Shigematsu (1967)	New York City, U.S.	No consistent case-control differences demonstrable for any food items
Wynder et al. (1969)	Japan	Colon cancer patients had diet lower in rice and higher in fruit and milk than controls
Haenszel et al. (1973)	Hawaii, U.S.	Excess bowel cancer risk for Hawaiian Japanese who regularly ate only Western-style meals. Bowel cancer patients ate meats, legumes, and starches more frequently; beef and string beans were major contributors to meat and legume effects
Bjelke (1973)	Norway	Relatively low intake of fish, vegetables, vitamin A and high intake of "processed" meats by colon and rectal cancer patients. A negative association with coffee was specific for colon cancer. Patients with cancer of the low rectum had diets deficient in fruits, berries, and vitamin C and in this respect closely resembled the diets of stomach cancer patients
Bjelke (1973)	Minnesota, U.S.	Total group of colorectal cancer patients had lower intakes of vegetables, fruits, vitamins A and C, coffee, and crude fiber than controls. Lower intake of fruits and vitamin C most marked in patients with low rectum cancer.
Phillips (1975)	Seventh-Day Adventists	Higher proportion of colon cancer cases gave history of past use of meat, heavy use of dairy products, except milk, and other high-fat foods compared to Adventist controls. Classification based on current use of meat did not discriminate between cases and controls.

had a more Westernized diet and ate less rice and more fruit and milk than did controls. However, detection of case-control differences would be difficult in locales presenting a homogeneous background of diet practices. The study of the Hawaiian Japanese—a population undergoing displacement from low to high colon cancer risk and in varying stages of transition from a Japanese to Western-style diet—was the first to uncover important correlations between individual foods and bowel cancer (Haenszel *et al.*, 1973). The detection of positive findings was probably facilitated by the more favorable setting of greater heterogeneity in diet provided by a migrant population.

The Hawaiian Japanese study collected extensive data on individual food items, and the data analysis was carried out in a manner that permitted the computation of relative risks for individual foods (meats, legumes, starches, etc.) adjusted for other dietary factors. The capsule summary in Table XXIV is supplemented by the accompanying tabulation of adjusted relative risks for selected meats.

	Beef	Pork, total	Chicken
Unadjusted	2.2^a	1.5	1.43
Adjusted for			
Beef	—	1.20	1.20
Pork, total	2.1^a	—	1.34
Chicken	2.1^a	1.45	—

[a] Risks significantly different from unity at the 1% level.

Beef exhibited the most pronounced case-control difference and was the only meat that yielded a significantly elevated risk for the summary contrast of above-average vs below-average use. The risk estimates for pork and chicken were substantially reduced by control for beef, while control for pork and chicken had minimal effect on the result for beef. The case-control differences in total meat use thus appeared to be concentrated in some facets of beef consumption. The introduction of information on past history of use strengthened the association between beef and bowel cancer, but left unchanged the results for other meats.

The other major findings can be summarized as follows:

1. More bowel cancer patients than controls had abandoned the practice of eating at least one Japanese-style meal daily.

2. Patients ate meat, legumes, and starches more frequently, the disparity between patients and controls being less pronounced for

starches than for meat and legumes. When the relative risks for individual meats and legumes were adjusted for consumption of other foods within the same category, beef and string beans were identified as major contributors to the meat and legume effects.

3. The case-control differences for meat (beef) and legumes (string beans) persisted among both Issei (migrants) and Nisei (U.S.-born offspring); the excess frequency in consumption of starches was limited to Nisei.

4. Individual meats, legumes, and starches displayed gradients in risk rising with frequency of use.

5. Separate, independent effects for beef, string beans, and starches were suggested; the case-control contrasts were strengthened by the consideration of various combinations of beef, string beans, and starches.

6. The associations with beef and string beans were enhanced in the subset of patients whose tumors were in the sigmoid and adjacent colon.

The risk differentials of the magnitude found in this study, up to 3-fold and greater, compared favorably with those found in case-control studies of other cancer sites and other etiologies (cigarette smoking and lung cancer excepted). It is worth noting that the foods implicated in the bowel cancer study were entirely different from those incriminated in the companion stomach cancer study (Haenszel *et al.*, 1972).

No single case-control study can be viewed as definitive, and the findings must be viewed in the context of other evidence. The interpretation by Haenszel *et al.* of the Hawaiian Japanese study relied on collateral evidence from several sources. Their reading of the geographic comparisons was that consumption of meat and refined carbohydrates and mortality from bowel cancer and arteriosclerotic heart disease all appear in relatively affluent populations. In the search for promising lines of investigation they viewed meats (beef) as a more likely etiologic candidate than starches for the following reasons:

1. There is a stronger and more coherent pattern of associations for meat than for starches in the Hawaiian Japanese data.

2. Meat provides a striking example of a change in food practices between Japan and Hawaii—the rise in beef consumption—to parallel the upward displacement of bowel cancer risk among Japanese migrants.

3. An epidemiologic observation exists on an unusual congruence of high meat and low refined carbohydrate consumption; it argues for attention to meat in perference to refined carbohydrates. Argentina has

a high meat (beef) intake, and the fraction of calories from refined carbohydrates is relatively low (Puffer and Griffith, 1967). Corresponding to this, Argentina presents a major exception to the usual configuration of a positive association between bowel cancer and atherosclerosis: Mortality from bowel cancer in Argentina is as high as that in the United States, but mortality from arteriosclerotic heart disease is moderately low in Argentina (Puffer and Griffith, 1967). Uruguay also has had a high per capita meat consumption (Food and Agriculture Organization of the United Nations, 1958), and Doll (1969) projects a bowel cancer incidence rate higher than that for U.S. whites. The death rate from arteriosclerotic heart disease in Uruguay, while high for Latin America, is only about half that of the United States (World Health Organization, 1973).

4. Similar, if less striking, contrasts are found elsewhere among countries of high bowel cancer incidence. Doll (1969) considers Scotland to have the world's highest bowel cancer incidence rate and the highest death rate, certainly much higher than that of England to the south. The Scots eat less meat than the English but currently 20% more beef (National Food Survey Committee, 1971). [They also eat more carbohydrates (bread) and have more coronary heart disease.] New Zealand has the highest bowel cancer incidence rates as reported in Doll et al. (1970) and also has ranked high—far above the United States—in beef consumption (Food and Agriculture Organization of the United Nations, 1958). Beef consumption has dropped substantially in Australia between 1955 and 1965 (Food and Agriculture Organization of the United Nations, 1958, 1971), and the bowel cancer mortality in Australia, which was as high as that in New Zealand, is now 10% lower (Segi and Kurihara, 1972). The search for parallels is much less successful in regions of lower incidence and lower beef intake. However, no populations with a high beef intake and a low rate of bowel cancer have been found.

Bjelke's (1973) case-control studies were also carried out within the context of a migrant population setting. Bjelke had observed that most cancer epidemiological studies are directed to the detection of initiating or promoting factors and that, in the preoccupation with initiating–promoting agents, the search for protective effects is neglected. His concern with protective effects enabled him to note the lower intake of vegetables, fruits, and crude fiber among patients in his Norway and Minnesota series. Bjelke felt that the negative association of colorectal cancer with total vegetable intake was consistent with data from India reported by Paymaster et al. (1968).

Past history of food use is more relevant to the etiology of bowel cancer than current status, and the intriguing feature of the small Seventh-Day Adventist study (Phillips, 1975) was its ability to detect a higher frequency of use of meat, poultry, and fish by cases 20 years earlier, while responses on current practices failed to discriminate. Although precise determinations of frequency of use 20 years earlier are not possible, the pedigree of historical data in this situation is good. Among Seventh-Day Adventists one can assess reliably the vegetarian vs nonvegetarian status in the distant past, since members can recall distinctly the change from nonvegetarian to vegetarian status which often took place after they joined the church.

Investigators have utilized intercountry variation in bowel cancer and per capita food consumption as consistency checks on dietary hypotheses. Other axes of comparisons used for this same purpose include region, race, farm vs nonfarm, urban vs rural, social class, time trends. Howell (1975) in her review concentrated on diet information contained in the Department of Agriculture publications with special attention to race, region of country, and farm vs nonfarm and concluded that the pattern of variation for beef consumption in the available contrasts coincided better with the variation in bowel cancer that did pork, poultry, or fish. However, the available consistency checks do not invariably lead to the same conclusions. Enstrom (1975a) in matching the time trends and socioeconomic, urban–rural, and regional gradients in beef and fat consumption with the corresponding information on bowel cancer felt that the data were incompatible and argued against an etiological role for beef and fat consumption. The more telling points in Enstrom's critique were an upward trend in per capita beef consumption over the past 25 years in contrast to the relatively stable colorectal cancer incidence and a rise in per capita beef consumption with income in contrast to the minimal socioeconomic gradients in risk. Enstrom (1975b) also pointed to the deficit of colon cancer among Mormons, who have no religious proscription against the use of meat, as favoring other hypotheses.

Ad hoc modifications of hypotheses to blunt specific citations of inconsistencies are possible. For example, the force of some of Enstrom's criticisms would be lessened if the association were dependent on specific beef or cattle characteristics. For example, beef will differ in fat content depending on age, on how long it was range fed and whether it was grain fed in a feeding lot. Or if there is a certain level of beef consumption beyond which there is no increased carcinogenic risk, this might explain the failure to detect social class gradients in risk for bowel cancer within the United States. The latter explanation cannot be dismissed, since in Cali (Colombia) (Haenszel *et al.*, 1975) the gradient in bowel cancer correlates well with social class differences in meat (beef) consumption, the latter being almost absent in the diet of the lower social classes. Other loopholes in consistency checks and data interpretation could be advanced, but their elaboration does not appear to be a profitable exercise.

The review on the role of diet has focused on information collected from patient interviews and data from vital statistics and nutritional survey sources. The most defensible position to take with respect to the observations on dietary factors is that etiologic leads have been generated, but that the evidence does not suffice to choose among them with certainty. New information is required that must be sought either by animal experimentation or by more refined epidemiological studies. It would be better not to multiply indefinitely the type of exploratory epidemiological studies conducted in the recent past, but to wait until animal work suggested by leads from epidemiological studies can in turn produce more sharply defined ideas on carcinogenic mechanisms. When ideas on mechanisms are developed or refined, it should then be possible to design new studies to test and elaborate them.

Reliance on prospective studies would improve the accuracy of the diet information by permitting current collection of diet histories from members of defined cohorts, whose subsequent morbidity and mortality experience could be monitored. Such studies have been initiated in Norway (for a representative male population sample) and in the United States (for a Hawaiian Japanese male cohort), but sufficient time has not elapsed for the collection of suggestive, let alone definitive, results. To reduce the time interval between exposure and response, large-bowel cancer might be replaced by a different observational end point, and for this purpose adenomatous polyps could be used as a marker. While the introduction of adenomatous polyps as an end point in ongoing cohort studies is conceptually feasible, this would create operational and logistical difficulties. The alternative of a case-control study contrasting the diet of polyp-bearers and non-polyp-bearers might be more manageable.

C. ALCOHOL

One of the first indications of a possible association between alcohol consumption and large-bowel cancer came from a report by the Registrar General of England and Wales (1962) that pinpointed buccal cavity, esophagus, intestines, and rectum (but not stomach) as the sites in the digestive tract displaying excess risks for persons engaged in the alcoholic-beverage trades. Precisely the same site profile of elevated risks was also observed among migrants from Ireland to the United States (Haenszel, 1961), for whom a high rate of alcohol consumption had been suggested by vital statistics and mental hospital sources; the death rate from alcoholism among the Irish in Boston had been extremely high (Davis, 1913), and the Irish had accounted for a disproportionate number of first admissions for alcoholic psychoses in New York State mental hospitals (Malzberg, 1935, 1936). More recently, E. Bjelke (Personal communication, 1974) noted the same configuration of excess risks for digestive tract neoplasms (the ratio of observed to expected deaths for large bowel being 1.7) among waiters in Norway during the years 1961–1971.

These impressions and leads have been elaborated by systematic geographical correlations of cancer mortality and alcohol consumption within the United States in international comparisons of 24 countries. Breslow and Enstrom (1974) reported a strong correlation ($r = 0.78$) between beer and rectal cancer in the U.S. male data, which was reproduced in the more heterogeneous data for 24 countries. In the latter set of data there was a strong correlation ($r = 0.83$) between beer and rectal cancer accompanied by a somewhat weaker association with colon cancer ($r = 0.58$). In both sets of data the relationship appeared to be limited to beer drinking; no association with wine and hard liquors was demonstrable.

The leads derived from observations of population aggregates have not been consistently confirmed by case-control studies. In studies conducted in 6 areas of England and Wales, Stocks (1957) reported large-bowel cancer and beer drinking to be associated, but other work in Finland (Pernu, 1960), Hawaii (Haenszel et al., 1973), and the continental United States (Higginson, 1966) failed to detect a relationship, and another U.S. study yielded inconclusive results due to the widely divergent experience of the two control populations (Wynder and Shigematsu, 1967).

Histories of alcohol use are difficult to elicit, and erroneous responses by cases and controls may have diluted or concealed any associations that might exist. To circumvent this problem, investigators in Finland (Hakulinen et al., 1974) and Norway (E. Bjelke, personal communication, 1974b) assembled rosters of individuals known to use alcohol to excess and monitored their subsequent cancer morbidity and mortality. The Norwegian male cohort has experienced a 40–50% excess in observed cases, and deaths for large-bowel cancer over the numbers expected and the results for Finland pointed in the same direction. The effects are small and require confirmation by continued surveillance, but the consistency between the two sets of data encourages the belief that an association does, in fact, exist. Similar findings are emerging from a prospective study of 12,000 men in Norway done as part of a comprehensive study of the cancer experience of Norwegian migrants to the United States, which show a positive gradient in risk of colorectal cancer with increased frequency of use of beef and hard liquors (Bjelke, 1975). The latter investigation also agrees with the population aggregate studies in describing the stronger relationship to be with beer consumption.

D. Bowel Habits; Laxatives

Bowel habits as related to size and frequency of stools has been the subject of interpopulation comparisons, but little information on this subject has been collected in case-control studies of large-bowel cancer patients. Pernu (1960) and Higginson and Oettlé (1960), who investigated this point, were unable to demonstrate important case-control differences in history, duration, and severity of constipation. Wynder and Shigematsu (1967) included this topic in their interviews but found no marked case-control differences in lifetime patterns of frequency of bowel movements. The latter authors in their analysis also reviewed their data for individual bowel segments but found no consistent associations between tumor localization and degree of constipation.

Boyd and Doll (1954) collected histories on use of laxative agents and reported an excess use of liquid paraffin among patients with gastrointestinal cancers, but not for other laxatives. Neither Higginson and Oettlé (1960) nor Wynder and Shigematsu (1967) were able to replicate the findings of Boyd and Doll.

E. Obesity

Obesity is intimately related to diet and caloric intake, and associations of obesity with large-bowel cancer may arise indirectly via other diet-related factors. For example, while it is true that the Hawaiian Japanese are more obese than people in Japan (Kagan et al., 1974), it does not necessarily follow that obesity per se is implicated in the higher large-bowel cancer rates of the Hawaiian Japanese. The role of body weight has been investigated by a few authors. Sommers (1964) reported overweight male and female subjects to be overrepresented in an autopsy series of colon and rectum cancer, when compared with both autopsy controls and data on life insurance policyholders. Wynder and Shigematsu's case-control study in New York City (1967) contrasted the weights of patients and controls as of 2 years prior to diagnosis and found the patient series to have a significant excess of individuals 20% or more overweight. This feature was more evident among males for whom the association was concentrated in the tumors presenting in the cecum-sigmoid segments. The smaller weight differential between female cases and controls was not accompanied by any pronounced link with tumor localization. Wynder and Shigematsu (1967) noted that the weights of their controls agreed well with baseline data assembled by the Metropolitan Life Insurance Company.

More recently, Bjelke (1973) has examined the data from studies conducted in Norway and Minnesota (the latter series containing a substantial representation of migrants from Scandinavia and their descendants). In Norway no noteworthy differences between colon and rectum patients and controls were found for either sex in weight or weight adjusted for height (bulk index expressed as weight/height^2). In Minnesota the cases displayed the higher mean values for weight and bulk index, particularly for males. The case-control study effects are not large, and too much emphasis should not be placed on any single result, but the consistency between the New York and Minnesota results in describing males to exhibit the stronger relationship between obesity and large-bowel cancer and the failure to detect an effect for either sex in Norway or Japan (Wynder et al., 1969) raise the possibility that the "obesity" effects are related to some more specific factors to which American men are more heavily exposed.

F. Associations with Other Diseases

The association of bowel cancer with the presentation of other diseases has been investigated in a variety of ways. The approach most extensively employed has been to plot and correlate the death rates for specific causes reported from countries throughout the world. Wynder et al. (1967) have summarized many of the available mortality data from national vital statistics offices on this subject. A substantial body of data has also been derived from study of the distribution of multiple primary cancer sites in individual patients as revealed by the surveillance of diagnosed cancer patients and determination of the incidence rate for a second primary cancer. Closely allied to the multiple primary approach are autopsy studies on the joint presentation of two or more pathological conditions and the calculation of whether their concordance is greater than expected based on the null hypothesis that the conditions are distributed independently. A more recent source of data comes from the constellation of morbid conditions entered on the death certificate for individual decedents. Coding of data on "multiple" causes of death is a relatively recent innovation and was not widely adopted by vital statistics offices until the 1960 decade.

Numerous authors have studied the covariation of site-specific cancer mortality among countries, and these efforts have been extended to consider associations with cardiovascular diseases as well (Wynder *et al.*, 1967; Segi *et al.*, 1960; Lea, 1967). The descriptive efforts include the preparation of graphs and the computation of Pearsonian product–moment correlation coefficients undertaken with the thought that the relationships revealed might yield clues helpful for formulating ideas on etiologic factors. Leaving aside the positive correlation between cancer of the colon and rectum (already commented on in the presentation of tumor registry data) the best-known examples of diseases associated with bowel cancer are: an inverse relationship with stomach cancer, positive associations with cancers of the female breast, endometrium, and ovary, and a positive association with arteriosclerotic heart disease (Wynder *et al.*, 1967). Associations with cancer of the stomach, bladder, lung, and pancreas have also been described (Bjelke, 1973). Bjelke pointed out that in his data the inverse relationship with stomach was confined to colon; for rectum he found a weak positive association with stomach. A similar anatomic distinction was noted for breast cancer, the association with breast being stronger for colon than rectum.

The scattergram depicting the joint distribution of mortality from colon and female breast cancer prepared by Wynder *et al.* (1967), shown in Fig. 24, suggests a rather well defined, regular relationship. The points for most countries (with the possible exception of Israel) did not deviate markedly from the expected values predicted by the fitted regression line. The positive geographical association with breast cancer suggested to Wynder *et al.* a role for dietary factors, possibly in the terms of fat intake that may influence the internal hormonal environment of the host.

Interest in the association of mortality from colon cancer and arteriosclerotic heart disease arises from the thought that the intake of saturated fats may be implicated in the etiology of the two diseases. The sex-specific nature of the relationships is worth noting. While the two diseases are strongly correlated for each sex (see Fig. 25), the rise in mortality of colon cancer per unit rise in mortality of arteriosclerotic heart disease is greater for females.

Although many authors have directed attention to the association of arteriosclerotic heart disease and colon cancer, it is not so well known

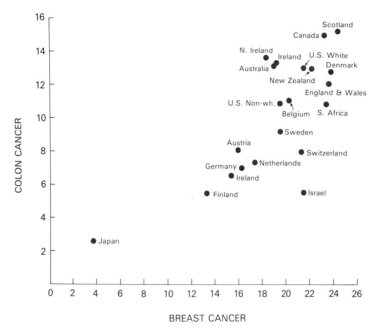

FIG. 24. Joint distribution of age-adjusted mortality rates per 100,000 for cancer of the colon and breast. 21 countries, 1960–1961. Source: Wynder *et al.* (1967).

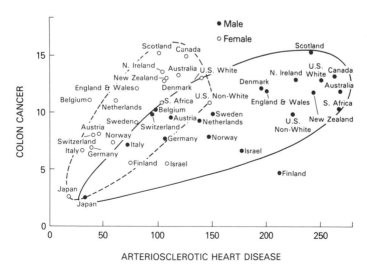

FIG. 25. Joint distribution of age-adjusted mortality rates per 100,000 for colon cancer and arteriosclerotic heart disease, by sex. 21 countries, 1960–1961. Source: Wynder *et al.* (1967).

that the international comparisons also depict an inverse association between cerebrovascular accidents and colon cancer, with Scotland, Norway, Italy, and Israel representing the only deviants from the regression curve. The attention of Haenszel and Kurihara (1968) was drawn to this inverse relationship when they considered the nature of the changes that had taken place in the mortality of the Japanese migrating to the United States with reference to the displacement of risks from the prevailing level in Japan to the host population level. They noted a rather complete transition in risks among Issei migrants for cerebrovascular accidents from the high risks in Japan to the characteristic low risks for U.S. whites. Colon cancer also showed a rather complete transition in the opposite direction. Stomach cancer and coronary heart disease represented examples of incomplete displacements in risk, and classification by degree of displacement in risk yielded two pairs: more or less complete transition—colon cancer, cerebrovascular accidents; incomplete transition—stomach cancer, coronary heart disease. Within each pair the changes occurred in the opposite direction and in this sense corresponded to the inverse relationships for these pairs of diseases noted in international comparisons of mortality. The singular aspect of the Japanese migrant experience has been the maintenance of an inverse relationship between colon cancer and cerebrovascular accidents despite the transformation in risks within a single generation from the characteristic level for Japan to that for U.S. whites. The maintenance of the inverse relationship under such radically changed conditions reinforces the belief that the negative association represents a real phenomenon, even though a plausible mechanism for relating the two disease complexes remains to be identified.

The literature on multiple primary cancers has been reviewed by Moertel (1966) and Schoenberg *et al.* (1969). The results bearing on the synchronous presentation and diagnosis of two or more primary sites of cancer in the same individual are more difficult to interpret and evaluate than those that come from surveillance of individuals with cancer of some specific site to determine the incidence rate for a second primary cancer. The question of interest is whether the risk of a second primary cancer of a specific site in a defined group of patients is the same, greater, or less than the risk of developing a first cancer at the site in question in the cancer-free population. Studies of second primary cancers are usually restricted to anatomic site groups different from that harboring the first primary and normally require that an interval of about 5 years elapse after the diagnosis of the first primary before a new primary is accepted for tabulation. The observed number of second primaries is compared with the number expected as determined by the site-, sex-, and age-specific incidence reported by population-based tumor registries.

Utilizing the material from the Connecticut Tumor Registry for female patients admitted to Connecticut hospitals between 1935 and 1962, Schoenberg et al. updated studies by Greenberg (1963) and Bailar (1963) on subsequent primary cancers in women with cancer of the breast or genital organs and found the ratio of observed to expected secondary primaries of the colon to be 1.5 or greater for patients whose index cancers were located in the breast, corpus uteri, ovary, and cervix uteri. Only patients with cancers of the cervix and corpus uteri displayed an excess of second primaries located in the rectum; for those sites the ratio of observed to expected rectal cancers exceeded 2:1. The results of Schoenberg et al. have not been consistently replicated by other investigators. In follow-up of patients with carcinoma of the corpus uteri seen in a Boston hospital over a 40-year period, MacMahon and Austin (1969) found no excess of bowel cancer. Schottenfeld and Berg (1971) in their report on second primary cancers in female patients with cancer of the breast and genital organs seen at Memorial Sloan-Kettering Cancer Center in New York City described an excess of colon cancers among women previously diagnosed as having cancer of the corpus uteri or ovary, but not for women with cancer of the breast or cervix uteri. The latter authors did note an excess of rectal tumors for women whose first primary was in the cervix or corpus uteri. Given the small numbers of observations, the individual study results are subject to sizable sampling errors. The findings for colon and rectum from the three studies cited have been summarized by Bjelke (1973), and Table XXV has been abstracted from that source.

The reverse approach has also been employed. Starting with women whose index cancer presented in the large bowel, Schottenfeld et al. (1969) found an excess of second primary cancers of the breast and female genital organs. The ratio of observed to expected cases of breast cancer were 2.1 for the index patients with colon cancer and 1.7 for patients with cancer of the rectum. The corresponding ratios for second primaries of the female genital organs were 2.1 and 0.8, respectively, for the index patients with colon and rectal cancer. Neither Schottenfeld et al. nor Moertel distinguished between colon and rectum in their observations on second primary cancers for index patients with bowel cancer.

Greenberg (1963) reported an excess number of second primary breast cancers in patients whose first primary cancer was located in the colon. The association in his data was specific for colon and not present

TABLE XXV

RATIO OF OBSERVED TO EXPECTED SECOND PRIMARY CANCERS OF THE
COLON AND RECTUM FROM THREE SERIES OF WOMEN WITH INDEX
CANCERS OF THE BREAST AND FEMALE REPRODUCTIVE ORGANS

Site of first primary	Reporting author[a]	O/E[b] second primary	
		Colon	Rectum
Breast	Schoenberg *et al.*	1.5	0.9
	Schottenfeld and Berg	0.9	1.2
	Total	1.3	1.0
Cervix uteri	Schoenberg *et al.*	1.6	2.2
	Schottenfeld and Berg	1.0	2.1
	Total	1.4	2.2
Corpus uteri	Schoenberg *et al.*	1.6	2.4
	Schottenfeld and Berg	1.9	1.8
	MacMahon and Austin	0.9	0.9
	Total	1.3	1.6
Ovary	Schoenberg *et al.*	2.4	0
	Schottenfeld and Berg	3.3	0
	Total	2.5	0

[a] Sources: Schoenberg *et al.* (1969); Schottenfeld and Berg (1971); MacMahon and Austin (1969).
[b] O, observed; E, expected.

in patients whose first primary was located elsewhere in the digestive tract. Bjelke (1973) followed up this observation and abstracted from the Norwegian Cancer Registry information on all other primary cancers recorded for women first diagnosed and reported to the registry as colon cancer cases. Pending a more precise life table analysis of the experience for the index series of colon cancer patients, Bjelke in an initial analysis compared the percent site distribution of second (or coprimary) tumors with the percent site distribution of first primaries in Norwegian women as of 1959–1961 and found an apparent excess of cancers of the breast and corpus uteri, in addition to the anticipated excess of second primary cancers in the colon and rectum. While Bjelke's series exhibited a relative preponderance of cancers of the breast and corpus uteri among the extracolonic primaries in women with colon cancer in conformity with other reports, his distributions of the extracolonic primaries did not differ markedly between women whose tumors were located in the right and left colon. In this respect his observations did not coincide with Schottenfeld *et al.* (1969) in finding that patients with cancer in the right colon had the highest risk of subsequent extracolonic primary or of Schoenberg *et al.* (1969) that tumors of the right colon are more strongly associated with cancer of the breast and corpus uteri. After review of the separate data for women over and under age 70, Bjelke did suggest that an association between colon and breast cancer might be confined to tumors occurring among the older women.

Studies of multiple primaries leave little doubt about the associations among cancers of the breast, endometrium, and ovary, but the same high degree of certainty and assurance does not prevail for the association of colorectal tumors with breast and endometrial cancers. The fact that the same sources fail to reveal any association among stomach, breast, and endometrial cancers is a point in favor of accepting the findings for bowel cancer, even though the small sizes of the study series, the uncertainties in calculating the control numbers of expected cancers, and the difficulties of distinguishing between a second primary and a recurrence of the primary tumor preclude firm judgments. One can interpret the studies of second primaries as supporting the site-specific associations revealed by the international comparative studies without accepting the data on second primaries as independent evidence on the presence of site-specific associations.

Entries of a combination of conditions or diseases on the death certificate are subject to various complicating factors, and they may reflect no more than the probability of joint recognition, quite independent of whether the conditions are in fact associated. The only intensive study of this data source in relation to bowel cancer has been carried out in Norway by Bjelke (1973) using the death certificates filed in 1956–1965. The Norwegian statistical office was one of the first to code systematically information on multiple conditions entered on the death certificate (Norges Offisielle Statistikk, 1962). Bjelke looked at the behavior of individual cancer sites in relation to 13 contributory conditions and arrived at the following tentative conclusions. Colon and rectum cancer displayed different patterns of associations with contributory diseases; colon, but not rectum, appeared to be associated with the presentation of arteriosclerotic heart disease. This result is consistent with some of the findings suggested by the correlation studies of geographic variation and the investigations of multiple primary cancer sites.

Since elevated serum cholesterol levels have been shown to be predictive for higher risks of myocardial infarctions (Kannel *et al.*, 1971;

Rhoads *et al.*, 1976), the observed association of large-bowel cancer with arteriosclerotic heart disease in geographical comparisons prompts the question whether the former disease is also related to serum cholesterol. Rose *et al.* (1974) postulated that a high fatty acid intake, favoring a high serum cholesterol level, could form more bile salts, increase the substrate available for carcinogen-forming bacteria, and hence increase the risk for colon cancer. Since serum cholesterol can be determined by a simple screening test, hypothesized relationships between serum cholesterol and bowel cancer are amenable to test by straightforward case-control study methods. Four such studies have reported serum cholesterol to be significantly lower in colon cancer patients than controls in contrast to the findings made for patients with coronary artery disease (Rose *et al.*, 1974; Bjelke, 1974; Pearce and Dayton, 1971; Leren, 1970). There are three studies which describe serum cholesterol and colon cancer to be positively associated (Report of a Research Committee to the Medical Research Council, 1968; Turpeinen *et al.*, 1968; National Diet-Heart Study Final Report, 1968). The role of cholesterol in the etiology of bowel cancer remains uncertain, and the subject needs further investigation. Ederer *et al.* (1971) analyzed the data from 5 of the above trials of serum cholesterol-lowering diets, and their review led them to conclude that serum cholesterol-lowering diets do not affect bowel cancer risk.

Autopsy studies have the potential of generating additional data on associations of morbid conditions. Several autopsy studies have investigated separately the prevalence of intestinal metaplasia of the gastric mucosa and the prevalence of intestinal polyps, which are suspect precursor states of stomach and bowel cancer. From simultaneous observations on the presence of both conditions in the same individual, information on the association of the two conditions is provided automatically. Such a study has recently been completed in Costa Rica, and the findings suggest that the two conditions present independently in individual subjects (J. C. Salas, personal communication, 1976) and thus do not support an inverse association of stomach and bowel cancer inferred from studies of the geographical distribution of the two diseases. The same approach could be extended to studies of other conditions, such as atherosclerosis of the coronary arteries and intestinal polyps. An autopsy study to see whether the positive association of arteriosclerotic heart disease and bowel cancer noted in the geographical variation in risk of the two diseases can be reproduced in studies of related precursor conditions in individuals has been initiated in New Orleans, but no study findings are available to date (P. Correa, personal communication, 1976).

G. Blood Group

Vogel and Krüger (1968) have made a thorough review of the extensive literature on ABO-blood group and disease. From the composite data, they estimated an 11% excess of colorectal patients of blood group A compared to blood group O. The association with blood group A is definitely weaker than that described by numerous reports for stomach cancer, for which Vogel and Krüger report a typical A : O ratio of 1.22. The recent studies in Norway and Minnesota did not detect consistent or marked case-control differences in ABO distribution for large-bowel cancer (Bjelke, 1973).

H. Marital Status

It is well known that unmarried persons have a less favorable mortality experience than married persons. The authors who have investigated this subject have considered the following points: (1) selective factors that cause persons at greater risk to early death to avoid marriage; (2) errors in the reporting of marital status on death certificates and census returns; (3) the disadvantageous environment associated with the unmarried state (Shurtleff, 1956; Sheps, 1961). To control for the influence of health-related factors that operate against the remarriage of widowed and divorced persons, the customary practice is to compare the experience of the "never-married" and "ever-married" in investigations of the effects of marital status.

The cause-specific contrasts of mortality by marital status for the United States as of 1949–1951 and 1959–1961 included some data on digestive-tract cancers (National Office of Vital Statistics, 1956; Klebba, 1970). For the group of digestive-tract cancers the age-adjusted mortality in 1959–1961 was about 20% higher among never-married than ever-married white men, but among white females approximately equal rates for both marital groups prevailed. The excess risks of digestive system cancers among the never-married were smaller than those for total mortality among whites and nonwhites of both sexes. The 1947 U.S. cancer morbidity survey (Dorn and Cutler, 1959) reported a 10% excess incidence for all cancer sites combined among never-married white females and a more substantial differential in the same direction for nonwhite females, accompanied by the well-established excess risks for breast cancer among single females and a similar, but smaller, excess for uterine corpus and ovary (Table XXVI). The marital status differential for total digestive system was minimal. This and the other sources cited above provided no informa-

TABLE XXVI

AGE-ADJUSTED INCIDENCE RATES PER 100,000 FOR SELECTED SITES OF CANCER
BY RACE AND MARITAL STATUS. UNITED STATES MORBIDITY SURVEY, 1947[a]

	White		Nonwhite	
Site	Never married	Ever married	Never married	Ever married
All sites	353	326	396	289
Digestive system	79	80	93	67
Breast	98	70	66	54
Corpus uteri	13	10	24	10
Ovary	21	14	15	11

[a] Source: Dorn and Cutler (1959).

tion on risk differentials specific for large bowel and their relationship
to the typical patterns presented for breast and other reproductive
organs. Given the parallels in interpopulation variation in risks of
breast and large-bowel cancer (Wynder et al., 1967), more precise
information on marital status differentials for large-bowel cancer might
provide clues as to whether some of the reproductive and hormonal
factors thought to be involved in breast cancer play a role in the etiology of large-bowel cancer.

Some data on this point have been provided by Fraumeni et al.
(1969), who examined unpublished 1959–1961 U.S. mortality data and
were able to report that large bowel differed from other digestive tract
sites with respect to variation by marital status. The rates for single
women exceeded those for the ever-married at every age for colon and
rectum while higher mortality for the ever-married prevailed after age
55 for stomach and after age 45 for biliary passages and liver. As an
indicator of the "environmental" effects of marital status on cancer
risks, studies of women in religious orders offer certain advantages,
since they represent well-defined groups who in most orders remain
unmarried and celibate throughout life. Such an observational setting
minimizes the selective factors that affect the composition of the unmarried general adult female population. Fraumeni et al. (1969)
analyzed the mortality experience of white, U.S.-born, never-married
Sisters in 41 religious communities and found the nuns to have
slightly lower rates for digestive site cancers in the age span 40–69
years than did the control population of white females. After age 70 the
relationship was reversed and nuns had the higher rates. More detailed inquiry pinpointed deaths from cancer of the colon, but not

rectum, as responsible for the excess risk observed among older nuns. The authors concluded that the single-married differential for large-bowel cancer presented by the general population experience was consistent with the excess frequency of such cancers in their cohort of nuns. They reviewed the variety of host factors that have pointed to an endrocrinologic influence in the etiology of reproductive-organ cancers and quoted Sommers (1964) as stating that "similar factors may occur in colonic cancer, as suggested by a reported association with obesity, pancreatic islet-cell hyperplasia, adrenal cortical hyperplasia and adenomas, and ovarian cystadenomas."

Bjelke (1973) subsequently reviewed the available Norwegian incidence data for females by marital status and calculated never-married/ever-married ratios for colon and rectum by broad age groups. It is difficult to reconcile the data from Norway with the U.S. findings. The two series available to Bjelke (Norway, 1953–1962; Oslo, 1961–1965) depicted a deficit in rectal cancer among the never-married and a minimal difference in risk by marital status for colon cancer; no excess risk for colon cancer among never-married females over age 70 was present. In the Oslo series an excess number of tumors presenting in the left colon including rectosigmoid among the never-married was suggested, but the possibility that this represented nothing more than chance variation could not be ruled out.

I. REPRODUCTIVE HISTORY

Interpopulation comparisons showing a positive correlation between the risks for cancer of the breast and of the large bowel suggest that a review of the epidemiology of large-bowel cancer should touch on the reproductive history parameters investigated with respect to breast cancer. This topic has not been actively pursued, and the only evidence on this point comes from work in Norway and Minnesota (Bjelke, 1973). These studies found no case-control differences in menarchal or menopausal ages or in age at first childbirth (adjusted for parity). In both the Norwegian and Minnesota series, the relationship with parity differed by anatomical location, with the risk of colonic cancer decreasing and the risk of rectal cancer increasing among women of high parity.

A provocative finding emerging from the Norway–Minnesota studies was the possible interaction of parity and blood group; the combined data described women of group O who had borne 3 or more children to have about half the colon cancer risk of other ever-married women in group A (Bjelke, 1973). No such effect was noted for women with fewer children. Since the effect was reproduced in both localities and a possible biological mechanism (immunization from ABO-incompatible or cross-reactive fetal tissues during pregnancy) was identified, Bjelke felt that this remained a subject for further investigation. Given the small size of the study samples, the parity effects observed may reflect nothing more than the vagaries of sampling variation due to the fractionation of a limited amount of data by repeated cross-classification. Bjelke's observations must be replicated and confirmed in other settings before they can be accepted as established fact.

J. Immunology; Carcinoembryonic Antigens (CEA)

The immunologic aspects of bowel cancer have received some attention in recent years, stimulated by the finding of Gold and Freedman (1965) of an antigen in extracts from colon cancer tissues. This antigen was absent in normal adult intestinal mucosa but was present in primitive endoderm and was therefore named carcinoembryonic antigen of the digestive system (CEA). Thompson et al. (1969) described a radioimmunoassay for CEA in the serum and reported positive results in 97% of a series of colon cancer patients. CEA has been isolated in a pure state as a glycoprotein with a molecular weight of 200,000. From fluorescent and electron microscopy studies, it has been concluded that CEA is synthesized in the cytoplasm of the mucosal cell, rapidly accumulates in the apical portion of the cell membrane, and is then excreted to the glandular lumen. An intense fluorescent stain is found in well-differentiated adenocarcinomas, whereas anaplastic carcinomas stain very weakly. There are cross reactions between CEA and blood group antibodies, and it has been proposed that CEA is a precursor of blood-group substances.

The discovery of CEA raised hopes for the development of new and effective tools in cancer diagnosis. These expectations have been moderated by the accumulated experience of several years, which has been the subject of several recent reviews (Neville and Laurence, 1974; Go, 1976; Herberman, 1976; Reynoso et al., 1972). The high accuracy of CEA as a diagnostic test for bowel cancer reported in the early papers was apparently due to the fact that most of the cases studied represented advanced disease with extensive metastases. In such cases CEA is not only very frequently detected, but is present at very high levels in the blood, especially with liver metastasis. In cancer localized to the mucosa and submucosa without invasion of the muscularis (Dukes A), the percentage of positive tests drops to 30–

40%. Even in recurrences when the tumor is localized to the bowel wall, the test is usually negative. Such findings rule out CEA as a method for screening populations for asymptomatic localized cancers.

CEA levels play a useful role in the follow-up of colon cancer patients. The blood level of the antigen reverts to normal in a few days after complete removal of the tumor. A limited drop to an intermediate level is indicative of incomplete excision. The CEA results are not totally reliable in the first 3 months after surgery, since small rises have been found that are not accompanied by tumor recurrence (Herberman, 1976). After 3 months the correlation of CEA level with tumor recurrence is much better, especially when three consecutive values taken at monthly intervals are available.

Preoperative CEA levels have prognostic value. Patients with localized disease as assessed by clinical methods exhibit a higher recurrence rate when a high preoperative CEA level is found than when the preoperative CEA level is low. It has been suggested that in these cases CEA is an indicator of "hidden" spread of tumors (Neville and Laurence, 1974).

CEA is of limited help in the search for the primary site of a metastatic carcinoma. The antigen is found in about 50% of tumors of the breast, stomach, lung, and other solid tumors. Above-normal levels have also been detected in heavy smokers and patients with cirrhosis, pancreatitis, uremia, peptic ulcer, intestinal metaplasia of the stomach, and ulcerative colitis. In tissues, CEA has been found in intestinal polyps, colonic inflammatory mucosa, and normal intestinal mucosa of children. CEA have also been reported in cancerous tissues from the breast, liver, and lung as well as in body fluids exposed to cancer tissue. In colonic washings high levels were found in patients with colon cancer and/or colon polyps, intermediate levels in ulcerative colitis and lower levels in normal subjects (Winawer, 1975).

A fraction of CEA, named CEA-S, has been isolated by Edgangton (Herberman, 1976). Preliminary results suggest that CEA-S can detect a higher proportion of patients with gastrointestinal cancer and still be characterized by a low incidence of false positives. The sensitivity and specificity of the CEA test can also be improved if tests for other tumor-associated antigens are performed simultaneously.

K. APPENDECTOMY

When McVay (1964) reported that a significant excess of colon cancer patients gave a history of appendectomy in his case-control study, he suggested that the relationship might be explained by immunologic factors. The exciting possibility of an immunologic link encouraged other investigators to try to reproduce McVay's findings, with mixed results. Bierman's data cited by Wynder and Shigematsu (1967) pointed in the same direction as McVay's, but other reports failed to reproduce the association of appendectomy with large-bowel carcinoma (Gross, 1966; Howie and Timperley, 1966). Gross extended his study to include tonsillectomies and found no case-control difference for that procedure. Hyams and Wynder (1968) made a systematic study of appendectomies in relation to age, sex, birthplace, socioeconomic class, and other demographic variables and reported the distribution of appendectomies to be significantly correlated with these factors. The equivocal observations on the subject of appendectomy and large-bowel cancer have not encouraged further efforts to delineate this association. Hyams' results make it clear that future studies would need to control for confounding demographic variables in assessing the significance of any association between appendectomy and large-bowel cancer.

L. FAMILIAL AGGREGATION

The literature on entities intimately linked to high bowel cancer risks, such as familial adenomatous polyposis coli, an autosomal dominantly inherited disease, is reviewed in Section III, M. While the significance and relevance of these entities to the presentation of bowel cancer in individual patients is clear, the epidemiology of bowel cancer suggests that only a minor fraction of bowel cancers can be linked to these and other precursor states, and the question arises concerning the presence of other familial differences in bowel cancer susceptibility for which no obvious mechanisms of inheritance are demonstrable. Observations on familial aggregation are required for studies of both genetic and environmental factors. Any advance in identification of susceptible families and individuals would represent a breakthrough in the study of environmental agents, since the contrasts normally yielded by case-control and prospective studies may be diluted by negative findings for nonsusceptible individuals. If the latter could be identified and removed from the comparisons, the contrasts in risk might be greatly magnified, thus permitting reduced study sizes and more straightforward analyses of results. While studies of familial aggregations of bowel cancer and other diseases are obviously indicated, it should be stressed that demonstration of familial aggregation is a necessary, but not sufficient, condition for the presence of genetic variability. Familial aggregation can also reflect common environmental exposures, and for sites in which dietary factors are suspect, a common pattern of dietary habits.

Although the caveats on the difficulties in distinguishing between genetic, environmental, and chance effects need to be borne in mind, numerous observations on "cancer families" strongly suggest a genetic basis for familial aggregation of bowel cancer not related to familial polyposis. Carcinoma of the colon has been reported frequently in "cancer families," in association with endometrial carcinoma and multiple primary malignancies (Lynch *et al.*, 1966). Moreover, clusters of bowel cancer cases have been described in other families unaccompanied by malignancies of associated sites (Ceulemans, 1958; Kluge, 1964; Macklin, 1960; Peltokallio and Peltokallio, 1966). The kindreds displaying a high incidence of bowel neoplasms do not show a high degree of inbreeding, and Burdette (1970) stated that they do not show excessive consanguinity. The study from Finland (Peltokallio and Peltokallio, 1966) had described three families with multiple occurrences of colon carcinoma; in one family the malignancy was present in members from three generations, and the striking feature was that the majority of affected individuals were diagnosed before 30 years of age. The observation that relatives of colon cancer probands have an earlier age of onset of the disease had been made earlier by Moertel *et al.* (1958). The impression of a young age at diagnosis of bowel cancer in cancer families is consistent with the observations of Wynder and Shigematsu (1967), who were impressed by the high frequency with which colorectal cancer patients under 40 years of age studied by them gave a history of large bowel cancer in a parent or sibling. Lovett (1976) also noted that index cases under age 40 gave a higher proportion, 67.5%, of positive family histories compared to 25% for all probands studied. While the mode of inheritance cannot be clearly inferred from the collective observations of cancer families, Lynch and Krush (1967) on review of the data felt that an autosomal dominant factor appeared likely.

More precise studies to quantitate the degree of familial aggregation have relied on comparisons of the presentation of disease in relatives of affected index patients (probands) with relatives of index controls, although sometimes the cases observed among relatives of probands have been contrasted with an expected number calculated from the age- and sex-specific incidence or mortality rates for the general population in the area where the families reside. The findings from proband studies of bowel cancer conducted by Macklin (1960), Woolf (1958), Lovett (1976), and Bjelke (1973) are summarized in Table XXVII. The studies differ in detail with respect to scope of coverage (first-degree

TABLE XXVII

OBSERVED AND EXPECTED CASES OF CANCER OF THE LARGE BOWEL
(COLON AND RECTUM) AMONG RELATIVES IN FOUR PROBAND STUDIES

Author[a]	Relatives	Cases of large-bowel cancer among relatives of index cases with large-bowel cancer	
		Observed	Expected
Macklin	Total relatives	108	45.0
	1st degree	31	9.7
	Other	77	35.3
Woolf	1st degree	26	8.0
Lovett	1st degree	41	11.7
Bjelke	1st degree	17	8.8
	Total 1st degree	115	38.2

[a] (Sources: Macklin, 1960; Woolf, 1958; Lovett, 1976; Bjelke, 1973).

relatives only or inclusion of uncles, aunts, cousins, grandparents),
period of surveillance, exclusion of families with multiple polyposis,
etc., but collectively they are in close agreement in describing a 3-fold
excess of colorectal cancer risk among relatives of the probands. The
excess risk was specific for bowel cancer and was not accompanied by
any excess for stomach or other sites. Table XXVIII presents additional
details on the findings for first-degree relatives from the four studies.
Although the numbers are small and subject to sampling variation, the

TABLE XXVIII

OBSERVED AND EXPECTED CASES OF CANCER OF THE LARGE-BOWEL
(COLON AND RECTUM) AMONG FIRST DEGREE RELATIVES IN
FOUR PROBAND STUDIES COMBINED

Relatives	Cases of large-bowel cancer among relatives of index cases with large-bowel cancer	
	Observed	Expected
Fathers	28	9.8
Mothers	32	9.3
Brothers	28	10.5
Sisters	28	8.6
	116	38.2

data suggest the same 3-fold excess of colorectal cancer for siblings and parents of the affected subjects. Bowel cancer in this respect differs from stomach cancer, where the proband studies have described the excess risk to be greater for siblings than parents. In Macklin's series, which provided the most data on non-first-degree relatives, the excess risks for uncles, aunts, and cousins was smaller, slightly greater than double the rate for controls.

Burdette (1970, 1971) reported a 6-fold excess of bowel cancer among parents of probands, a ratio substantially greater than those yielded by the other study series. His presentation, however, provided no details on the derivation of the numbers of cases expected, and in the absence of such information his findings should be treated with reserve.

McConnell's (1966) assessment of the studies by Macklin, Moertel, and Woolf is that they leave little doubt about a genetic component in bowel cancer distinct from and additional to that due to familial polyposis or ulcerative colitis and that the weight of the evidence is in favor of this component being polygenic.

Proband studies may overestimate the degree of familial aggregation. The bias in such studies arises from the fact that relatives of index cases do not constitute a random sample of families, since they come to the investigator's attention through the presence of an affected individual within the family, so that families with more than one affected individual may have an enhanced probability of being represented in a series of index cases. Aspects of index case selection that may inflate estimates of familial aggregation of disease have been discussed by Haenszel (1959), and methods of compensating for this bias through procedures developed for studies of family size and birth order (Greenwood and Yule, 1914) were suggested. However, an abundance of collateral evidence (persistence of excess risk among the several subcategories of relatives and over several generations, younger ages of diagnosis for cases among proband relatives) suggests that the aggregation depicted by proband studies reflect something more than statistical artifacts introduced by selection biases associated with the identification of index cases. We caution only that the degree of familial aggregation may be overstated in the studies cited, not that it is not present. This particular type of bias is not present in the sib-pair comparisons reported by Chen et al. (1961).

A different approach to familial aggregation was taken by Chen et al. (1961), who studied the site distributions of 180 sibling pairs dying of cancer assembled from over 4000 death certificates stating cancer to be the underlying cause of death filed in a U.S. (Maryland) county between 1900 and 1960. Six sibling-pair concordances for colorectal cancer were found compared with the expected number of 2.4 calculated on the assumption that the cancer sites for individuals were independently distributed. Under these conditions the probability of observing 6 or more matches by chance would be slightly less than 0.035. While the number of observations is too small to permit definite conclusions, the result points in the same direction as the proband studies and can be construed as consistent with them in suggesting a 2- to 3-fold excess risk among relatives of index cases.

Contrasts in site-specific concordance between monozygous and dizygous twins in theory could play a valuable role in assessing the importance of genetic factors in individual susceptibility to bowel cancer with exposure to a suitable environment. However, twin studies to date have contributed little to the evaluation of inherited factors in the causation of bowel cancer. The logistical difficulties of assembling a sufficient number of twin pairs to yield at least 1 concordant pair of monozygous or dizygous twins are obvious, and even the sizable Danish (Harvald and Hauge, 1963) and Swedish (Cederlöf et al., 1970) twin series have yielded too few cases for a meaningful analysis of concordance.

The presentation of bowel cancer in husband–wife pairs should reflect the influence of common environmental exposures (disregarding the effects of assortative mating), and such observations could thus provide a useful check on the findings on associations observed in parent–child and sib–sib comparisons. If a genetic model is correct, the excess margin of risk for the spouse of a proband should be less than that for a first-degree relative. Little information is available on the distribution of bowel cancer among spouse pairs. Chen et al. (1961) observed no sets of husbands and wives with bowel cancer against an expected value of 1.3. Bjelke (1973) found 3 spouses of index cases with colorectal cancer to have the disease compared to an expected value of 1 based on control experience. Segall's (1965) data suggested an increased mortality from colon cancer among both wives and husbands of index patients who died from this condition. From the scanty evidence available we must conclude that no inferences on the magnitude of concordance of large bowel cancer among spouse pairs are possible.

Placed in the perspective of the total epidemiological picture of bowel cancer, the results from the proband studies and allied investigators do not suggest genetically determined susceptibility to be of critical importance in fixing the level of bowel cancer risk in high-incidence populations for those bowel cancers not associated with familial polyposis or other polyp-promoting conditions. Genetic susceptibility may be of importance in the etiology of subsets of bowel cancers, and an important criterion for suspecting a role of genetic factors is the presentation and diagnosis of bowel cancers at a young age, under 30 years.

To date no studies have been mounted that attempt to investigate the joint contributions of genetic and environmental factors. Conceptually, the latter could be undertaken within groups of kindreds thought to be at high risk to bowel cancer. This would require expansion of work along lines described by Lynch *et al.* (1974), who through large-scale population screening have attempted to define substantial numbers of kindreds presenting high risks for specific cancer sites. This approach poses difficulties since chance factors alone can yield kindreds with 2 or more members positive for colorectal cancer or other specific diseases and to distinguish families truly at high risk from other families presenting 2 or more observed cases requires collection and collation of other detailed evidence supporting the presumption of genetic factors.

M. PRECANCEROUS CONDITIONS

In terms of cancer incidence, the most important condition implicated in colon carcinogenesis is the adenomatous polyp. It is the one entity suspected to be a precursor of the great majority of cases of colon cancer and for that reason is reviewed in a separate section. There remains a group of nosologic entities—the familial polyposis complex and the chronic idiopathic colitis complex—which, although relatively rare, carries an excessive risk of developing colon cancer.

1. *Familial Polyposis*

Although patients with multiple polyps of the colon have been on record in the medical literature for over 250 years (Menzel, 1721; Wagner, 1832; Rokitansky, 1839; Lushka, 1861), only recently have the different diseases responsible for the presence of multiple intestinal polyps become more clearly defined as a result of more precise histologic definition of the different types of polyps and of genetic studies of the affected families. There remain some points of confusion, and the process of characterization of the different nosologic entities continues. To a great extent advances in knowledge of these syndromes have been made by contributions from the staff of St. Marks Hospital in London (Lockhart-Mummery, 1925; Dukes, 1930, 1952; Veale, 1965; Morson and Bussey, 1970; Bussey, 1975). Bussey (1975) has classified the intestinal polyposis syndrome in the following categories:

Inflammatory: Colitis polyposa
                       Bilharzial polyposis
                       Benign lymphoid polyposis
Hamartomatous: Peutz–Jeghers syndrome
                       Multiple juvenile polyposis
                       Neurofibromatous polyposis
                       Lipomatous polyposis
Neoplastic: Adenomatous polyposis coli
                          (including Gardner's syndrome)
                       Minor or recessive adenomatous polyposis
                       Lymphosarcomatous polyposis
                       Leukemic polyposis
Miscellaneous: Metaplastic polyposis
                       Cronkhite–Canada syndrome
                       Pneumatosis cystoides intestinalis

The list may in the future prove to be incomplete. New eponyms, such as Turcot's syndrome and Oldfield's syndrome, as well as new clusters of family tumors (Fraumeni *et al.*, 1968; Lindberg and Kock, 1975) may be added to the list if further research proves that they are more than variants of the familial adenomatous polyposis syndrome. We review briefly the relationship with colon cancer for those syndromes in which objective evidence of an association has been reported.

2. *Familial Adenomatous Polyposis Coli*

This autosomal-dominant inherited disease, if untreated, carries a lifetime risk of 100% for carcinoma of the large bowel. Estimates of the incidence of the disease have varied from 1 in 6850 (Pierce, 1968) to 1 in 29,000 (Neel, 1954) but most estimates have arrived at a figure close to 1 case per 8000 live births (Reed and Neel, 1955). The intestinal tumors are morphologically indistinguishable from the adenomatous polyps, the exceptional feature being the extraordinary number of polyps, counted in thousands for the great majority of cases. About one-fourth of the cases represent new mutations. Slightly less than half of the offspring of patients with the disease eventually develop the syndrome, and this has been explained on the basis of a penetrance of about 80% (Morson and Bussey, 1970). There is a slight excess of males attributable to the fact that new mutations in males outnumber those in females by a ratio of 3 to 2 (Bussey, 1975).

The disease is seldom diagnosed in the first decade of life and the average age at diagnosis is around 35 years. A few cases are diagnosed late, and 10% of the cases are diagnosed after age 50. Special attention has been given to polyposis families in whom the average age at diagnosis of polyposis is 25 years. Since the average age at diagnosis of cancer in polyposis patients is around 39 years, this suggests that once the polyps are well established the progression of some polyps to carcinoma may take only a few years. Although each individual malignant tumor is similar to those found in nonpolyposis families, the multiplicity rate is greater in polyposis families: 47% of polyposis patients with carcinoma will have multiple tumors, as opposed to 4% for nonpolyposis patients with colorectal cancer. This may explain in part the lower average age at death from cancer in polyposis cases, 42 years vs about 70 years in nonpolyposis patients (Bussey, 1975).

The treatment of familial adenomatous polyposis has been abdominal colectomy with ileorectosigmoidostomy. It has been observed that after such procedures the rectal polyps tend to regress and disappear, and this has given rise to speculations about the role of environmental and host factors in polyp causation (Cole and Holden, 1959). Rectal polyps present at time of operation or appearing after surgery have been fulgurated or resected in an attempt to prevent the appearance of rectal cancer. Long-term follow-up of a series of patients at the Mayo Clinic has shown that the risk of rectal cancer remains high, 5% in patients followed for 5 years, 13% at 10 years, and 42% at 20 years (Moertel, 1973). This experience is at variance with that of St. Marks Hospital (London), where only 2 of 86 patients followed up to 25 years have developed rectal cancer after colectomy and ileorectal anastomosis. In such cases the rectal stump was kept free of polyps by fulguration (Morson, 1974). In patients without rectal polyps before or at the time of operation, no rectal cancer has developed after surgery and it would seem that colectomy and ileorectal anastomosis is adequate treatment for those patients. A similar experience has been reported for patients whose rectal polyps regressed spontaneously after colectomy and ileorectal anastomosis (Williams and Fish, 1966). Modern surgical techniques have improved to the point where some authors recommend total colectomy and permanent ileostomy as the treatment of choice for intestinal polyposis (Moertel, 1973).

3. Minor or Recessive Adenomatous Polyposis

Most cases of familial adenomatous polyposis have 1000 or more polyps, and a few have as few as 200. At the other extreme of the spectrum, most patients with adenomatous polyps have fewer than 10

polyps. A few cases with between 20 and 70 polyps have been identified and tentatively classified as "minor" or "recessive" adenomatous
polyposis. This classification is based on the theory proposed by Veale
(1965), who postulated that a recessive gene (p) may occupy the same
locus (x) of the dominant (P) gene of familial polyposis. The hypothetical combination of genes may explain some peculiarities in the distribution of number of polyps and age of appearance of polyposis
symptoms, but more data are needed to define more precisely the
cancer risk of individuals in this category.

4. Gardner's Syndrome

Gardner (1951) identified a family in which adenomatous polyps
were associated with osteomas of the skull and mandible and with
epidermoid cysts. Later reports have described other tumors associated with the syndrome in members of such families, although not all
present in the same individuals, and it has been stated that the syndrome is a familial rather than an individual member characteristic
(Bussey, 1975). Other lesions so far reported include: abnormal denti-
tion, impacted supernumerary and permanent teeth, early caries, den-
tigerous cysts, and abnormal bone structures of the mandible (Gardner, 1969); desmoid tumors of the abdominal wall and the peritoneal
cavity sometimes preceded by surgical trauma and other times leading
to intestinal or urinary obstruction (MacAdam and Goligher, 1970);
periampullary carcinoma of the duodenum with invasion of the head
of the pancreas and generalized abdominal carcinomatosis (Bussey,
1972). Approximately 18% of the families with adenomatous polyposis
will present features of Gardner's syndrome in at least one family
member. Utsunomiya and Nakamura (1974) have described a high
frequency of bone opacity of the mandible in adenomatous polyposis
patients. These findings indicate a close relationship between
adenomatous polyposis and Gardner's syndrome, and future genetic
studies should clarify their mutual association.

5. Turcot's Syndrome

There have been several reports of association of familial adenomatous polyposis with malignant central nervous tissues tumors, especially medulloblastomas (Turcot et al., 1959; Crail, 1949; Camiel et
al., 1968). The central nervous tissue tumors usually cause death of the
patient before the polyposis becomes far advanced, although in these
patients the polyposis has become manifest early in life and one patient developed carcinoma of the colon at the early age of 15 years
(Turcot et al., 1959).

6. Other Associated Tumors

A variety of other tumors has been found in families whose members have been affected by adenomatous polyposis. In one such family, cases of osteosarcoma, liposarcoma, and malignant lymphoma (reticulum cell sarcoma) have been found (Fraumeni et al., 1968). A variety of tumors in other parts of the gastrointestinal tract, including adenomas of the small intestine and stomach, has been occasionally found in polyposis families (Bussey, 1975). Association of gastric carcinoma and intestinal polyposis has been reported in one family, but the number of polyps in most of these cases was too small to meet the criteria for familial polyposis (Lindberg and Kock, 1975).

7. Peutz-Jegher's Syndrome

This autosomal dominantly inherited syndrome involves mainly the small intestine, but in almost half of the cases it is associated with polyps of the large intestine. The polyps are of the hamartomatous type and have a branching architecture with smooth muscle fibers in the certral core and orderly cell differentiation in the crypt of Lieberkühn and the villi of the mucosa of the polyp. From this histologic configuration no malignant transformation is usually expected and no premalignant meaning had been assigned to the syndrome. With the passage of years, however, more and more reports of adenocarcinoma, several involving the large bowel, arising in patients with Peutz-Jegher's syndrome have appeared in the medical literature (Shivata and Phillips, 1970; Salas and Miranda, 1974). As is usually the case, the advanced tumors had destroyed any evidence of a polyp, making it impossible to determine whether the cancer originated in the polyp. In the Peutz-Jegher's syndrome, the carcinomas may have arisen from the truly adenomatous polyps that are occasionally seen accompanying the hamartomatous proliferations. Morphologic observations made by one of us (P. C.) suggest that, in the surface of Petz-Jegher's hamartomatous polyps, true adenomatous changes may originate.

8. Juvenile Polyposis

This familial syndrome is characterized by hamartomatous "retention" polyps, and so far no case of carcinoma of the large intestine has been unequivocally linked to it. Since the syndrome has in the past been confused with adenomatous polyposis, mention of this point is pertinent to this discussion. There are reports that suggest the presentation of juvenile and adenomatous polyps in different members of the same family (Veale et al., 1966).

9. *Ulcerative Colitis*

This chronic, relapsing, idiopathic inflammatory condition of the large bowel carries a lifetime risk of cancer of approximately 57% (DeDombal *et al.*, 1966). The risk is practically nil in the first 10 years of the disease, but increases with time thereafter. Since this disease is much more common than familial polyposis, it accounts for many more cases of colorectal carcinoma. Most of the colorectal cancers observed before age 45 are preceded by ulcerative colitis (Edwards and Truelove, 1964). The cancer risk rises when the symptoms of colitis are continuous instead of relapsing and when the disease presents in early life. The tumors are flat, infiltrating adenocarcinomas and generally more poorly differentiated than those not associated with ulcerative colitis. A multicentricity rate of 52% has been reported, much higher than for noncolitis cases (Moertel, 1973). These features account in part for the bad prognosis; the reported 5-year survival rate is approximately 15%. There is no evidence that the carcinomas originate in the pseudopolyps frequently seen in ulcerative colitis. Many foci of atypical hyperplasia and carcinoma *in situ* are seen concomitantly with infiltrating carcinomatous lesions (Morson and Bussey, 1970). Atypical epithelial hyperplasia may be observed in rectal biopsy material, and this feature has been used as an indicator of colectomy to prevent the appearance of infiltrating malignant lesions (Morson and Tang, 1967). Rectal cancer has occurred after ileorectal anastomosis (MacDougall, 1964). In such cases the inflammatory changes persist after colectomy. The extent of rectal mucosa involvement may determine the type of surgical treatment.

10. *Crohn's Disease*

This transmural, chronic, granulomatous inflammation affects primarily the small bowel but may also involve the large intestine (granulomatous colitis). There have been reports of carcinoma of the small intestine associated with Crohn's disease (Morowitz *et al.*, 1968). Since small intestinal carcinoma is a very rare disease, its association with Crohn's disease is at least suggestive of a premalignant role. The association of large-bowel cancer with granulomatous colitis is less well established, since only a few cases have been reported and the relatively high frequency of large-bowel cancer makes an origin independent from the granulomatous lesion a more likely explanation. Contrary to what is observed in ulcerative colitis, no correlation has been found between the chronicity of the inflammatory lesion and the appearance of carcinoma (Jones, 1969). Epithelial atypical hyperplasia is less common in Crohn's disease than in ulcerative colitis. It is not possible at present to adequately assess the relationship between granulomatous colitis and colon cancer, and further observations are needed.

N. Polyp–Cancer Relationship

This subject constitutes an old medical controversy familiar to many readers. Recent advances in our knowledge of the pathology and epidemiology of polyps have clarified considerably some of the obscure points of the controversy.

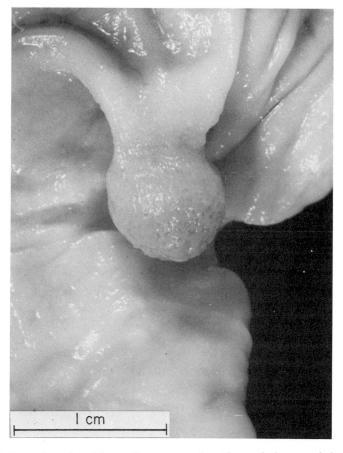

Fig. 26. Juvenile polyp. The surface is smooth with regularly spaced depressions corresponding to the openings of dilated glands. A pedicle is partially formed.

There are three well recognized common histologic types of large-bowel polyps: juvenile, hyperplastic, and adenomatous. Juvenile (or retention) polyps (Figs. 26 and 27) are characterized by cystically dilated glandular cavities surrounded by abundant stroma and have a smooth surface lined by a single-layered columnar epithelium. Hyperplastic (or metaplastic) polyps (Figs. 28 and 29) are characterized by lengthening of the epithelial tubules and pseudopapillary infoldings of epithelial cells projecting into the glandular lumen. Adenomatous polyps (Figs. 30 and 31) are crowded accumulations of

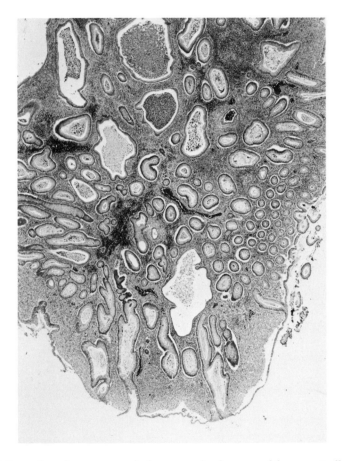

FIG. 27. Juvenile polyps composed of mucous glands, some of them cystically dilated by retained secretion, separated by abundant stroma. Some of the glands are open to the surface, which otherwise is lined by columnar epithelium. ×18.

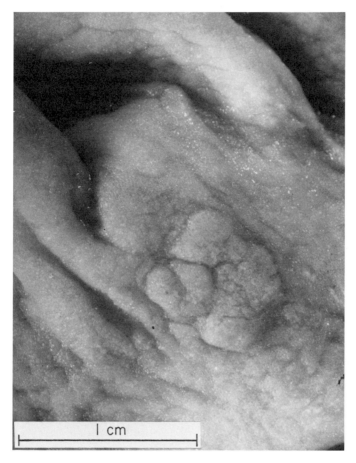

FIG. 28. Hyperplastic polyp formed by a flat, sessile, papular elevation of the mucosa.

tubular glands with little stroma between them, their surface is composed of the same type of glands found in the deeper portions of the polyp. Some of the adenomatous polyps have areas of villous or papillary architecture, the villi being lined by the same type of epithelial cells lining the tubular glands. Pure villous adenomas are also found and are universally recognized as having marked propensity for malignant transformation. Little epidemiologic information is available on pure villous adenomas, in part owing to their low frequency in autopsy material.

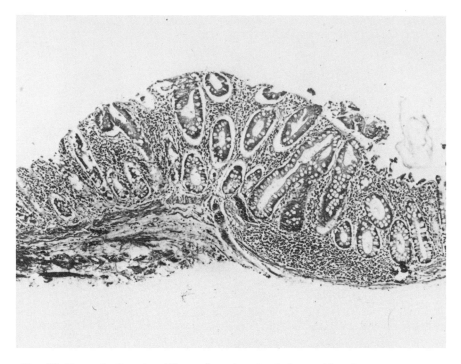

FIG. 29. Hyperplastic polyp. The surface elevation is due to dilated, tortuous, mature glands with epithelial intraluminal folds. ×58.

1. *Juvenile Polyps*

Most of the claims of a malignant potential for juvenile polyps date back to the time when their distinction from adenomatous polyps, familial polyposis, villous adenoma, and Peutz-Jaeger's polyps was not well documented. The prevalence of juvenile polyps is summarized in Table XXIX, which shows data for three different series: two from autopsies and one from surgical pathology material. These polyps are rare during the first year of life; the highest prevalence occurs from 1 to 7 years of age and drops sharply after adolescence, being infrequent in adults. They are more frequent in boys than in girls and are more often single than multiple. Since most of these polyps are not resected, the low prevalence in adults indicates that they are self-amputated or regress spontaneously, well-known events in this condition (Roth and Helwig, 1963; Andren and Frieberg, 1956). Their overall prevalence (both sexes combined) ranges from around 1% in autopsy series from

United States (Helwig, 1946) to around 5% in Colombia (Correa *et al.*, 1972). Although the number of autopsy series available for comparison is limited, the data suggest higher prevalence in populations at low risk to colon cancer.

Table XXX compares findings on polyp location from a surgical pathology series in the United States (Roth and Helwig, 1963) and an autopsy series in Colombia (Correa *et al.*, 1972). The surgical series reports an excess of juvenile polyps (70%) in the rectum, while the autopsy series describes a more even distribution throughout the large bowel with lesser concentration in the rectum.

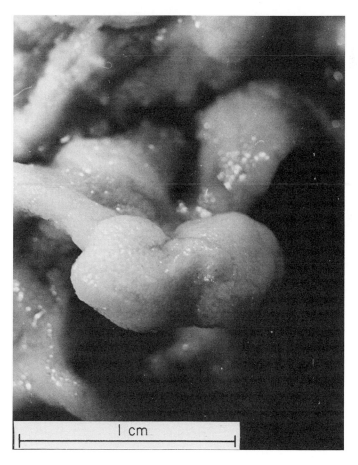

FIG. 30. Adenomatous polyp. A protruding solid mass of tissue whose surface has many tiny and closely packed small depressions.

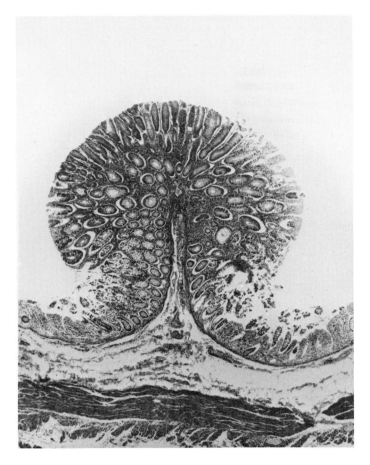

FIG. 31. Adenomatous polyps formed by closely packed tubular glands that fill almost all the space available from base to surface. ×25.

The scanty epidemiologic data available suggest that these lesions obey noncongenital environmental factors operating selectively or exclusively during childhood and are apparently not related to the causation of large-bowel cancer. A few retention polyps have been observed among more numerous adenomatous polyps and carcinomas induced by azoxymethane in rats (Ward *et al.*, 1973b). This observation may indicate a relationship between juvenile polyps and cancer not yet revealed by studies in humans. Follow-up of patients in whom juvenile polyps were resected should be attempted.

TABLE XXIX

DISTRIBUTION OF JUVENILE POLYPS BY AGE AND SEX

Autopsies—Colombia (Correa et al., 1972)			Autopsies—U.S.A. (Helwig, 1946)			Surgical pathology AFIP—U.S.A. (Roth and Helwig, 1963)	
Age	Number of specimens	Prevalence rate	Age	Number of specimens	Prevalence rate	Age	Number of cases
0–14	Males 208	6.3	0–1	Males 161	0	0–1	1
	Females 170	2.9		Females 123	0	1–4	58
						5–9	39
15–44	Males 348	3.5	1–10	Males 56	5.3	10–14	1
	Females 209	3.4		Females 29	0	15–19	17
						20–24	19
45–64	Males 279	1.4	11–20	Males 49	0	25–29	8
	Females 95	1.0		Females 31	6.4	30–35	8
						35+	7
65+	Males 126	0.8				Total boys 0–10 Years	62
	Females 59	0				Total girls 0–10 Years	37
						Total males 11+ Years	55
						Total females 11+ Years	4

TABLE XXX
LOCATION OF JUVENILE POLYPS

Segment	AFIP, U.S.A. surgical pathology[a] (%)	Cali autopsies[b] (%)
Cecum	0.6	9.3
Ascending	1.2	14.8
Transverse	3.6	20.4
Descending	2.4	9.3
Sigmoid	11.0	18.5
Rectum	72.0	27.8
Unspecified	7.8	—
Number of polyps	166	54

[a] Roth and Helwig (1963).
[b] Correa et al. (1972).

2. Hyperplastic Polyps

Most investigators of the role of hyperplastic polyps have concluded, mainly on morphological grounds, that they are not precancerous (Morson, 1962; Lane et al., 1971). Some studies, based on interpopulation comparisons of frequency and anatomic distribution, have raised the question of a possible role for hyperplastic polyps in large-bowel carcinogenesis (Stemmermann and Yatani, 1973). More extensive data on interpopulation variation in prevalence of hyperplastic polyps from autopsy series have recently become available (Stemmermann and Yatani, 1973; Correa et al., 1972, 1977; Sato, 1974; Sato et al., 1976), and the results are summarized in Table XXXI.

As seen in Table XXXI, some populations at high risk to colorectal cancer display a high prevalence of hyperplastic polyps, and some populations with low colorectal cancer risks also have very low polyp-prevalence rates. The correlation between the two conditions, however, has many inconsistencies. There is a 3- to 4-fold difference in prevalence of hyperplastic polyps between Hawaii-Japanese and New Orleans males, and the excess cancer incidence in Hawaii when compared to southern U.S. cities is about 30% (Cutler and Young, 1975). The difference in colorectal cancer mortality between Akita and Miyagi prefectures of Japan is not accompanied by different rates of hyperplastic polyps (Sato et al., 1976). The prevalence of hyperplastic polyps, but not cancer incidence, differs between Japan and Colombia. The available data, therefore, cannot be construed as supporting a premalignant role for hyperplastic polyps. The wide range of inter-country variation in polyp prevalence and the differences between migrant and nonmigrant Japanese would implicate environmental fac-tors in the causation of hyperplastic polyps, but such factors seem to be independent from those associated with colorectal cancer (Correa *et al.*, 1977). The anatomic localization of hyperplastic polyps is characterized by concentration in the rectum and lower sigmoid, especially in the lower rectum as illustrated by Fig. 32 reporting the data on hyperplastic and adenomatous polyps for New Orleans. This anatomic distribution is not congruent with the distribution of the "epidemic" type of colon cancer, which in high risk populations shows a predominance of tumors in the intermediate segments of the large bowel (Haenszel and Correa, 1971; J. W. Berg and W. Haenszel, personal communication, 1976).

3. *Adenomatous Polyps*

Interpopulation comparisons of the prevalence of adenomatous polyps correlate better with measures of the frequency of colorectal cancer (Table XXXI). People of Japanese extraction living in Hawaii have the highest polyp prevalence on record and very high colon

TABLE XXXI
AGE-ADJUSTED PREVALENCE RATE OF COLORECTAL POLYPS

Population	Colon cancer incidence	Prevalence rate (%)	
		Hyperplastic	Adenomatous
		Males	
Hawaii-Japanese	Very high	71	63
New Orleans White	High	15	33
New Orleans Black	High	14	35
Japan (Akita)	Intermediate	2	35
Japan (Miyagi)	Low	2	13
Colombia (Cali)	Low	11	10
		Females	
Hawaii-Japanese	Very high	51	49
New Orleans White	High	21	19
New Orleans Black	High	8	29
Japan (Akita)	Intermediate	4	19
Japan (Miyagi)	Low	1	11
Colombia (Cali)	Low	10	10

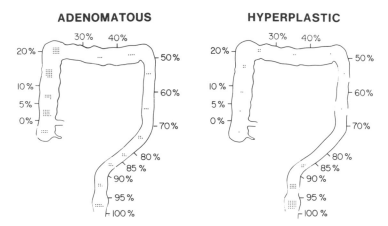

FIG. 32. Anatomic distribution of adenomatous and hyperplastic polyps in New Orleans white males. Source: Correa *et al.* (1977).

cancer incidence. New Orleans whites and blacks have rates for both adenomatous polyps and cancer somewhat lower than those of Hawaii-Japanese, but much higher than those of residents of Miyagi (Japan) or Colombia (Correa *et al.*, 1977). The Japanese experience indicates that race is not an overriding determinant of the risk of either cancer or adenomatous polyps, and the data for blacks support this contention. African blacks have very low colon cancer incidence (Burkitt, 1971a), and American blacks currently have very high incidence rates (Cutler and Young, 1975). Parallel observations have been made for adenomatous polyps. No adenomatous polyps were found in a series of 14,000 autopsies of South African Bantu (Bremner and Ackerman, 1970). Williams *et al.* (1975) found only 1 adenomatous polyp in 40 intestinal polyps surgically removed in Ibadan, Nigeria, compared with 65 adenomatous polyps in 83 polyps surgically removed from black residents of Washington, D.C. (Williams *et·al.*, 1975).

Figure 32 reveals the different anatomic distribution of adenomatous and hyperplastic polyps in the New Orleans data. The proportion of adenomatous polyps in the sigmoid and upper rectum is higher in New Orleans (17.5%) than in Cali (10%), a finding that coincides well with the greater concentration of cancers in the same anatomical regions in New Orleans compared to Cali (Correa, 1975). The average size of adenomatous polyps was greater in New Orleans (6.5 mm) than in Cali (3.5 mm). Polyp size increased with age and with distance from the ileocecal valve. The multiplicity rate is greater in males than females and greater in New Orleans than Cali. The age-adjusted multiplicity rate was 14% for New Orleans males, 8.5% for New Orleans females, 5% for Cali males, and 2% for Cali females.

Cali also provides an example of parallel findings on socioeconomic class variation for adenomatous polyps and colon cancer. In that community, a substantial deficit for both conditions in the lower social classes has been reported (Haenszel et al., 1975).

An increase in cancer incidence has been documented in the United States since 1940 (Axtell and Chiazze, 1966). A series of independent autopsy studies in the United States date back to 1946, when the prevalence of "adenomas" was reported by Helwig (1947). Although there are differences in methodology among the studies, rough comparisons of prevalence over subsequent time intervals can be drawn. Table XXXII documents a steady increase in polyp prevalence with time similar to the time trends observed for colon cancer incidence.

The significance of the geographical associations in the distributions of adenomatous polyps and cancer is enhanced by the greater size and multiplicity of polyps in populations at higher risk to bowel cancer, a feature consistent with the observations that larger and more numerous polyps have a greater tendency to malignant transformation (Silverberg, 1970). Sato and co-workers in Japan (1976) have shown in Akita prefecture, where colon cancer is more frequent, the size of polyps and the frequency of multiple polyps to be greater than in neighboring Miyagi prefecture (13.7% prevalence of multiple polyps vs 7.5%). They also evaluated the degree of histologic (architectural) and cytologic atypia in adenomatous polyps and found 23% of polyps from Akita to have moderate or severe atypia while only 12.7% of those from Miyagi showed these changes.

Japanese (Sato et al., 1976) and Swedish (Ekelund and Lindstrom, 1974) investigators have reported that polyps of the distal (sigmoid)

TABLE XXXII
AGE-ADJUSTED PREVALENCE RATES OF ADENOMATOUS
POLYPS IN THE UNITED STATES

Author	City	Males	Females
Helwig (1947)	St. Louis, Missouri	17	13
Blatt (1961)	New Rochelle, New York	33	27
Arminski and McLean (1964)	Detroit, Michigan	33	30
Correa et al. (1977)	New Orleans, Louisiana[a]	33	19
Stemmermann and Yatani (1973)	Honolulu, Hawaii	63	49

[a] Whites only.

colon have more advanced atypical and dysplastic changes than those of the proximal (cecum) colon. This feature would be consistent with a model postulating that the distal colon receives a greater dose of carcinogen than the proximal colon (Haenszel and Correa, 1971).

4. Pathology of the Polyp-Cancer Sequence. Patient Follow-up

Excellent descriptions of the pathologic anatomy of adenomatous polyps are available in the literature (Helwig, 1947; Morson and Bussey, 1970). They include illustrations of all degrees of cellular differentiation, from the very mature tubular and benign-appearing polyps to the very atypical, anaplastic, and malignant-appearing epithelium. The presence within some polyps of groups of glands with the morphologic characteristics of adenocarcinomas, including the capacity to invade the lamina propria has been documented and, infrequent but well illustrated, case reports of metastasis from such foci are available.

The more undifferentiated polyps exhibit the stronger associations with the presence of cancer. The well-differentiated tubular adenoma is associated with cancer in only about 5% of the cases. Villous adenoma, on the other hand, is associated with cancer in 40% of the cases and adenomatous polyps with severe atypia in 34% of the cases (Morson, 1974).

The experience accumulated with the follow-up of large numbers of patients with polyps and some aggregates of patients with familial polyposis has thrown considerable additional light on the polyp–cancer sequence (Morson, 1974; Bussey, 1975).

In a series of 2305 patients with early rectal cancer, Morson (1974) found that the evidence of tumor origin in adenomatous polyps was greatest (66%) when the lesions were limited to the submucosa, intermediate (18%) when limited to the muscle, and minimal (7%) in cases with extramural spread. Given the higher growth rate of cancer cells and their capacity to invade neighboring tissues, it should be expected that the cancer growth destroys the original polyp tissue. Since the smaller and more localized malignant tumors are most of the time found in intimate association with polyps, Morson's observations constitute good evidence that most cancers in surgical series originate in polyps. In 3 out of 4 patients who refused treatment for adenomatous polyps of the rectum and were followed for more than 10 years, cancer developed in the site of the previously diagnosed, but untreated, polyps. Similar conclusions on site relationship can be deduced from a 15-year follow-up of patients with adenomatous polyps removed after sigmoidoscopy (Prager *et al.*, 1974). In that study the observed number of colon cancers was twice that expected, but the cancers found were limited to those segments that could not be reached by proctosigmoidoscopy and not previously surveyed and treated. Brahme and co-workers (1974) utilizing radiological methods followed 115 polyp-free subjects and an equal number of polyp patients and found 21% of the patients followed for 8 or more years developed new polyps and 2.7% developed carcinoma, a statistically significant excess compared to the corresponding figure of 7% and 0% for the polyp-free controls followed for approximately the same length of time.

Further evidence on the effect of polyp removal is provided by familial polyposis patients for whom periodic fulguration of rectal polyps after ileorectal anastomosis has prevented the appearance of carcinoma in the rectal stump.

O. INTESTINAL FLORA AND FECAL CHEMISTRY

The role of the intestinal flora in the etiology of large-bowel cancer has come under closer scrutiny since Laqueur demonstrated that the plant product cycasin, not carcinogenic in itself, was hydrolyzed by the intestinal bacteria of experimental animals with release of its aglycon (methylazoxymethanol or MAM), an active carcingoen. Colon cancer has been induced in experimental animals by feeding cycasin, but its occurrence is prevented when the action of the intestinal flora is suppressed by means of germfree experiments or surgical bypass of the fecal stream (Laqueur, 1970; Gennaro et al., 1973). There may be several pathways by which intestinal bacteria may act as mediators in chemical reactions leading to the production of ultimate carcinogenesis. Germfree mice are resistant to the carcinogenic effect of dimethylbenz[a]anthracene, which in normal mice is a potent carcinogen (Roe and Grant, 1970). The carcinogen ethionine is synthesized by Escherichia coli (Fisher and Mallette, 1961).

Attention has been focused especially on the possible role of bacteria in altering the structure of fecal steroids. The classic work of Kennaway and co-workers called attention to the similarities in the chemical structures of bile salts and some well known carcinogens, such as methylcholanthrene (Badger et al., 1940). The same group demonstrated that a normal constituent of bile salts, deoxycholic acid, can be converted chemically to the potent animal carcinogen 20-methylcholanthrene (Cook and Haselwood, 1933).

Aries et al. (1969) found that the nonsporing anaerobes (bacteroides and bifidobacteria) were the dominant flora in fecal samples from English and Ugandan subjects and that the English had 30 times more

bacteroides than Ugandans. There were greater numbers of streptococci, enterococci, lactobacillus, and yeasts in the Ugandan
specimens as compared to the English. Hill *et al.* (1971) confirmed
these results and further reported that the total fecal steroid concentration was 7 times greater in subjects from the United States and England than in subjects from India and Uganda. He also found greater
conversion of fecal cholesterol to coprostanol and coprostanone in the
U.S. and English subjects. Acid steroid concentration (from bile salts)
was 11 times greater among English and Americans than Ugandans
and Indians. The same groups of Westerners subject to high colon
cancer risk showed more complete degradation of their bile acids; a
higher proportion of nonsporing fecal anaerobes in these populations
were able to perform bile degradation reactions. Hill (1974) reported
that feces from U.S. and English subjects contained greater numbers
of nuclear dehydrogenating bacteria (NDC), and *Clostridium paraputrificum* group, than their counterparts from African and Asian countries. The implication was that high colon cancer risk might be associated with higher fecal steroid concentrations and with more complete
degradation of steroids by intestinal bacteria such as *Clostridium
paraputrificum.*

Hill's case-control study (Hill *et al.*, 1971) investigated the level of
fecal bile acids and presence of clostridia able to desaturate the bile
acid nucleus (NDC) and reported the presence of NDC in 82% of
bowel cancer patients compared to 43% of the controls. He also noted
the combination of high fecal bile acids and presence of NDC to
characterize 70% of the large-bowel cancer patients compared to 9%
of the controls, suggesting important etiologic roles for both bile acids
and NDC. Hill's observations on NDC have not been confirmed as yet
by other investigators. Finegold *et al.* (1975) studied feces from 25
subjects with colonic polyps and matched controls and compared 2
Japanese-American groups with distinctive Japanese- and Western-
style diets, and in neither study did he replicate Hill's findings on
NDC. Nor was he able to reproduce the type of differences, in distribution of bacteroides and bifidobacteria between high- and low-risk
populations described by Aries *et al.* (1969).

Moore and Holdeman (1975) collected fecal samples from individuals in five populations at three distinct levels of bowel cancer—high-
risk: Hawaiian Japanese from whom adenomatous polyps had been
removed; moderately high-risk: normal Hawaiian Japanese and North
Americans; low-risk: rural Japanese and Africans of the Tswana tribe.
This was supplemented by experiments on the effects of extreme
changes in diet. Moore concurs with Finegold in his inability to corre-

late individual genera or species of bacteria with bowel cancer risk. Specifically, he was unable to detect in his high-risk groups the type of clostridia that Hill found to oxidize bile salts to carcinogens anaerobically. Moore characterizes the differences in intestinal flora between low-risk native populations and the higher-risk groups of polyp patients, Hawaiian Japanese, and North Americans as follows. Individuals from the low-risk native groups tended to maintain high concentrations of few species, whereas individuals from high-risk populations presented a more heterogeneous flora. Most of the species encountered in North American polyp patients were also seen in the flora of Japanese and African natives, and there was little difference in the overall composite distribution of number and type of species in the two types of populations.

The predominance of 2 or 3 species in individuals from low-risk populations suggested that they had a more uniform intestinal physiology. The role of diet in altering the composition of intestinal flora has been amply demonstrated in rats (Onderdonk et al., 1974; Weinstein et al., 1974), and Moore believes that the discrepancies among the metabolic epidemiology studies in man based on observations at a point in time or over a short time-interval may merely indicate that most diets exert little effect on the distribution of bacteria until the host's intestinal physiology changes in response to diet. He is inclined to emphasize individual physiology as a controlling factor in composition of the flora. Moore also believes that some of the differences in fecal floras described by the early surveys may be an artifact of procedures used to transport specimens from the several study areas to the laboratory for analysis, and he has adopted the practice of initiating culture work within a few minutes of sample collection in each study location.

Studies of familial polyposis families (Bone et al., 1975) have reported that patients in whom polyposis had already developed did not degrade cholesterol in significant proportions, therefore suggesting, contrary to the previous English–Africans comparisons, that in these patients it is the lack of conversion of steroids that is associated with the high risk. The same study found that half of the children of polyposis families have the same inability to convert cholesterol and suggested that this may be a marker of risk. This interpretation of the results has been challenged by Hackman et al. (1976) on the basis of finding a fair number (27%) of healthy subjects who show the same lack of cholesterol conversion. It should be remembered in this context that some products of bile manipulation, such as methylcholanthrene, are potent carcinogens to some experimental animals, but their carcinogenic role in primates has not been proved. Some indirect evidence does exist in humans for the carcinogenic role of some steroid hormones, particularly estrogens in the case of breast cancer.

The models of tumorigenesis developed by pioneer investigators in this field represent a good beginning, but their modification and elaboration will require additional studies in carefully chosen observational settings and the accumulation and collation of data from a variety of sources. The latter should include longer-term prospective studies of defined cohorts.

P. Effect of Diet on Intestinal Microenvironment

The investigators active in the field of metabolic epidemiology hold substantially identical views on probable pathways for tumorigenic activity, although there is some divergence of views on details. Burkitt *et al.* (1972) have emphasized the fiber content of the diet in modulating the sequence of events leading to bowel cancer. Wynder and colleagues (Wynder and Reddy, 1973; Wynder and Shigematsu, 1967) were impressed by the correlation between dietary fat intake and colon cancer and reasoned that the dietary fat content raised both the concentration of anaerobic bacteria and the amount of bile acid and cholesterol substrates in the gut, thus enhancing production of the bile acid and cholesterol metabolites which may be the proximate carcinogens. Reddy *et al.* (1975a) have reviewed the evidence that a high fat intake not only changes the composition of bile acids and neutral sterols but also modifies the distribution of intestinal flora, which may in turn produce tumorigenic substances from bile acids and neutral sterols (Hill *et al.*, 1971; Reddy and Wynder, 1973; Wynder and Reddy, 1973).

Reddy and Wynder (1973) have reported the daily fecal excretion of cholesterol metabolites, coprostanol, and coprostanone to be higher among Americans eating a Western diet than among Seventh-Day Adventists and American vegetarians eating a diet without meat but with vegetable protein. The fecal bacteria of Americans on a conventional mixed Western diet also contained more β-glucuronidase activity. The intestinal bacteria of Americans eating a normal Western diet appeared to be more active in hydrolyzing glucuronidase conjugates than those of the other groups. Similar contrasts of fecal contents in terms of bacteria, cholesterol, and bile acid metabolites carried out by them on patients characterized by colon cancer, polyps, familial polyposis, and ulcerative colitis showed a higher fecal excretion of cholesterol metabolites and bile acids among colon cancer patients than among controls, but familial polyposis patients did not differ from the control experience with respect to total neutral sterol and bile acid excretion. The pattern of cholesterol excretion was unique in indicating familial polyposis patients to excrete more cholesterol and less coprostanol and coprostanone, and a decrease in microbial conversion of cholesterol and primary bile acids in these patients was suggested.

Hill (1975) after review of several observational and experimental studies of the effect of changes in amounts of dietary fat and dietary meat was inclined to conclude that it is the fat, not the protein component, in the meat that determines the effects on the fecal acid steroids. Studies of the effects attributable to amount of dietary fiber are more difficult to assess, and Hill believes that few generalizations are possible concerning fiber effects; the source and dose of fiber must be specified for meaningful statements on this subject.

IV. Experimental Aspects of Colorectal Cancer

Extensive work has been done in the experimental aspects of colon cancer covering several areas, such as cell replication, animal models, experimental tumors, and testing of epidemiologic hypothesis.

A. CELL REPLICATION

The early steps in the development of the intestinal neoplasia have been clarified to a great extent by the use of isotope markers. Tritiated thymidine has been administered to patients scheduled for colonic surgery in whom colonic biopsies at different time intervals have been taken (Deschner and Lipkin, 1966; Cole and McKalen, 1963). These studies have shown that in the early stages of the neoplastic process active DNA synthesis and mitosis, normally limited to the deeper portions of the crypts, is abnormally present in the most superficial portions of the mucosa. This shift in the location of cell division has been observed in patients with familial polyposis (Cole and McKalen, 1963) as well as in patients with adenomatous polyps and villous adenomas (Deschner and Lipkin, 1966). These findings strongly suggest that changes in the microenvironment at the level of the mucosal surface determine that the normal cessation of mitotic activity of the superficial cells does not take place. This represents the earliest detectable change in the neoplastic process, results in an overproduction of cells, and interferes with the normal desquamation of the epithelial elements. The new cells eventually protrude into the lumen of the bowel, giving rise to such lesions as the adenomatous polyps and the villous adenomas. It has been suggested that the former represents neoplastic stimulus concentrated on a few glands whereas the villous adenoma occurs when an extensive area encompassing many glands is subjected to the environmental carcinogenic stimulus (Cole and McKalen, 1963).

B. Spontaneous Tumors

Carcinomas of the colon and rectum occur spontaneously in several animal species, but in none with the frequency observed today in the human populations of the United States and Western Europe. The one species who shares more intimately the human environment, the dog, shows the highest frequency of spontaneous tumors of the large intestine. Lingeman and Garner (1972) have made a thorough review of the subject and report remarkable similarities between the spontaneous tumors of the dogs and those of humans. As in man, canine tumors are more frequent in the distal colon and may originate from adenomatous polyps; rectal tumors predominate in males while tumors of the other segments show no sex predominance; tumors of dogs and man have similar histologic patterns and similar patterns of invasion and metastasis. Tumors of rodents are similar to those of dogs but are definitely less frequent. A few "outbreaks" have been reported in mice (Rowlatt et al., 1969) and rats (Helsop, 1969). The canine model seems to represent the "epidemic" type of human colon cancer which predominates in Europe and North America and is probably determined by environmental factors. The "endemic" type, predominant in Africa and other populations at low risk, is better represented by the spontaneous tumors of highly inbred rats, all of which have been found in the ascending colon (Miyamoto and Takizawa, 1975). This suggests that the human "endemic" cancers may be genetically determined.

C. Experimental Tumors

There have been numerous successful attempts to induce intestinal carcinomas in experimental animals with a variety of chemical compounds, mainly aromatic amines, polycyclic hydrocarbons, and nitrosamines, summarized recently by Wynder and Reddy (1973). Lorenz and Stewart (1940) produced intestinal adenocarcinomas in mice with 1,2,5,6-dibenzanthracene and 20-methylcholanthrene. Positive results were obtained by several investigators after the administration of 2-acetylaminofluorene to mice and rats (Bielschowsky, 1944; Cox et al., 1947; Foulds, 1947). Other chemicals known to induce intestinal carcinomas in experimental animals are: 1,2-dimethylhydrazine (Druckery *et al.*, 1967; Ward, 1974), bracken toxin (Pamukcu and Price, 1969), cycasin (Laqueur, 1965), N-2-fluorenyl acetamide (Morris *et al.*, 1961), and several nitroso compounds (Druckery *et al.*, 1964; Herrold, 1969; Schoental, 1965; Ward, 1975). Spjut and Spratt (1965) injected rats with 3,2-dimethyl-4-aminobiphenyl and obtained adenomatous polyps and adenocarcinomas that morphologically were similar to the human counterpart. There were also epidemiologic similarities between the lesions in rats and those in humans: concentration in the distal segments, sex distribution, increased frequency with age. Findings of this type justified the extensive use of the rat model for the exploration of the human risk factors. Ward *et al.* (1973a) induced intestinal neoplasms in rats with azoximethane and found dose-related differences in the localization of tumors equivalent to what is known of the localization of tumors in human populations with low and high incidence of colon cancer.

D. Testing of Hypothesis

After the demonstration by Laqueur (1965) and Laqueur and Matsumoto (1966) of the need of intestinal bacteria for the carcinogenic role of cycasin and his identification of methylazoximethanol as the proximate carcinogen, a number of synthetic analogs of the aglycon have been studied, mainly 1,2-dimethylhydrazine and azoximethane. The same experiments raised the possibility that human tumors might follow a similar pathway in which a carcinogen precursor is modified by the intestinal bacteria to yield the metabolite with direct carcinogenic potential. Cleveland *et al.* (1967) injected 3,2-dimethyl-4-aminobiphenyl to rats with surgically defunctionalized segments of the intestine and concluded that the chemical, after absorption from the injection site, is modified by the liver and excreted in the bile to induce neoplasia by direct contact with the intestinal mucosa. Similar results were obtained by Gennaro *et al.* (1973) with azoximethane. Ward *et al.* (1973a,b) tested the hypothesis, put forward by Burkitt, that the high rates of colon cancer in Western populations are due to the low amount of bulk in the diet. Rats were injected with azoximethane, fed low-residue diets, and compared with rats on the same diet with added 20% and 40% cellulose. The group on 20% cellulose had slightly greater frequency of colon tumors than the other two groups. In these animals, tumors of the small intestine showed a better correlation with the amount of bulk. Nigro *et al.* (1975) induced tumors in rats by azoximethane injection and compared animals fed excessive beef fat and animals on a normal diet. The animals given high-fat diet developed more intestinal tumors of greater size and with more metastasis than the animals on a normal diet. Reddy *et al.* (1975b) have found that high-fat diets make rats more susceptible to tumor induction with 1,2-dimethylhydrazine than rats on normal diet.

V. Discussion and Summary

A. Epidemiology of Bowel Cancer and Adenomatous Polyps

The epidemiology of large-bowel cancer is characterized by (1) large intercountry differences in risk, (2) anatomic- and segment-specific patterns of risk, (3) sex-specific patterns of risk, and (4) a disease response modulated by events in adult life linked with migration to a new environment. These features are consistent with a predominant role for environmental factors in the etiology of bowel cancer, although the weak associations with occupation and smoking history suggest that many environmental exposures are unrelated to this disease. The role of genetic factors in the subset of cases linked to familial polyposis is unequivocal, and documentation of familial aggregation for other bowel cancers suggests a genetic basis for individual variability in disease susceptibility. The major point, however, is that the observed magnitude of familial aggregation cannot account for the interpopulation differences in risk without the introduction of extreme, and probably unrealistic, assumptions on population variability in the distribution of "susceptible" families and individuals.

The concentration of bowel cancer in the economically developed countries of North America and Western Europe coincides well with the distribution of high-fat, high-protein diets and suggests large-bowel cancer to be a disease of affluence. This also correlates well with the distribution of endocrine-dependent tumors (breast, endometrium, ovary, prostate) and arteriosclerotic heart disease, which presents high risks in affluent populations. Although low risks prevail in the non-white populations of Africa and Asia, other evidence would rule out race as an important variable. U.S. blacks exhibit rates much higher than those reported by registries in Nigeria and other African countries, and this disparity has been magnified by the sharp rise in colon cancer incidence among U.S. blacks during the past two decades. The Jamaican registry covering primarily a black population also reports incidence well above the African level. The upward displacement of bowel cancer risks, particularly for the segments proximal to the rectosigmoid junction, among Japanese migrants to approximate those of the U.S. white host population argues against racial factors. The divergent results from Israel showing Jews from North America and Europe to have higher risks than Jews from Asia and North Africa provide additional evidence against important racial-genetic determinants.

Several epidemiological features that differentiate colon and rectum can be cited:

1. The divergent time trends in high- and intermediate-risk countries. Colon cancer rates have tended to rise, while those for rectum have remained stationary or declined. The U.S. blacks with a rise of 110% in colon cancer incidence between 1948 and 1970 illustrate this point well. The differences in time trends extend to individual segments. In Connecticut during recent years the most pronounced increases have occurred in cecum and ascending colon.

2. Colon and rectum tend to display different socioeconomic class gradients, the evidence from high-risk populations suggesting for colon a direct, but weak, relationship and for rectum an inverse relationship with level of risk. In one low-risk population studied this distinction has been more sharply defined; the data for Cali describe the excess incidence for the higher socioeconomic classes to be concentrated in the region from the ascending to rectosigmoid colon, and accompanied by minimal social class differences for rectum.

3. The concomitance in geographic distribution of risk with endocrine-dependent tumors and arteriosclerotic heart disease is more clearly defined for colon than rectum.

4. An association with alcohol consumption appears to be limited to an excess liability to rectal cancer among beer drinkers. No convincing evidence linking colon cancer with alcohol has been reported.

The incidence rates for colon and rectum in individual countries are obviously correlated (Fig. 3), but there are enough departures from a regular relationship to support the conjecture that tumor location might discriminate among populations at different levels of risk. More refined observations have demonstrated tumor location to be an important discriminator. Cancer registries arrayed in order of total bowel cancer incidence showed a rise in sigmoid–cecum ratios, steeper for males than females, as one progressed from low- to high-risk populations, and more recent studies based on careful measurements of tumor location in 2 high- and 2 low-risk populations have pinpointed the sigmoid colon and the region immediately distal (8–16 cm above the anus) as the segments in which the elevated incidence in concentrated. A more uniform distribution of incidence by bowel segment is a distinguishing characteristic of low-risk populations.

The findings on tumor localization suggest this to be a more promising variable than histology in epidemiological studies. Bowel tumors are predominantly adenocarcinomas, and work to date has not uncovered correlations between histologic characteristics and interpopulation differences in risk. The segment-specific differences raise the question whether large-bowel cancer represents a single disease or whether several etiologies are involved.

Numerous sex differences in the presentation of bowel cancer appear in data by geographic area, age, anatomic location, and time periods. Male dominance is firmly established, especially for rectum, in the high-risk populations of North America and western Europe. The sex ratios in risk become more variable in Africa, Asia, and Latin America. The slopes of the age-specific incidence curves for both colon and rectum are consistently higher for males than females in virtually all populations, and this phenomenon is related to male dominance in risk after age 60 or 65. Male dominance at older ages is not expressed to the same degree in all populations, but for a large subset of populations in the high-, intermediate-, and low-risk ranges this is an obvious feature.

Systematic segmental differences in sex ratios have been depicted by the U.S. cancer morbidity survey, which showed the high male-female ratio of incidence for rectum to become progressively smaller in the more distal segments. Data from other sources, including the Connecticut Tumor Registry, appear to be consistent with the survey findings. In recent years the incidence of male colon cancer has been more volatile and risen more rapidly than the corresponding female rates in several populations, as described in Fig. 15. The U.S. black experience between 1948 and 1970 provides a dramatic illustration of this point. The upward trend in male colon cancer would suggest that the response to changed environmental conditions is first expressed by males. The U.S. Japanese experience supports this conjecture. As of 1960 the colon rates for female Japanese migrants had lagged behind the male rates in making the transition from the low risks prevailing in Japan to the elevated level characteristic of the host U.S. white population. Subsequently, the female Japanese rates have continued to rise, and now the rates for both male and female Japanese migrants closely approximate the corresponding U.S. white experience.

The epidemiological characteristics of bowel cancer on review form a distinctive configuration, a key element being the interrelationship among the magnitude of the incidence rates, the sex–age patterns of incidence, and anatomic localization of tumors.

The controversy concerning the premalignant role of adenomatous polyps is gradually being resolved in the affirmative. The accumulation of new evidence indicates that we can no longer assume that adenomatous polyps are unrelated to large-bowel cancer. From an epidemiologic point of view, the association between adenomatous polyps and colon cancer is reinforced by the following characteristics:

1. The incidence of colon cancer closely parallels the prevalence of adenomatous polyps in all populations so far studied.

2. Whites, blacks, and orientals have a low prevalence of adenomatous polyps while living in areas of low colon cancer frequency, but display high polyp prevalence if they migrate to areas of high colon cancer risk. The difference in adenomatous polyp prevalence between migrant and native Japanese is consistent with the differences in colon cancer incidence in the two groups.

3. The frequency of both conditions has increased over time in the United States, presumably in response to environmental changes that may be related to improving socioeconomic conditions. The latter is suggested by the inverse socioeconomic gradient found for both conditions in Cali, Colombia, a city in a developing country that has large social class differences in diet.

4. In the populations studied, the risk of colon cancer increases with the size and multiplicity of polyps, thus suggesting a dose-effect relationship.

5. Males tend to present more multiple polyps in the sigmoid colon and adjacent segments, a feature that agrees with and reinforces the excess male cancer incidence rather consistently observed for that portion of the large bowel.

6. The inference of a causal relationship between adenomatous polyps and bowel carcinoma is reinforced by observations on the cancer experience of polyp patients. Prospective studies in the United States (Prager *et al.*, 1974) and Sweden (Ekelund and Lindstrom, 1974) have shown persons with adenomatous polyps to be at higher risk to colon cancer. Also, rectal cancer can be prevented by fulguration of adenomatous polyps, and the number of more proximal cancers in the rectosigmoid region seems to have been reduced by resection of polyps reached through the sigmoidoscope.

Collectively, these features depict a strong, consistent association between adenomatous polyps and colon cancer. Studies of the pathology of both lesions would support a causal interpretation of the association in most cases: the polyp is a prerequisite to cancer when the malignancy starts in the polyp. There are, however, well documented cases where the cancer did not arise in a polyp, and in this situation the association would be indirect and mediated via two independent responses to a common agent. The distinction in pathways is relevant to the question of control strategies. The hope of preventing all (or a large proportion) of the cases of cancer by polyps resection seems to be unrealistic, since most patients in whom colon cancer is diagnosed are found to have malignant tumor at the time of the first medical examination of the large bowel. The ideal cancer prevention, therefore, should include prevention of polyps by removal of the polyp-producing factor, and if that can be accomplished the distinction between direct and indirect association becomes irrelevant.

B. Etiologic Model

The more recent information provided by cancer registries, summarized in Fig. 1 and 6 (Waterhouse *et al.*, 1976) confirms the interactions between risk level, sex ratios, and anatomic localization which led us to formulate our epidemiologic model (Haenszel and Correa, 1971). The components of the model remain valid:

1. In low-risk populations, where the disease is "endemic," there is a preponderance of female cases and a relatively uniform distribution of cases throughout the length of the colon with little or no concentration of left-sided tumors in the sigmoid colon.

2. When a new etiologic factor is introduced in a low-risk population, the transition from an "endemic" to an "epidemic" phase is first expressed as a rise in sigmoid cancer among older males. This was clearly observed in the data for Japanese migrants to Hawaii as of 1958–1965.

3. A rise in female sigmoid cancer follows later, as shown by the most recent data for Hawaii-Japanese as of 1966–1972.

4. When the epidemic is well established, a rise in cecum and ascending cancer, first noticed in males, is accompanied by similar shifts in the frequency of descending and transverse cancers. This is what has been observed in recent years in Connecticut.

We postulated that the model could fit a hypothesis based on the presence of a carcinogen in the intestinal contents which become increasingly concentrated as it travels from the ileocecal valve to the rectum. Animal models give ample support for such hypothesis, as discussed earlier in relation to the role of intestinal bacteria in metabolizing precursors to ultimate carcinogens and in relation to cell kinetics studies calling for a local carcinogen to explain the abnormal rate of DNA synthesis in surface epithelium of early neoplastic lesions.

The sex ratio of incidence rates continues to be a puzzling

phenomenon since it shows differences among populations, by anatomic localization and between different time periods (Correa and Haenszel, 1975). We postulate that cecum cancer is predominant in females in low-risk populations and that this predominance probably accounts for the female excess in colon cancer in such populations.

If the base-line rates of low-risk populations estimate an "endemic" component present in other populations including those in the "epidemic" phase, the rates for low-risk populations could be subtracted from the latter to estimate the additional "epidemic" components. The effect of this would be to enhance the male contribution to the "epidemic" component and to yield incidence curves that would display the more normal male predominance for most non-sex-related cancers. This, however, falls short of explaining the time trends in the late stages of an epidemic, when females finally attain a high rate of increase. The earlier male response to carcinogens characterizes populations in transition and seems to be part of a biologic phenomenon responsible for higher rates and poorer survival in males for most cancers common to both sexes.

In order to assess the sex ratios in populations at or near the peak of the epidemic, we have to consider the findings on precursor lesions. We have discussed the evidence for a premalignant role of adenomatous polyps, which to us appears beyond dispute. The male–female ratios of the frequency of the precursor, however, diverge from the sex ratio of the cancers. There is a male excess in the prevalence of adenomatous polyps in all populations, including those at low-, intermediate-, and high-risk. We consider this to be the "normal" behavior of the biologic response to a carcinogen and to represent well the situation in experimental models and observations on humans. The sex difference in colon cancer incidence is of a lower order of magnitude than that observed for adenomatous polyps. We have, therefore, a male-predominant precursor apparently leading to a sexually more evenly distributed cancer.

Several hypotheses could be explored in search for answers to the riddle. A greater dose of the carcinogen in females might be postulated, but the male excess of the precursor argues strongly against that explanation. Given the known greater susceptibility of males to carcinogens, it seems that polyp prevalence in humans favors the notion that the dosage is about equal for both sexes. It could be postulated that there is an equal dose of initiators for both sexes, but a greater dose of promoters for the female. Against this argument is the finding of greater "promoter" effect is males, as represented by their greater liability to multiple polyps. A greater dose of "initiator" in females seems likewise ruled out by the greater prevalence of single polyps in males. Another possibility is that females are more susceptible to colon cancer than males, but this runs contrary to observations of greater male susceptibility to most nonendocrine cancers, with the exception of the biliary tract.

Our knowledge of the prevalence of polyps may be incomplete since all the available data come from populations at low risk (Japan, Latin America), in transition (Hawaiian Japanese), or somewhat under epidemic peak values (New Orleans).

We know of no recent polyp prevalence data in populations that have been at an epidemic peak for a prolonged time period, such as Connecticut, Canada, Scotland, or New Zealand. If there should prove to be no male predominance in prevalence of adenomatous polyps in such populations, an equal dose of carcinogen or a loss of natural resistance to carcinogens in females at the peak of the epidemic could then be entertained. An equal prevalence of polyps in both sexes in populations at highest risk is not predicted from extrapolations of the sex ratios of adenomatous polyps in Table XXXI, which shows no consistent gradient in sex ratios by level of colon cancer risk.

We seem, therefore, to be in need of the complementary action of an additional tumorigenic stimulus, a cocarcinogen with preference for females. One possibility in this regard is suggested by the positive and statistically significant correlation between incidence rates for large-bowel cancer and for cancer of the female breast (Berg, 1975). Large-bowel cancer shares with endocrine-dependent cancers (breast, endometrium, ovary, prostate, testis) several epidemiologic characteristics summarized recently by Berg (1975). This group of cancers are diseases of affluence, most probably related to affluent nutrition. It has been postulated that affluent nutrition increases the breast cancer rates by altering the endocrine status and balance (Wynder et al., 1960), and this hypothesis has found support in studies of the endocrine profile of young Hawaiian Japanese women, who in this respect more closely resemble U.S. white women than women in Japan (Dickinson et al., 1974). Along these lines it has been reported that breast cancer correlates positively with body size (deWaard and Halejijn, 1974), which is correlated with growth hormone, which in turn is influenced by the level of dietary protein (Merimec and Fineberg, 1973). Based on these ideas it may be suggested that the lack of a pronounced male excess in colon cancer incidence in high-risk populations is due to an extra female component in cancer rates given by response of the colon to endocrine-related carcinogenic factors. It may be that the colon epithelium responds to the same (or similar) carcinogens responsible for breast cancer, mainly its postmenopausal component. This hypothesis finds some support in experimental carcinogenesis. Excessive fat in the diet of experimental animals raises the rate of cancer induction for both the colon (Nigro *et al.*, 1975; Reddy *et al.*, 1975b) and breast (Carroll *et al.*, 1968).

C. Mechanisms of Action

Some tentative speculations about the mechanisms of action are suggested by the joint consideration of human and experimental data.

All indications are that we are dealing with a direct carcinogen that comes into contact with the large-bowel mucosa and, therefore, is probably carried by the fecal content. This carcinogen seems to be diet-dependent. But a carcinogen directly ingested with food is not a good prospect because in that case it should also produce tumors in the upper gastrointestinal tract. The fact that populations at high risk to esophageal and gastric cancer usually do not have high risk to large-bowel cancer speaks in favor of different etiologies for tumors in the upper and lower digestive tract. There are some indications that this carcinogen(s) may be contained in the bile: some experimental colon carcinogens are excreted with the bile (Cleveland *et al.*, 1967). It has been suggested that there is a precarcinogen in the normal components of bile, namely the bile acids, which supposedly are transformed to ultimate carcinogens by intestinal bacteria (Wynder, 1975; Reddy *et al.*, 1975a; Hill, 1975). This hypothesis has not been proved or rejected, but the prospects of its being correct do not appear good when one recalls the very low rates of colon cancer in many populations whose members presumably experience the daily delivery of bile acids in substantial amounts to the intestinal lumen. Another candidate along these lines of thought would be cholesterol, which is diet-dependent and excreted with the bile. The expected higher conversion of cholesterol to its metabolites in the intestinal lumen of cancer patients or in high-risk populations has not been confirmed. To the contrary, familial polyposis patients show a lack of conversion of fecal cholesterol to its metabolites (Bone *et al.*, 1975). We are, therefore, at the stage where convincing proof on the identity of any precarcinogen excreted in or with the bile is lacking.

Once our hypothetical carcinogen reaches the large bowel it results in excessive replication of the normally dormant epithelial cells of the surface of the intestinal glands. This continued replication is the result of a mutation, since the daughter cells inherit the loss of obedience to the normal regulatory mechanisms of cell growth. Further mutations bring about other abnormalities of cell replication, such as polyploidy and finally the capacity to invade the submucosa and other tissues. Since the differences between populations at high and low colon cancer risk are not only in the prevalence of single polyps, but also in the multiplicity and in atypia, it follows that not only initiator effect (first polyp) but also promoter effect (multiplicity and atypia) are greater in high-risk populations. This speaks in favor of a constant or repeated supply of carcinogen over a long time period. A carcinogen carried in bile would fit this requirement. In this case, as in most experimental models, initiator and promoter effects seem to be executed by the same chemical substance.

Our hypothetical direct carcinogen seems to induce adenomatous polyps before it induces cancer. This is inferred by several facts, such as the greater numbers of polyps than cancer, the earlier appearance of polyps in the host, and the fact that many cancers have been seen arising in well-formed adenomatous polyps. Adenomatous polyps fit in many ways the previously proposed model for colon cancer (Haenszel and Correa, 1971), especially the "epidemic" component. In common with the "epidemic" component, adenomatous polyps increase in frequency with age, and in high-risk populations they are more concentrated in the intermediate segments of the large intestine. The one epidemiologic characteristic that the two conditions do not share, as noted above, is the lack of sex differential for cancer in high-risk populations. It may be that this effect is not mediated through adenomatous polyps. We do not favor this explanation because it is not supported by the observations on the pathology of the polyp–cancer sequence. An alternative explanation is that the high-fat diet (or whatever other factor is responsible for this effect) somehow alters the capacity of the tissue to resist invasion. This sort of explanation may also be responsible for the increase in breast cancer observed in Japanese migrants to Hawaii. Some evidence that this occurs in other endocrine tumors is provided by Akazaki and Stemmermann (1973), who reported the Japanese in Japan and the United States to have almost the same autopsy prevalence of latent prostatic carcinoma, the differences being that the U.S. Japanese displayed a much higher proportion of biologically aggressive lesions, "proliferative" in Akazaki's terminology. The excessive incidence of clinically overt prostatic cancer in U.S. Japanese and U.S. whites might, therefore, be explainable on the basis of a greater proportion of latent carcinomas finding their way to invade other tissues, as opposed to an excess of new neoplastic foci.

D. FUTURE WORK

1. A direct approach to the problem, at the risk of being simplistic, consists of searching for a carcinogen in the stools of patients with cancer or adenomatous polyps. Even better candidates for this approach are the familial polyposis patients. The obvious difficulty with this approach is that the amounts of carcinogen expected are minute, and they may also be unstable. Modern chemical techniques applied to concentrates of stools may offer new hope of finding the culprit. Other hopeful new developments are the growing realization that most carcinogens are mutagens linked with improvements in technology of tests for mutagenesis. These tests could detect strong carcinogens in concentrations of parts per million, but it may be that the hypothetical carcinogen present in stool is in concentrations of parts per billion, thus suggesting the probable need for concentration and extraction.

2. Analytical epidemiology has two relatively new options: the identification of a precursor and the availability of populations at low, intermediate, and high risks. Study of patients with precursor lesions may point to diet and other etiologic factors present before habits are changed by the patient as a result of the necrosis and ulceration of the intestinal mucosa brought about by a carcinomatous growth. The study of the diet of cancer and control patients in populations at differing colon cancer risk levels may offer an opportunity to search for items associated with the disease (or with absence of the disease) which may coincide with items that represent additions or deletions to the diet of populations whose cancer risk is changing rapidly (i.e., Hawaiian Japanese) or in populations whose risk is not increasing in spite of changes toward a more affluent type of diet (i.e., Puerto Rico).

3. There are available today very good experimental models of colon carcinogenesis in which many of the suspected factors could be tested. These models could also give some clues as to the general group of chemical substances which should be suspected in humans and tested by chemical means.

4. Reddy et al. (1975a) have suggested that identification of chemical or bacterial indicators may discriminate between high- and low-risk populations and between colon cancer patients and controls. They believe that this will be a more rewarding immediate, short-term goal than precise identification and quantification of bacteria and intraluminal compounds. Their candidates for possible indicators are β-glucuronidase and 7α-dehydroxylase activities, fecal clostridia, and lithocholic and deoxycholic acid.

5. Some of the leads uncovered by work since 1960 pose questions that can be pursued in animal experiments and by collection of more refined clinical observations. Past history would not have led one to expect prompt and timely exchange and interplay of information among epidemiologists, experimentalists, and clinicians, but recent events in large-bowel cancer have not followed the standard script. Epidemiological observations were being accumulated at a time when institutional forces in the United States and elsewhere favored interdisciplinary collaboration. The U.S. National Cancer Institute in 1971 established an intramural program with the mission of developing and supporting multifaceted etiological investigations of large-bowel cancer and subsequently extended the scope of this interdisciplinary approach by funding the National Large Bowel Cancer Project. Within less than 10 years, studies embracing such diverse topics as cell kinetics, enzyme systems, intestinal flora, fecal chemistry, and mutagenic activity of stools have been launched. Advances in fiberoptic technology and development of the colonoscope enlarge the possibilities for studies of antecedent conditions.

6. Comparative data on intra- and interpopulation variations in risk should incorporate dietary and metabolic information (cholesterol, bile acid metabolites, type and enzyme potential of intestinal flora).

7. The most promising lead identified by epidemiologic studies relates to diet, particularly high-meat, high-saturated fat diet. Favorable observational settings are present with unusual and extreme contrasts in food consumption such as migrant populations, Seventh-Day Adventists. Especially designed diet studies in volunteers could also be helpful if conducted for an extended period of time. The role of beef in the etiology of bowel cancer is sufficiently prominent to warrant planning of dietary intervention studies with "prudent" diets in both cancer and premalignant conditions.

8. The development of prospective studies would improve in accuracy of diet information by permitting current collection of diet histories from members of defined cohorts, whose subsequent morbidity and mortality experience could be monitored. Such studies have been initiated in Norway for a representative sample of the male population and in the United States for Hawaiian Japanese.

ACKNOWLEDGMENTS

The staff of the Biometry Branch, National Cancer Institute, gave valuable help in the preparation of this review paper, and the authors thank in particular Mrs. Frances B. Locke for her work in review of the literature and preparation of text figures and tables, and Ms. Carol Webber for typing the several drafts of the manuscript. This work was supported in part by Contract NO1-CP-53521, National Cancer Institute.

References

Akazaki, K., and Stemmermann, G. N. (1973). *J. Natl. Cancer Inst.* **50**, 1137–1144.
Andren, L., and Frieberg, S. (1956). *Acta Radiol.* **46**, 507–510.
Aragón, L. A. (1964). "Estimación del consumo de algunos alimentos basicos en la ciudad de Cali," Tesis de Grado. Cali Universidad del Valle, Facultad de Ciencias Economicas, Cali, Colombia.
Aries, V., Crowther, J. S., Drasar, B. S., Hill, M. J., and Williams, R. E. O. (1969). *Gut* **10**, 334–335.
Arminski, T. C., and McLean, D. W. (1964). *Dis. Colon Rectum* **7**, 249–261.
Armstrong, B., and Doll, R. (1975). *Int. J. Cancer* **15**, 617–631.
Axtell, L. M., and Chiazze, L. (1966). *Cancer* **19**, 750–754.
Badger, G. M., Cook, J. W., Hewett, C. L., Kennaway, E. L., Kennaway, N. M., Martin, R. H., and Robinson, A. M. (1940). *Proc. R. Soc. London, Ser. B* **129**, 439–467.
Bailar, J. C., III. (1963). *Cancer* **16**, 842–853.
Berg, J. W. (1972). *Lancet* **2**, 486.
Berg, J. W. (1975). *Cancer Res.* **35**, 3345–3350.
Bielschowsky, F. (1944). *Br. J. Exp. Pathol.* **25**, 1–4.
Bjelke, E. (1973). "Epidemilogic Studies of Cancer of the Stomach, Colon, and Rectum: With Special Emphasis on the Role of Diet," 1–5. University Microfilms, Ann Arbor, Michigan.
Bjelke, E. (1974). *Scand. J. Gastroenterol.* **9**, Suppl., 1–235.
Bjelke, E. (1975). *Pro. Int. Cancer Congr., 11th, 1974* Excerpta Med. Found. Int. Congr. Ser. No. 354, Vol. 6, pp. 324–330.
Blatt, L. J. (1961). *Dis. Colon Rectum* **4**, 277–282.
Bone, E., Drasar, B. S., and Hill, M. J. (1975). *Lancet* **1**, 1117–1120.
Boyd, J. T., and Doll, R. (1954). *Br. J. Cancer* **8**, 231–237.
Boyd, J., Landman, M., and Doll, R. (1964). *Gut* **5**, 196–200.
Brahme, F., Ekelund, G. R., Nordem, J. G., and Wenkest, A. (1974). *Dis. Colon Rectum* **17**, 166–171.
Bremner, C. G., and Ackerman, L. V. (1970). *Cancer* **26**, 991–999.
Breslow, N. E., and Enstrom, J. E. (1974). *J. Natl. Cancer Inst.* **53**, 631–639.
Burbank, F. (1971). *Natl. Cancer Inst., Monog.* **33**, 1–593.
Burdette, W. J. (1970). *In* "Carcinoma of the Colon and Antecedent Epitehlium" (W. J. Burdette, ed.), pp. 78–102. Thomas, Springfield, Illinois.
Burdette, W. J. (1971). *Cancer* **28**, 51–59.
Burkitt, D. P. (1970). *Lancet* **2**, 1237–1240.
Burkitt, D. P. (1971a). *Cancer* **28**, 3–13.
Burkitt, D. P. (1971b). *J. Natl. Cancer Inst.* **47**, 913–919.
Burkitt, D. P., Walker, A. R., and Painter, N. S. (1972). *Lancet* **2**, 1408–1412.
Bussey, H. J. R. (1972). *Proc. R. Soc. Med.* **65**, 294.
Bussey, H. J. R. (1975). "Familial Polyposis." Johns Hopkins Univ. Press, Baltimore, Maryland.
Camiel, M. R., Mule, J. E., Alexander, L. L., and Benninghoff, D. L. (1968). *N. Engl. J. Med.* **278**, 1056–1059.
Carroll, K. K., Gammel, E. B., and Plunkett, E. R. (1968). *Can. Med. Assoc. J.* **98**, 590–593.

134   P. CORREA AND W. HAENSZEL

Cederlöf, R., Floderus, B., and Friberg, L. (1970). *Acta Genet. Med. Gemellol.* **19,** 69–74.
Cederlöf, R., Friberg, L., Hrubec, Z., and Lorich, U. (1975). "The Relationship of Smoking and Some Social Covariables to Mortality and Cancer Morbidity." Dept. Environ. Hyg. Karolinska Institute, Stockholm.
Ceulemans, G. (1958). *J. Int. Coll. Surg.* **30,** 649–652.
Chapman, I. (1963). *Ann. Surg.* **157,** 223–226.
Chen, W. Y., Crittenden, L. B., Mantel, N., and Cameron, W. R. (1961). *J. Natl. Cancer Inst.* **27,** 875–892.
Cleave, T. L., Campbell, G. D., and Painter, N. W. (1969). "Diabetes, Coronary Thrombosis and the Saccharine Disease." Bristol.
Clemmesen, J. (1965a). *Acta Pathol. Microbiol. Scand., Suppl.* **174,** I.
Clemmesen, J. (1965b). *Acta Pathol. Microbiol. Scand., Suppl.* **174,** II.
Clemmesen, J. (1969). *Acta Pathol. Microbiol. Scand., Suppl.* **209,** III.
Clemmesen, J. (1974). *Acta Pathol. Microbiol. Scand., Suppl.* **247,** IV.
Clemmesen, J., and Nielsen, A. (1951). *Br. J. Cancer* **5,** 159–171.
Cleveland, J. C., Litvak, S. F., and Cole, J. W. (1967). *Cancer Res.* **27,** 708–714.
Cohart, E. M., and Muller, C. (1955). *Cancer* **8,** 379–388.
Cole, J. W., and Holden, W. D. (1959). *Arch. Surg. (Chicago)* **79,** 385–392.
Cole, J. W., and McKalen, A. (1963). *Cancer* **16,** 998–1002.
Connecticut State Dept. of Health. (1969). "Annual Reports, 1963–1968."
Connecticut State Dept. of Health. (1973). *Conn. Health Bull.* 1–5.
Connecticut State Dept. of Health. (1966). "Cancer in Connecticut—Incidence and Rates, 1935–62."
Cook, J. W., and Haselwood, G. D. A. (1933). *Chem. Ind. (London)* **11,** 758.
Cook, P. J., Doll, R., and Fellingham, S. A. (1969). *Int. J. Cancer* **4,** 93–112.
Correa, P. (1975). *Cancer Res.* **35,** 3395–3397.
Correa, P., and Haenszel, W. (1975). *In* "Cancer Epidemiology and Prevention" (D. Schottenfeld, ed.), pp. 386–403. Thomas, Springfield, Illinois.
Correa, P., and Llanos, G. (1966). *J. Natl. Cancer Inst.* **36,** 717–745.
Correa, P., Duque, E., Cuello, C., and Haenszel, W. (1972). *Int. J. Cancer* **9,** 86–96.
Correa, P., Strong, J., Reif, A., and Johnson, W. (1977). *Cancer* **39,** 2258–2264.
Cox, A. J., Wilson, R. H., and DeEds, F. (1947). *Cancer Res.* **7,** 647–657.
Crail, H. W. (1949). *U.S. Navy Med. Bull.* **49,** 123–128.
Creagan, E. T., and Fraumeni, J. F., Jr. (1972). *J. Natl. Cancer Inst.* **49,** 959–967.
Curwen, M. P. (1954). *Br. J. Cancer* **8,** 181–198.
Cutler, S. J. (1975). *In* "Cancer Epidemiology and Prevention" (D. Schottenfeld, ed.), pp. 375–385. Thomas, Springfield, Illinois.
Cutler, S. J., and Lourie, W. I. (1963). *Natl. Cancer Inst., Monogr.* **15,** 281–299.
Cutler, S. J., and Young, J. L., Jr., eds. (1975). *Natl. Cancer Inst., Monogr,* **41,** 1–454.
Davis, W. H. (1913). *Bull. Am. Acad. Med.* **14,** 19–54.
DeDombal, F. T., Watts, J. McK., Watkinson, G., and Goligher, J. C. (1966). *Br. Med. J.* **1,** 1442–1447.
de Jong, U. W., Day, N. E., Muir, C. S., Barclay, T. H. C., Bras, G., Foster, F. H., Jussawalla, D. J., Kurihara, M., Linden, G., Martínez, I., Payne, P. M., Pedersen, E., Ringertz, N., and Shanmugaratnam, K. (1972). *Int. J. Cancer* **10,** 463–477.
Deschner, E. E., and Lipkin, M. (1966). *J. Natl. Cancer Inst.* **36,** 849–857.
DeWaard, F., and Halejijn, B. (1974). *Int. J. Cancer* **14,** 153–160.
Dickinson, L. E., MacMahon, B., Cole, P., and Brown, J. B. (1974). *N. Engl. J. Med.* **29,** 1211–1213.
Doll, R. (1969). *Br. J. Cancer* **23,** 1–8.

Doll, R., and Hill, A. B. (1964). *Br. Med. J.* **1**, 1399–1410.

Doll, R., Payne, P., and Waterhouse, J., eds. (1966). "Cancer Incidence in Five Continents," Tech. Rep. Int. Union Against Cancer, Berlin and New York.

Doll, R., Muir, C., and Waterhouse, J., eds. (1970). "Cancer Incidence in Five Continents," Vol. II. Int. Union Against Cancer, Berlin and New York.

Dorn, H. F., and Cutler, S. J. (1959). *U.S., Public Health Serv., Public Health Monogr.* **56**.

Drexler, J. (1967). *Arch. Intern. Med.* **119**, 503–509.

Drexler, J. (1968). *Arch. Intern. Med.* **121**, 62–66.

Drexler, J. (1971). *Arch. Intern. Med.* **127**, 466–469.

Druckery, H., Steinhoff, D., Preussmann, R., and Ivankovic, S. (1964). *2. Krebsforsch* **66**, 1–10.

Druckery, H., Preussmann, R., Matzkies, F., and Ivankovic, S. (1967). *Naturwissenschaften* **54**, 285–286.

Dublin, L. I. (1922). *Sci. Mon.* **14**, 94–104.

Dublin, L. I., and Baker, G. W. (1920). *Q. Publ. Am. Stat. Assoc.* **17**, 13–44.

Dukes, C. E. (1930). *J. Pathol. Bacteriol.* **35**, 323–332.

Dukes, C. E. (1952). *Ann. Eugen. London* **17**, 1–29.

Dunham, L. J., and Bailar, J. C., III. (1968). *J. Natl. Cancer Inst.* **41**, 155–203.

Ederer, F., Leren, P., Turpeinen, O., and Frantz, I. D. (1971). *Lancet* **2**, 203–206.

Edwards, F. C., and Truelove, S. C. (1964). *Gut* **5**, 1–22.

Eisenberg, H., Mork, T., and Connelly, R. R. (1964). *Natl. Cancer Inst., Monogr.* **15**, 301–319.

Ekelund, G., and Lindstrom, C. (1974). *Gut* **15**, 654–663.

Enstrom, J. E. (1975a). *Br. J. Cancer* **32**, 432–439.

Enstrom, J. E. (1975b). *Cancer* **36**, 825–841.

Finegold, S. M., Flora, D. J., Attebery, H. R., and Sutter, V. L. (1975). *Cancer Res.* **35**, 3407–3417.

Fisher, J. F., and Mallette, M. F. (1961). *J. Gen. Physiol.* **45**, 1–13.

Food and Agriculture Organization of the United Nations. (1958). "Food Balance Sheets 1954–56." FAO, Rome.

Food and Agriculture Organization of the United Nations, (1971). "Food Balance Sheets 1964–66." FAO, Rome.

Foulds, L. (1947). *Br. J. Cancer* **1**, 172–176.

Fraumeni, J. F., Jr., Vogel, C. L., and Easton, J. M. (1968). *Arch. Intern. Med.* **121**, 57–61.

Fraumeni, J. F., Jr., Lloyd, J. W., Smith, E. M., and Wagoner, J. K. (1969). *J. Natl. Cancer Inst.* **42**, 455–468.

Gardner, E. J. (1951). *Am. J. Hum. Genet.* **3**, 167–176.

Gardner, E. J. (1969). *Proc. Utah Acad.* **46**, 1–11.

Gennaro, A. R., Villanueva, R., Sukonthaman, Y., Vathanophas, V., and Rosemond, G. P. (1973). *Cancer Res.* **33**, 536–541.

Go, V. L. W. (1976). *Cancer* **37**, 562–566.

Gold, P., and Freedman, S. O. (1965). *J. Exp. Med.* **122**, 467–481.

Graham, S., Levin, M., and Lilienfeld, A. M. (1960). *Cancer* **13**, 180–191.

Greenberg, R. A. (1963). *Conn. Health Bull.* **77**, 257–268.

Greenwald, P., Korns, R. F., Nasca, P. C., and Wolfgang, P. E. (1975). *Cancer Res.* **35**, 3507–3512.

Greenwood, M., and Yule, G. U. (1914). *J. R. State. Soc.* **77**, 179–197.

Gregor, O., Toman, R., and Prusova, F. (1969). *Gut* **10**, 1031–1034.

Gross, L. (1966). *Cancer* **19**, 849–852.

Guralnick, L. (1963a). "Vital Statistics Special Reports," Vol. 53, No. 3. US Govt. Printing Office, Washington, D.C.

Guralnick, L. (1963b). "Vital Statistic Special Reports," Vol. 53, No. 5. US Govt. Printing Office, Washington, D.C.

Hackman, A. S., Wilkins, T. D., Finegold, S. M., and Sutter, V. L. (1976). *Lancet* 1, 752.

Haenszel, W. (1959). *J. Natl. Cancer Inst.* 23, 487–505.

Haenszel, W. (1961). *J. Natl. Cancer Inst.* 26, 37–132.

Haenszel, W. (1971). *Isr. J. Med. Sci.* 7, 1437–1450.

Haenszel, W., and Correa, P. (1971). *Cancer* 28, 14–24.

Haenszel, W., and Dawson, E. A. (1965). *Cancer* 18, 265–272.

Haenszel, W., and Kurihara, M. (1968). *J. Natl. Cancer Inst.* 40, 43–68.

Haenszel, W., Marcus, S. C., and Zimmerer, E. G. (1955). *V.S., Public Health Serv., Public Health Monogr.* 37, 1–85.

Haenszel, W., Kurihara, M., Segi, M., and Lee, R. K. C. (1972). *J. Natl. Cancer Inst.* 49, 969–988.

Haenszel, W., Berg, J. W., Segi, M., Kurihara, M., and Locke, F. B. (1973). *J. Natl. Cancer Inst.* 51, 1765–1779.

Haenszel, W., Correa, P., and Cuello, C. (1975). *J. Natl. Cancer Inst.* 54, 1031–1035.

Hakulinen, T., Lehtimaki, L., Lehtonen, M., and Teppo, L. (1974). *J. Natl. Cancer Inst.* 52, 1711–1714.

Hammond, E. C. (1966). *Natl. Cancer Inst., Monogr.* 19, 127–204.

Harvald, B., and Hauge, M. (1963). *J. Am. Med. Assoc.* 186, 749–753.

Helsop, B. F. (1969). *Lab. Invest.* 3, 185–195.

Helwig, E. B. (1946). Am. J. Dis. Child. 72, 289–295.

Helwig, E. B. (1947). *Surg., Gynecol. Obstet.* 84, 36–49.

Herberman, R. B. (1976). *Cancer* 37, 549–562.

Herrold, K. McD. (1969). *Pathol. Vet.* 6, 403–412.

Higginson, J. (1966). *J. Natl. Cancer Inst.* 37, 527–545.

Higginson, J. (1967). *Natl. Cancer Inst., Monogr.* 25, 191–198.

Higginson, J., and Oettlé, A. G. (1960). *J. Natl. Cancer Inst.* 24, 589–671.

Hill, M. J. (1974). *Am. J. Clin. Nutr.* 27, 1475–1480.

Hill, M. J. (1975). *Cancer Res.* 35, 3398–3402.

Hill, M. J., Drasar, B. S., Aires, V., Crowther, J. S., Hawksworth, G., and Williams, R. E. O. (1971). *Lancet* 1, 95–100.

Howell, M. A. (1974). *Br. J. Cancer* 29, 328–336.

Howell, M. A. (1975). *J. Chronic Dis.* 28, 67–80.

Howie, J. G. R., and Timperley, W. R. (1966). *Cancer* 19, 1138–1142.

Hyams, L., and Wynder, E. L. (1968). *J. Chronic Dis.* 21, 391–415.

Interdepartmental Committee on Nutrition for National Defense. (1961). "Nutritional Survey. Colombia." US Govt. Printing Office, Washington, D.C.

Järvi, O. (1962). *Proc. Finn. Acad. Sci. Lett.* pp. 151–187.

Jones, J. H. (1969). *Gut* 10, 651–654.

Jussawalla, D. J., and Jain, D. K. (1976). "Cancer Incidence in Greater Bombay, 1970–1972." Indian Cancer Society—Bombay Cancer Registry, Bombay.

Kagan, A., Harris, B. R., Winkelstein, W., Johnson, K. G., Kato, H., Syme, S. L., Rhoads, G. G., Gay, M. L., Nichaman, M. Z., Hamilton, H. B., and Tillotson, J. (1974). *J. Chronic Dis.* 27, 345–364.

Kahn, H. A. (1966). *Natl. Cancer Inst., Monogr.* 19, 1–126.

Kannel, W. B., Castelli, W. P., Gordon, T., and McNamara, P. M. (1971). *Ann. Intern. Med.* 74, 1–12.

King, H., and Haenszel, W. (1973). *J. Chronic Dis.* 26, 623–646.

Klebba, A. J. (1970). "National Center for Health Statistics," Ser. 20, Nos. 8a and 8b. US Govt. Printing Office, Washington, D.C.

Kluge, T. (1964). *Acta Chir. Scand.* **127**, 392–398.
Lane, N., Kaplan, H., and Pascal, R. (1971). *Gastroenterology* **60**, 537–551.
Laqueur, G. L. (1964). *Fed. Proc., Fed. Am. Soc. Exp. Biol.* **23**, 1386–1388.
Laqueur, G. L. (1965). *Virchows Arch. A* **340**, 151–163.
Laqueur, G. L. (1970). *In* "Carcinoma of the Colon and Antecedent Epithelium" (W. J. Burdette, ed.), pp. 305–313. Thomas, Springfield, Illinois.
Laqueur, G. L., and Matsumoto, H. (1966). *J. Natl. Cancer Inst.* **37**, 217–232.
Lauren, P. (1965). *Acta Pathol. Microbiol. Scand.* **64**, 31–59.
Lea, A. J. (1967). *Ann. R. Coll. Surg. Engl.* **41**, 432–438.
Lemon, F. R., and Walden, R. T. (1966). *J. Am. Med. Assoc.* **198**, 117–126.
Lemon, F. R., Walden, R. T., and Woods, R. W. (1964). *Cancer* **17**, 486–497.
Leren, P. (1970). *Circulation* **42**, 935.
Levin, M. L., Haenszel, W., Carroll, B. J., Gerhardt, P. R., Handy, V. H., and Ingraham, S. C., II. (1960). *J. Natl. Cancer Inst.* **24**, 1243–1257.
Lilienfeld, A. M., Levin, M. L., and Kessler, I. I. (1972). "Cancer in the United States." Harvard Univ. Press, Cambridge, Massachusetts.
Lindberg, B., and Kock, N. G. (1975). *Cancer* **35**, 255–259.
Lingeman, C. H., and Garner, F. M. (1972). *J. Natl. Cancer Inst.* **48**, 325–346.
Lockhart-Mummery, P. (1925). *Lancet* **1**, 427–429.
Lombard, H. L., and Doering, C. R. (1929). *J. Prev. Med.* **3**, 343–361.
Lorenz, E., and Stewart, H. L. (1940). *J. Natl. Cancer Inst.* **1**, 17–39.
Lovett, E. (1976). *Br. J. Surg.* **63**, 13–18.
Lushka, H. (1861). *Pathol. Anat. Physiol. Klin. Med.* **20**, 133.
Lynch, H. T., and Krush, A. J. (1967). *Gastroenterology* **53**, 517–527.
Lynch, H. T., Shaw, M. W., Magnuson, C. W., Larsen, A. L., and Krush, A. J. (1966). *Arch. Intern. Med.* **117**, 206–212.
Lynch, H. T., Guirgis, H., Albert, S., and Brennan, M. (1974). *Cancer* **34**, 2080–2086.
Lyon, J. L., Klauber, M. R., Gardner, J. W., and Smart, C. R. (1976). *N. Engl. J. Med.* **294**, 129–133.
MacAdam, W. A. E., and Goligher, J. C. (1970). *Br. J. Surg.* **57**, 618–631.
McConnell, R. B. (1966). "The Genetics of Gastro-intestinal Disorders," Oxford Med. Publ., Oxford Monogr. Med. Sci. Oxford Univ. Press, London and New York.
McDonald, J. C., McDonald, A. D., Gibbs, G. W., Siemiatycki, J., and Rossiter, C. E. (1971). *Arch. Environ. Health* **22**, 677–686.
MacDougall, I. B. M. (1964). *Lancet* **2**, 655–658.
Macklin, M. T. (1960). *J. Natl. Cancer Inst.* **24**, 551–571.
MacMahon, B. (1960). *Acto Unio Int. Cancrum* **16**, 1716–1724.
MacMahon, B., and Austin, J. H. (1969). *Cancer* **23**, 275–280.
McVay, J. R., Jr. (1964). *Cancer* **17**, 928–937.
Malzberg, B. (1935). *Psychiatr. Q.* **9**, 538–569.
Malzberg, B. (1936). *Psychiatr. Q.* **10**, 127–142.
Mason, T. J., McKay, F. W., Hoover, R., Blot, W. J., and Fraumeni, J. F., Jr. (1975). "Atlas of Cancer Mortality for U.S. Counties: 1950–1969." US Govt. Printing Office, Washington, D.C.
Menzel, D. (1721). *Acta Med. Berl.* **9**, 78.
Merimec, T. J., and Fineberg, S. E. (1973). *Lancet* **2**, 120–122.
Milham, S. (1976). "Occupational Mortality in Washington State, 1950–1971," Vols. 2 and 3.
Miyamoto, M., and Takizawa, S. (1975). *J. Natl. Cancer Inst.* **55**, 1471–1472.
Moertel, C. G. (1966). *Recent Results Cancer Res.* **7**, 1–107.

Moertel, C. G. (1973). *In* "Cancer Medicine" (J. F. Holland and E. Frei, eds.), pp. 1519–1636. Lea & Febiger, Philadelphia, Pennsylvania.

Moertel, C. G., Bargen, J. A., and Dockerty, M. B. (1958). *Gastroenterology* **34**, 85–98.

Moore, W. E. C., and Holdeman, L. V. (1975). *Cancer Res.* **35**, 3418–3420.

Morowitz, D. A., Block, G. E., and Kirsner, J. B. (1968). *Gastroenterology* **55**, 397–402.

Morris, H. P., Wagner, B. P., Ray, F. E., Snell, K. C., and Stewart, H. L. (1961). *Natl. Cancer Inst., Monogr.* **5**, 1–54.

Morson, B. C. (1962). *Dis. Colon Rectum* **5**, 337–341.

Morson, B. C. (1974). *Proc. R. Soc. Med.* **67**, 451–457.

Morson, B. C., and Bussey, H. J. R. (1970). "Current Problems in Surgery," pp. 1–50. Yearbook Publ., Chicago, Illinois.

Morson, B. C., and Tang, L. S. C. (1967). *Gut* **8**, 423–434.

National Board of Health and Welfare. (1971). "Cancer Incidence in Sweden 1959–1965." Cancer Registry, Stockholm.

National Diet-Heart Study Final Report. (1968). *Circulation* **37**.

National Food Survey Committee. (1971). "Household Food Consumption and Expenditure: 1969," Annual report of the National Food Survey Committee. HM Stationery Office, London.

National office of Vital Statistics. (1956). *Vital Stat.–Spec. Rep.* **39**, 303–429.

Neel, J. V. (1954). *Am. J. Hum. Genet.* **6**, 51–60.

Neville, A. M., and Laurence, D. J. R. (1974). *UICC Tech. Rep.* No. 12.

Newill, V. A. (1961). *J. Natl. Cancer Inst.* **26**, 405–417.

New Mexico Tumor Registry. (1975). "Cancer in New Mexico, 1969–72."

Nigro, N. D., Singh, D. V., Campbell, R. L., and Pak, M. S. (1975). *J. Natl. Cancer Inst.* **54**, 439–442.

Norges Offisielle Statistikk. (1962). "Sunnhetstilstanden og Medisinalforholdene: 1937–1961." Statistisk Sentralbyra, Oslo, Norway.

Norwegian Cancer Society. (1959). "Cancer Registration in Norway, 1953–1954."

Norwegian Cancer Society. (1964). "Cancer Registration in Norway, 1959–61."

Norwegian Cancer Society. (1973). "Cancer Registration in Norway, 1969–71."

Onderdonk, A. B., Weinstein, W. M., Sullivan, N. M., Bartlett, J. G., and Gorbach, S. L. (1974). *Infect. Immun.* **10**, 1256–1259.

Painter, N. S., and Burkitt, D. P. (1971). *Br. Med. J.* **2**, 450–454.

Pamukcu, A. M., and Price, J. M. (1969). *J. Natl. Cancer Inst.* **43**, 275–281.

Paymaster, J. C., Sanghvi, L. D., and Gangadharen, P. (1968). *Cancer* **21**, 279–288.

Payne, P. M. (1963). "The South Metropolitan Cancer Registry," Bull. No. 1. Sutton, Surrey, England.

Pearce, M. L., and Dayton, S. (1971). *Lancet* **1**, 464–467.

Peltokallio, P., and Peltokallio, V. (1966). *Dis. Colon Rectum* **9**, 367–370.

Pernu, J. (1960). *Ann. Med. Intern. Fenn.* **49**, 1–117.

Phillips, R. L. (1975). *Cancer Res.* **35**, 3513–3522.

Pierce, E. R. (1968). *Dis. Colon Rectum* **11**, 321–329.

Prager, E. D., Swinton, N. W., Young, J., Veidenheimer, M. C., and Corman, M. N. (1974). *Dis. Colon Rectum* **17**, 322–330.

Puffer, R. R., and Griffith, G. W. (1967). *Sci. Publ., Pan Am. Health Organ.* **151**, 45–132.

Quisenberry, W. B., Bruyere, P. T., and Rogers, M. G. (1966). *Mil. Med.* **131**, 222–233.

Reddy, B. S., and Wynder, E. L. (1973). *J. Natl. Cancer Inst.* **50**, 1437–1442.

Reddy, B. S., Mastromarino, A., and Wynder, E. L. (1975a). *Cancer Res.* **35**, 3403–3406.

Reddy, B. S., Narisawa, T., Maronpot, R., Weisburger, J., and Wynder, E. L. (1975b). *Cancer Res.* **35**, 3421–3426.

Reed, T. E., and Neel, J. V. (1955). *Am. J. Hum. Genet.* **7**, 236–263.

Registrar General of England and Wales. (1956). "Studies on Medical and population Subjects, No. 13, Cancer Statistics for England and Wales, 1901–1955, A Summary of Data Relating to Mortality and Morbidity." HM Stationery Office, London.

Registrar General of England and Wales. (1962). "The Registrar General's Decennial Supplement, England and Wales, 1921, 1931, 1951, 1961, Occupational Mortality Tables." HM Stationery Office, London.

Registrar General of England and Wales. (1966). "Registrar General's Statistical Review of England and Wales for the Year 1965, Part I, Tables, Medical." HM Stationery Office, London.

Registrar General of England and Wales. (1971). "Registrar General's Statistical Review of England and Wales—Supplement on Cancer, 1965, 1966–1967, 1968–1970." HM Stationery Office, London.

Report of a Research Committee to the Medical Research Council. (1968). *Lancet* 2, 693.

Reynoso, G., Chu, T. M., Holyoke, D., Cohen, E., Nemoto, T., Wang, J. J., Chuang, J., Guinan, P., and Murphy, G. P. (1972). *J. Am. Med. Assoc.* 220, 361–365.

Rhoads, G. C., Gulbrandsen, C. L., and Kagan, A. (1976). *N. Engl. J. Med.* 294, 293–298.

Roe, F. J. C., and Grant, G. A. (1970). *Int. J. Cancer* 6, 133–144.

Rokitansky, C. (1839). *Med. Jahrb. K. K. Staates* 29, 88.

Rose, G., Blackburn, H., Keys, A., Taylor, H. L., Kannel, W. B., Paul, O., Reid, D. D., and Stamler, J. (1974). *Lancet* 1, 181.

Roth, S. I., and Helwig, E. B. (1963). *Cancer* 16, 468–479.

Rowlatt, U. F., Franks, L. M., Sheriff, M. U., and Chesterman, F. C. (1969). *J. Natl. Cancer Inst.* 43, 1353–1364.

Salas, J. C., and Miranda, M. G. (1974). *Acta Med. Costarric.* 17, 137–146.

Sato, E. (1974). *Gann* 65, 295–306.

Sato, E., Ouchi, A., Sasano, N., and Ishidate, T. (1976). *Cancer* 37, 1316–1321.

Schoenberg, B. S., Greenberg, R. A., and Eisenberg, H. (1969). *J. Natl. Cancer Inst.* 43, 15–32.

Schoental, R. (1965). *Nature (London)* 208, 300.

Schottenfeld, D., and Berg, J. (1971). *J. Natl. Cancer Inst.* 46, 161–170.

Schottenfeld, D., Berg, J. W., and Vitsky, B. (1969). *J. Natl. Cancer Inst.* 43, 77–86.

Schwartz, D., Flamant, R., and Lellough, J. (1961). *J. Natl. Cancer Inst.* 26, 1085–1108.

Schwartz, M. K. (1975). *Cancer Res.* 35, 3481–3487.

Segall, A. J. (1965). *Pap., 93rd Annu. Meet. Am. Public Health Assoc. 1965.*

Segi, M. (1960). "Cancer Mortality for Selected Sites in 24 Countries (1950–1957)." Tohoku Univ. School of Medicine, Sendai, Japan.

Segi, M., and Kurihara, M. (1963). "Trends in Cancer Mortality for Selected Sites in 24 Countries, 1950–1959." Dept. of Pbulic Health, Sendai, Japan.

Segi, M., and Kurihara, M. (1972). "Cancer Mortality for Selected Sites in 24 Countries, No. 6 (1966–1967)." Japan Cancer Society, Tokyo.

Segi, M., Fujisaku, S., Kurihara, M., Narai, Y., and Sasajima, K. (1960). *Tohoku J. Exp. Med.* 72, 91–103.

Segi, M., Kurihara, M., and Matsuyama, T. (1965). "Cancer Mortality in Japan (1899–1962)." Dept. of Public Health, Tohoku Univ. School of Medicine, Sendai, Japan.

Seidman, H. (1970). *Environ. Res* 3, 234–250.

Seidman, H. (1971). *Environ. Res.* 4, 390–429.

Selikoff, I. J., Hammond, E. C., and Seidman, H. (1973). *IARC Sci. Publ.* 8, 209–216.

Shamberger, R. J., and Frost, D. V. (1969). *Can. Med. Assoc. J.* 100, 682.

Sheps, M. C. (1961). *Am. J. Public Health* 51, 547–555.

Shivata, H. R., and Phillips, M. J. (1970). *Can. Med. Assoc. J.* 103, 285–287.

Shurtleff, D. (1956). *J. Am. Geriatr. Soc.* 4, 654–666.

140   P. CORREA AND W. HAENSZEL

Silverberg, S. G. (1970). *Surg., Gynecol. Obstet.* **131,** 103–114.
Smith, R. L. (1956a). *J. Natl. Cancer Inst.* **17,** 459–473.
Smith, R. L. (1956b). *J. Natl. Cancer Inst.* **17,** 667–676.
Smith, R. L. (1957). *J. Natl. Cancer Inst.* **18,** 385–396.
Sommers, S. C. (1964). *Dis. Colon Rectum* **7,** 262–269.
Spjut, H. J., and Spratt, J. S. (1965). *Ann. Surg.* **161,** 309–324.
Spratt, J. S., Ackerman, L. V., and Moyer, C. A. (1958). *Ann. Surg.* **148,** 682–698.
Staszewski, J. (1976). "Epidemiology of Cancer of Selected Sites in Poland and Polish Migrants." Ballinger, Cambridge, Massachusetts.
Staszewski, J., and Haenszel, W. M. (1965). *J. Natl. Cancer Inst.* **35,** 291–297.
Staszewski, J., McCall, M. G., and Stenhouse, N. S. (1971). *Br. J. Cancer* **25,** 599–610.
Steiner, P. E. (1954). "Cancer: Race and Geography." Williams & Wilkins, Baltimore, Maryland.
Stemmermann, G. N. (1966). *Cancer* **19,** 1567–1572.
Stemmermann, G. N., and Yatani, R. (1973). *Cancer* **31,** 1260–1270.
Stocks, P. (1957). *Cancer Res. Campaign, Annu. Rep.* **35,** Suppl. II.
Teppo, L., Hakama, M., Hakulinen, T., Lehtonen, M., and Saxén, E. (1975). "Cancer in Finland 1953–1970: Incidence, Mortality, Prevalence." Munksgaard, Copenhagen.
Thompson, D. M. P., Krupey, J., Freedman, S. O., and Gold, P. (1969). *Proc. Natl. Acad. Sci. U.S.A.* **64,** 161–167.
Turcot, J., Després, J. P., and St. Pierre, F. (1959). *Dis. Colon Rectum* **2,** 465–468.
Turpeninen, O., Miettinen, M., Kravonen, M. J., Roine, P., Pekkarinen, M., Lehtosuo, E. J., and Alivirta, P. (1968). *Am. J. Clin. Nutr.* **21,** 255–276.
Universitetsforlaget. (1972). "Trends in Cancer Incidence in Norway, 1955–1967." Moltzau, Oslo.
Utsonomiya, J., and Nakamura, T. (1974). *Br. J. Surg.* **62,** 45–51.
Veale, A. M. O. (1965). "Intestinal Polyposis," Eugen. Lab. Ser. 50. Cambridge Univ. Press, London and New York.
Veale, A. M. O., McCall, I., Bussey, H. J. R., and Morson, B. C. (1966). *J. Med. Genet.* **3,** 5–16.
Vogel, F., and Krüger, J. (1968). *Blut* **16,** 351–376.
Wagner, J. (1832). *Med. Jahrb. K. K. Staates* **11,** 274.
Ward, J. M. (1974). *Lab. Invest.* **30,** 505–513.
Ward, J. M. (1975). *Cancer Res.* **35,** 1938–1943.
Ward, J. M., Yamamoto, R. S., and Brown, C. A. (1973a). *J. Natl. Cancer Inst.* **51,** 1029–1039.
Ward, J. M., Yamamoto, R. S., and Weisburger, J. H. (1973b). *J. Natl. Cancer Inst.* **51,** 713–715.
Waterhouse, J., Muir, C., Correa, P., and Powell, J., eds. (1976). "Cancer Incidence in Five Continents," Vol. III. Int. Union Against Cancer, Berlin and New York.
Weinstein, W. M., Onderdonk, A. B., Bartlett, J. G., and Gorback, S. L. (1974). *Infect. Immun.* **10,** 1250–1255.
Williams, A. O., Chung, E. B., Agbata, A., and Jackson, M. A. (1975). *Br. J. Cancer* **31,** 485–491.
Williams, R. D., and Fish, J. L. (1966). *Am. J. Surg.* **112,** 846–849.
Winawer, S. J. (1975). *Natl. Large Bowel Cancer Proj. Newsl.* **3,** 7–9.
Woolf, C. M. (1958). *Am. J. Hum. Genet.* **10,** 42–47.
World Health Organization. (1972–1975). "World Health Statistics Annual 1968–1971." World Health Organ., Geneva.
World Health Organization. (1973). "World Health Statistics Report," Vol. 26. World Health Organ., Geneva.

Wynder, E. L. (1975). *Cancer Res.* **35**, 3388–3394.

Wynder, E. L., and Reddy, B. S. (1973). *J. Natl. Cancer Inst.* **50**, 1099–1106.

Wynder, E. L., and Shigematsu, T. (1967). *Cancer* **20**, 1520–1561.

Wynder, E. L., Bross, I. J., and Hirayama, T. (1960). *Cancer* **13**, 559–601.

Wynder, E. L., Hyams, L., and Shigematsu, T. (1967). *Cancer* **20**, 113–126.

Wynder, E. L., Kajitani, T., Ishakawa, S., Dodo, H., and Takano, A. (1969). *Cancer* **23**, 1210–1220.

Young, J. L., Jr., Devesa, S. S., and Cutler, S. J. (1975). *Cancer Res.* **35**, 3523–3536.

INTERACTION BETWEEN VIRAL AND GENETIC FACTORS IN MURINE MAMMARY CANCER

J. Hilgers and P. Bentvelzen

The Netherlands Cancer Institute, Amsterdam, and Radiobiological Institute TNO, Rijswijk, The Netherlands

I. Introduction

Genetic aspects of cancer are concerned with (1) the genetic or epigenetic change underlying the neoplastic conversion of a cell, (2) genetic susceptibility of the host to carcinogenic influences, or (3) cancer as a hereditary disease.

The latter concept originated from the familiar occurrence of various types of neoplasms in various animals; it has also been observed in the case of mammary cancer in man (Mühlbock, 1972; Heston, 1976). Early in this century, the familiar occurrence of mammary cancer was reported for mice (for review, see Heston and Vlahakis, 1967). The notion of genetic influences on the origin of the disease became even more apparent with the development of inbred mouse strains with great differences in mammary cancer incidence.

However, a highly significant difference in mammary tumor incidence was observed in reciprocal crosses between high- and low-cancer strains, indicating an extrachromosomal influence in the genesis of this disease (Jackson Laboratory Staff, 1933; Korteweg, 1934, 1935a). Bittner (1936a) demonstrated this extrachromosomal factor to be transmitted via the mother's milk. It soon became established that the factor was a virus that could be transmitted by means of cell-free extracts (Bryan *et al.*, 1942; Visscher *et al.*, 1942).

A similar development has occurred in the case of murine leukemia, where the finding of a virus by Gross (1951) was preceded by the development of high- and low-leukemia mouse strains and where the prevailing thought for a decade had been that genetic factors controlled the development of leukemia (Cole and Furth, 1941; MacDowell *et al.*, 1945).

While in the 1950s and 1960s the area of leukemia research was dominated by the viral concept, the genetic aspects have never been ignored in the murine mammary tumor area. In the early 1940s, Bittner (1940) and Andervont (1940) observed great differences between low-cancer mouse strains in susceptibility to the so-called milk factor introduced by foster-nursing on high-cancer strain females. The genetic nature of this resistance was clearly demonstrated by Heston *et al.* (1945).

It was found that, in several mouse strains that do not harbor the so-called milk factor, mammary tumors could be induced in relatively high incidence after appropriate hormone stimulation (Andervont and Dunn, 1948a; Heston *et al.*, 1950; Mühlbock and van Rijssel, 1954). However, viruslike particles that had the same morphology as particles thought to be milk agent were found in mammary tumors of some of these strains. This has led to considerable controversy between adherents of a viral etiology of these lesions (Dmochowski and Grey, 1957), and those who assume that these tumors develop owing to a combination of genetic and hormonal factors only (Heston, 1958). However, as early as 1948, Shabad (cited by Andervont, 1952) considered the possibility of an endogenous mammary tumor agent and that inbreeding through many generations might have promoted the concentration of this virus in certain lines of mice.

On the basis of studies on bacterium–phage interactions, Luria (1958) suggested that gene control and virus control over cellular functions are two aspects of the same genetic mechanism: "This concept removes any a priori incompatibility between a viral and a genetic theory of cancer etiology. It reduces the interpretation of virus-induced cancer to that of the control of cellular development and differentiation by genetic elements capable, either intrinsically or by association with other specialized genetic units, of assuming an infectively transmissible form."

Although research on viruslike particles in mammary tumors of the C3Hf mouse strain indicated the possibility of an endogenous virus, the real breakthrough came with the discovery by Mühlbock (1965) of very efficient male transmission of a virulent mammary tumor virus in the European mouse strain GR. Mendelian analysis of this phenomenon (Bentvelzen, 1968a) led to the hypothesis of genetic transmission of that virus in the GR strain.

Molecular hybridization studies have substantiated the view that every mouse carries genetic information for at least a part of a mammary tumor virus in its normal cellular DNA (Varmus et al., 1972, 1975; Scolnick et al., 1974).

The biology of the mammary tumor virus has been amply reviewed by, among others, Dmochowski (1953a), Blair (1968), Hageman et al. (1972), Bentvelzen (1972b, 1974a,b), and Nandi and McGrath (1973). The present review will focus on the genetics of susceptibility to mammary tumorigenesis under the influence of exogenous virus infections on the one hand, and of genetic control of release of endogenous viruses and subsequent tumorigenesis on the other. Some attention will also be given to those instances in which mammary tumors occur without clear demonstration of virus expression.

II. Transmission of MTV

The discovery of an extrachromosomal influence in murine mammary cancer and its subsequent designation as a milk factor has been narrated in extenso in various reviews (Dmochowski, 1953a; Blair, 1968; Nandi and McGrath, 1973). It is a curious note that this milk factor was the first virus to be universally accepted as a tumor virus and was discovered by the use of genetic techniques (Heston, 1972).

Although milk-borne transmission seems to be the most important route, other modes of transmission of this virus should not be neglected. A distinction must be made between horizontal and vertical transmission. In the first case, virus can be transmitted from one individual to another irrespective of relationship. Vertical transmission implies transfer from parents to offspring. Vertical transmission can be subdivided into chromosomal and extrachromosomal modes.

Special attention will be given to extrachromosomal male transmission, because of its historical relevance to the development of the concept of genetic or chromosomal transmission not only of MTV, but also of other RNA tumor viruses.

A. TRANSPLACENTAL TRANSMISSION

The general opinion is that the only route of nonchromosomal transmission in the female is via the mother's milk. This is based upon the observations that transfer of fertilized eggs from oviducts of high-cancer strain females into the uteri of pseudo-pregnant low-cancer strain females causes a significant decrease in mammary cancer incidence and a significant increase in the average age at which tumors develop (Boot and Mühlbock, 1956; Deringer, 1959, 1962). A noteworthy exception is the GR mouse strain (Zeilmaker, 1969). As no significant difference in tumor incidence was noted between lines derived from ova transfer or by cesarean section, it was concluded that no intrauterine transfer of the virus takes place. However, Fekete and Little (1942) found no mammary tumors in a DBA subline produced by transfer of ova into C57BL, while DBAf sublines produced by foster-nursing have a tumor incidence of 10% and 23%, respectively (Van Gulik and Korteweg, 1940; Murray, 1941b). This difference is even more remarkable when one considers that the mice in the experiments of Fekete and Little (1942) were breeders and the DBAf animals were virgins. Since biologically active virus can be demonstrated in placentas of high-cancer strain females (Mühlbock et al., 1952), it might be expected that placental transfer of the virus to the embryo could take place. No virus has been retrieved from embryos, but this can be due to limited sites of replication.

As far as we know, Fekete and Little (1942) and Zeilmaker (1969) were the only ones to have done the reciprocal experiment: transfer of low-cancer strain ova into high-cancer strain females. Fekete and Little (1942) observed that C57BL after transfer to DBA produced 50% mammary tumors in breeding females and 73% in a subsequent generation. They compared this with an approximate 10% tumor incidence in C57BL foster-nursed by DBA (Van Gulik and Korteweg, 1940; Murray, 1941b), but this is not warranted, as the latter observed only virgins. However, Mühlbock (1956) found a 2% tumor incidence in C57BL females foster-nursed on DBA. This would suggest a transplacental transfer of virus in the experiments by Fekete and Little (1942). Mühlbock and Dux (1972) reported a 52% tumor incidence in C57BLfDBA. This can be due to mutations in the virus or in the host (see Section III).

Zeilmaker (1969) observed no effect of transfer of (020×DBAf) F1 ova into GR females. The number of experimental animals was rather small, however, and he did not use the most susceptible genotype for the GR virus.

In our opinion, it cannot yet be excluded that transplacental transmission of MTV takes place, but, if so, then with low efficiency. Further studies seem to be necessary.

B. Extrachromosomal Male Transmission

In the crosses between C57BL and A mouse strains, Bittner (1942a) found no male influence on the development of mammary tumors in hybrid mice. However, he (1943) observed a higher incidence in the offspring of the mating ♀ C3Hf× ♂ C3H than in the ♀ C3Hf × ♂ C3Hf. Litter analysis of the progeny from the cross with the virus-carrying males revealed that the cancerous mice originated from the same litter. The cancerous litter always appeared after those in which no tumors developed. Strong (1943) obtained a 71% tumor incidence in the offspring of low-cancer strain females JK and high-cancer strain C3H males. In later studies by Bittner (1956, 1957), it became evident that this surprisingly high incidence must be due to transmission of MTV by the male parent. The first to realize that occasional male transmission might take place was Andervont (1945b).

An appreciable tumor incidence was found in crosses between low-cancer strain BALB/c females and agent-free C3Hf males, but the tumors appeared at a relatively late stage of 22–24 months of age. When BALB/c females were mated to virus-carrying C3H males, comparable tumor incidences were found, but some tumors appeared at a very young age of 6–10 months. The presence of the virus was confirmed by transfer of the agent by means of implantation of pieces of spleens into susceptible test mice, which developed mammary tumors before one year of age (Andervont and Dunn, 1953).

Foulds (1949) noticed that F_1 hybrids of C57BL females and high-cancer strain RIII males were heterogeneous: a minority, concentrated in certain litters, develop mammary tumors, carry the mammary tumor agent and transmit it to their offspring, which develop a high incidence of tumors. Since the incidence in F_1 hybrids produced by C57BL females and RIII males is reduced and delayed, the occasional early appearance in the aforementioned experiment has been attributed to the "erratic" transmission by the male parent.

Dmochowski (1953b) observed, however, that, in most families derived from the mating ♀ C57BL × ♂ RIII, many tumors developed after successive generations of inbreeding. Several tumors occurred at a young age. He claimed that many of these tumors contained the mammary tumor agent (milk factor) as revealed by bioassay of cell-free extracts in (C57BL × A) F_1 hybrid females. Biancifori et al. (1958) also noticed an increase in tumor incidence proportional to the number of generations of submating in one family derived from the cross ♀ C3Hf × ♂ BALB/cfC3H. In contrast to the F_1 generation, tumors in the later generations appeared at an extremely early age. Dmochowski (1953b) postulated that male transmission of the MTV occurs in all cases but that the quantity of virus is so small that only few tumors will appear in the early generations. During further inbreeding, the amount of virus slowly increases until sufficient virus has accumulated for the production of tumors.

Of importance in this respect is the finding of Andervont (1950) that several BALB/c mice infected with the mammary tumor virus did not develop mammary tumors, but could transmit the agent to the offspring, which developed the disease.

In two clear-cut instances of male transmission, Mühlbock (1952) found that this was associated with infection of the female and thereby her offspring. He did not obtain an indication for infection of the young *in utero* by sperm. Bittner (1952a, 1957) studied the transfer of MTV by so-called Z males (C3H/Bi), utilizing bioassays of cell-free tumor extracts as proof for the presence of virus. An important aspect of Bittner's work was the relatively high efficiency of male transmission in this system. In our opinion, this is due to the great susceptibility of the BALB/c strain on the one hand and tremendous virus production by the Z males on the other. Comparable differences in males with regard to efficiency of transmission were found by Severi *et al.* (1958) when C3H and BALB/cfC3H males were mated to CBA females. From Bittner's extensive studies in 1957 it becomes apparent that male transmission must be due to infection of the female, which then transfers the virus to the offspring and, furthermore, that this infection occurs only after repeated matings.

However, Dmochowski (1956) reported that, after the first mating of C57BL females with high-cancer strain RIII males, virus can be recovered from the mammary glands of the low-strain females.

Murray and Little (1967) detected male transmission in crosses between MA females and C3H males: 26% tumors were found at 17 months average age, and in the cross (MA × C3Hf)F_1, 17% tumors occurred at 27 months of age. This remarkable difference in average latency period can be due only to the induction of early tumors by male-transmitted exogenous MTV. Such a difference was not detected when C57BL females were mated to either C3H or C3Hf males. It is more than coincidental that Foulds (1949) and Dmochowski (1953b) found in crosses between C57BL females and RIII males that transmission of exogenous virus repeatedly occurs. Moore *et al.* (1974)

have shown that the C57BL strain is highly resistant to graded dilutions of C3H MTV, but quite susceptible to that from the RIII strain.

Peacock (1953) found that, when C3H males were kept with CBA females, 11 out of 82 hybrid offspring females developed mammary tumors, while 2 out of 82 contracted the disease when the C3H male was removed as soon as the CBA female was found to be pregnant. He suggested that oral contamination of the susceptible hybrid newborns with virus in the seminal fluid might occur during or soon after copulation that takes place within 24 hours of birth. Severi et al. (1958) obtained results in similar crosses which do not completely exclude such a postnatal paternal factor of mammary carcinogenesis in the hybrids. However, feeding of seminal fluid or testes from C3H mice to RIII females did not lead to an increase in tumors (Peacock, 1956).

Andervont obtained definite proof for in utero or "direct" infection of the offspring by the male. In one family, 2 (BALB/c × C3H) F_1 hybrids carried the virus and transferred that to their offspring, whereas one littermate and her descendants were virus-free. There was no evidence for infection of the BALB/c mother. As the pregnant females were removed from the male, cage transmission of the virus can be excluded. In retrospect on the basis of these findings, Andervont (1963) detected indications for in utero infection in his earlier studies (Andervont, 1945b; Andervont and Dunn, 1948b, 1953). Nevertheless, the "indirect" infection of offspring by the male via milk of the mother seems the most efficient.

Organ distribution studies of the virus demonstrated that it was present in two different secondary male genital organs: (1) the seminal vesicle as shown by bioassay (Andervont and Dunn, 1948b) and electron microscopy (Smith, 1966); and (2) the epididymis as demonstrated by bioassay (Mühlbock, 1950a) and electron microscopy (Smith, 1966; Bucciarelli et al., 1970). In recent quantitative immunological studies utilizing an immunofluorescence assay and a radioimmunoassay, Souissi et al. (1974) demonstrated MTV antigens to be present in the epididymis and the coagulating gland (see Fig. 1), but to be absent from the testis. The GR mouse strain proved to be an exceptionally highly positive strain with a content of antigen increasing from less than 100 ng at 2 months of age to over 10,000 ng per milliliter of tissue extract at 8 months of age or older. Other high-mammary cancer strain males were only occasionally positive in these tests.

It must be noted here that the virus is also expressed at an extremely early age (2 weeks) in mammary glands of the female mice of this strain (Shannon et al., 1974).

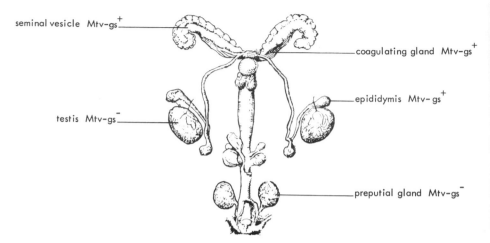

seminal vesicle Mtv-gs$^+$

coagulating gland Mtv-gs$^+$

epididymis Mtv-gs$^+$

testis Mtv-gs$^-$

preputial gland Mtv-gs$^-$

FIG. 1. Male genital tract of the mouse and mammary tumor virus antigen expression.

Bentvelzen (1968a) found that an occasional 020 female can become infected after repeated mating with GR males. Nandi and Helmich (1974) mentioned infection of BALB/c females after caging with GR males. R. Van Nie (unpublished results) noticed that BALB/c females become positive for MTV antigens in their milk when caged together with GR males, even when the relatively insensitive immunodiffusion test is used.

Bittner and Frantz (1954) found that vasectomized Z males, and Bentvelzen (1968a) that vasectomized GR males, could transmit the virus to females. This indicates that it is not the spermatozoa but the seminal fluid which harbors infectious virus. Females could also be infected when their uterine horns were removed leaving the ovaries intact. Therefore, the uterus does not seem to be necessary for male transmission. Smith (1966) found virus to be taken up by leukocytes present in the uterus of low-cancer strain females after mating to infected males. The leukocytes probably play a role in the further distribution of the virus in the female mouse, leading to infection of the mammary gland.

C. Horizontal Transmission

The transmission from one individual to another irrespective of relationship is a controversial issue at the moment in the case of the mouse mammary tumor virus.

Lathrop and Loeb (1913) placed mice from low-mammary cancer

families in cages with mice from mammary cancer stocks but found no indication for the infectivity of this malignancy.

Andervont *et al.* (1942) failed to obtain evidence that the virus is transmitted by bodily contact. Mühlbock (1950b) did not find virus in the urine or feces of tumor-bearing animals, although Squartini and Biancifori (1958) reported that the kidneys and urine contained virus as measured by bioassay a few days after infection. Peacock (1963) was unable to infect susceptible newborn mice by prolonged exposure to excreta of infected male mice.

Convincing evidence for horizontal transmission by means of arthropods has been presented by Pogossiantz (1956). Mouse or rat fleas which were first fed on high-cancer strain mice could transmit the virus to low-cancer strain females. The virus was probably present in a biologically active form in blood cells (Woolley *et al.*, 1941; Bittner, 1945).

Recently, Blair and Lane (1974a) and Blair *et al.* (1974) have reported that spleen cells from BALB/c females of over 14 weeks of age were consistently reactive against cultured primary syngeneic mammary tumor cells of the BALB/cfC3H subline in a microcytotoxicity assay. Blair and Lane (1975) reported that, in contrast to the cytotoxicity of BALB/cfC3H spleen cells, that of BALB/c cells could not be abrogated by incubation of tumor cells with BALB/cfC3H serum, suggesting a qualitatively different response. It did not prove to be dependent on T cells (Lane *et al.*, 1975). In a subsequent study, Blair and Lane (1974b) found that one 22-week-old BALB/c mouse reared in isolation did not show such immunological reactivity, while one colony-raised animal of the same age showed the same cytotoxicity as one female who had been caged with an infected female for 4 weeks. Since only one animal was used in each experimental group, we regard it highly premature to interpret these data as being indicative for horizontal transmission, especially outside of cages.

Lopez *et al.* (1976) claim that animals of a spatially isolated BALB/c colony display cellular immunity to a MTV-specific-antigen at a certain age. Their interpretation is that this is due to a (partial) switching on of endogenous BALB/c virus.

O. Stutman (personal communication) noticed that low-cancer strain female mice of a C3Hf subline caged with C3H females develop an appreciably higher mammary tumor incidence than controls kept in the same room. This strongly suggests that horizontal transmission may occur with low efficiency within the cage but not from cage to cage as suggested by Blair and Lane (1974b). A possible mode of transmission may be the saliva, since MTV particles are produced in the salivary gland of wild mice (Rongey *et al.*, 1975). Such particles have also been found in the salivary gland of several inbred mouse strains (F. De Groot and P. Bentvelzen, unpublished results).

D. DE NOVO APPEARANCE OF VIRULENT MTV

Bittner found in a foster-nursed A subline that the offspring of one female of the 8th generation produced many mammary tumors at early age, while only 0.3% mammary tumors were found in the other animals of that Af subline. The female harboring the virulent MTV developed a mammary tumor at 8 months of age. The few animals with late tumors proved to be virus-free.

Bittner (1956) demonstrated that a mammary tumor appearing in the 17th generation of the fostered Z(C3H/Bi) subline harbored a biologically active MTV.

Rudali *et al.* (1956) developed the high-cancer strain NLC from the mouse strain XVII in which mammary tumors are exceptional. The founder female of this new strain developed a virus-positive mammary tumor at relatively early age. By foster-nursing, it became established that the virus was exogenous.

In most laboratories, the CBA strain proves to be a low-mammary cancer strain (see Miller and Pybus, 1944). However, Gardner (1941) reported a 70% tumor incidence in forced-bred CBA females from his colony. Reciprocal crosses between his CBA line with the C57BL strain indicated the presence of an extrachromosomal factor. In a later paper, Gardner *et al.* (1959) report that, during the first two decades of inbreeding (done by L. C. Strong), the CBA was a low-tumor strain. However, mammary tumors began to appear in Gardner's colony, in 1935, and, in the 1950s, the CBA was a high-cancer strain in both Strong's and Gardner laboratories. According to Gardner, this alteration could be due to spontaneous acquisition of MTV. He mentioned that this interpretation must presuppose an original loss of the milk factor or fluctuation above and below effective levels, since the CBA and C3H are related on the maternal side with ancestors that develop mammary tumors. It is possible that the CBA sublines of Gardner and Strong picked up the virus by means of horizontal transmission and have transmitted it vertically since then to many generations. Mühlbock (1956) found, however, that the C3H milk factor is poorly replicated in his CBA subline. The virus disappears after a few generations of sib-mating. Therefore, if horizontal transmission were responsible for the change of the CBA into a high-cancer strain, genetic mutations of the host must have played an important additional role.

Müller and Zotter (1973) reported that their CBA/B1n subline carries a moderately oncogenic mammary tumor virus that can be completely eliminated by foster-nursing on low-cancer strain females. This indicates that this CBA subline carries an MTV that seems to be different from the C3H virus, since it has been vertically transmitted for many generations. It does not seem to be an endogenous virus.

Dmochowski (1956) claims the transformation of a C57BL and an RIIIf subline into high-cancer strains and bioassays was suggestive of the presence of a virus. Dmochowski himself, however, has considered the possibility of contamination, although he regarded this as highly unlikely. The alternative possibility that the virus could have arisen endogenously by some "accidental change in a normal cell component" was said to be well within the realm of speculation. With our present insight into endogenous mammary tumor viruses we no longer regard the latter possibility as so unlikely. This concept would explain the existence of many mouse strains of diverse genetic origin (C3H, DBA, A as some of the well-known American strains and WLL, LTS, RIII, DD, GR as some of the European strains) harboring the milk factor.

TABLE I

DISCOVERIES OF THE VARIOUS MODES OF TRANSMISSION OF MAMMARY
TUMOR VIRUS

Mode of transmission	Discovered by[a]
Extrachromosomal vertical	Jackson Laboratory staff (1933), Korteweg (1934)
a. Milk	Bittner (1936a), Andervont and McEleney (1938), Van Gulik and Korteweg (1940)
b. Transplacental[b]	Fekete and Little (1942)
c. Male (indirect) via infection of the mother	Andervont (1945b), Foulds (1949), Mühlbock (1952), Bittner (1952b)
d. Male (direct) *in utero*	Andervont (1963)
e. Male (direct) postnatally[b]	Peacock (1953)
Chromosomal vertical	
a. Male	Bentvelzen (1968a), Mühlbock and Bentvelzen (1968)
b. Female	Zeilmaker (1969)
Horizontal	
a. Arthropod-borne[b]	Pogossiantz (1956)
b. Cage[b]	O. Stutman (personal comm., 1975)

[a] For full reference see list at end of chapter.
[b] Not confirmed.

In one subline of the AKR strain, a moderate incidence of leukemia was noted and numerous B-type particles were found in the milk (Dmochowski *et al.*, 1968). Unfortunately, selection has been practiced against mammary tumors and in favor of the return of the high leukemia incidence characteristic of the AKR strain. Otherwise, an interesting genetic study could have been done on the *de novo* appearance of MTV and its interaction with endogenous murine leukemia virus (Dmochowski, 1971).

Fieldsteel *et al.* (1975) reported an unusually high incidence of spontaneous mammary carcinoma in their presumed MTV-free BALB/c colony. These tumors contained B-type particles. Since the foundation stock had been kept in separate quarters, horizontal transmission seems to be unlikely. This finding suggests that a virulent MTV has arisen *de novo* in this BALB/c subline.

In conclusion, the *de novo* appearance of virulent MTV in several low mammary cancer mouse strains may be explained by horizontal transmission, but also by accidental activation of an endogenous virus.

Table I shows the possible modes of MTV transmission and their discoverers. It does not seem to be superfluous to emphasize the complexity of problems concerning the natural history of MTV and other members of the oncornavirus group as is evident from the various possible modes of transmission.

III. Genetics of Susceptibility to Exogenous MTV

The great variation in mammary tumor incidence among several inbred mouse strains was originally attributed to genetically controlled differences in susceptibility to the disease. However, the discovery of the milk factor led to the opinion that chromosomal factors were immaterial in this respect (Murray and Little, 1935, 1936, 1939). Only Korteweg (1935b, 1936a,b) at that time realized that chromosomal factors in combination with the extrachromosomal factor determined the risk for the development of a tumor. In addition, he recognized that, even in the absence of the extrachromosomal factor, some tumors could develop, depending on a suitable genetic constitution.

An indication for the existence of an important genetic resistance to the milk factor becomes apparent from the work of Bittner (1940) in which he found that the C57BL strain could not be transformed into a high-cancer strain by foster-nursing on the high cancer strain A. Using four different low-cancer strains, Andervont (1940) noted a great variation in response to the milk factor of high cancer strain C3H: C57BL

6%, Y 14%, I 17%, and BALB/c 64%. A highly interesting finding, to be discussed in detail later, was that the hybrid of the two resistant strains C57BL and I were very susceptible to the C3H virus. The so-called "inherited susceptibility to MTV" was further demonstrated by a series of crosses between high- and low-cancer strains (Bittner, 1944a,b; Heston *et al.*, 1945).

A. RELATIONSHIP BETWEEN RESISTANCE TO AND REPLICATION OF MTV

Andervont (1945a) reported on the fate of C3H milk-borne virus in the initially low cancer strains BALB/c and C57BL. With two important exceptions, all BALB/c mice infected with the agent transmit the virus to the offspring, which in turn can transfer it to subsequent generations. It is noteworthy that the BALB/c strain can be transformed into a permanent high cancer strain. Andervont's original BALB/cfC3H subline has remained a high mammary cancer strain up to the present time. In contrast, the C57BL strain loses the agent within a few generations after foster-nursing. It is attractive to assume that resistance of the C57BL to tumor development in the presence of the milk factor is associated with poor replication of the virus. Similar observations were reported by Mühlbock (1952) and Bentvelzen (1968b), who did a semiquantitative study on the amount of virus present in C57BLfC3H by foster-nursing susceptible hybrid mice for various periods ranging from 1 day to 3 weeks.

Bittner (1952a,b) mated three I mice foster-nursed by C3H with virus-free C3Hf males. The incidences in the F_1 offspring were 10%, 25%, and 83%, respectively, indicating erratic transmission of the virus by the I females. Second-generation females of fostered I stock were unable to transmit the virus to their otherwise susceptible hybrid offspring. Andervont (1964) compared the transmission of the C3H virus in the C57BL and I strains. The virus disappeared most rapidly in the latter strain. In this case, resistance to MTV also parallels the poor replication of the virus.

The 020 and CBA strains are moderately susceptible to the milk factor derived from the DBA and C3H strains, respectively (Mühlbock, 1956). In both strains, the virus disappears rapidly within a few generations of sib-mating. In the same study, females of the IF strain proved to be susceptible to the C3H strain virus and to be able to transmit the virus for at least six generations.

When C3H newborn mice were kept for only 40 hours or less with their mother and then transferred to C57BL foster mothers, mammary tumor development ceased to occur after five generations of sib-mating on repeating this procedure. The same foster-nursing regimen had no effect in the case of the BALB/cfC3H. These results were interpreted as the gradual disappearance of the virus from the C3H strain (Andervont, 1949). It is now established that the C3Hf strain is relatively resistant to the C3H virus as compared to BALB/c (Bentvel-zen and Daams, 1969; Bentvelzen et al., 1970). This conclusion was made after end-point titrations of purfied C3H MTV preparations with regard to tumor induction after inoculation into 4-week-old mice.

Only a few studies have been made on the genetic control of propa-gation of exogenous mammary tumor virus (Heston et al., 1945, 1956, 1960). From a series of backcrosses of (C3H × C57BL)F_1 to C57BL in which a rapid disappearance of the virus was noted, the conclusion can be drawn that a small number of genes are concerned with the replica-tion of the virus (for a detailed review, see Bentvelzen, 1972b).

All available data strongly suggest that genetic resistance to mam-mary tumorigenesis under the influence of exogenous virus is, at least in part, due to interference with the replication of the virus. Since interference with replication has been deduced from transmission studies, the intracellular events of the replication cycle in the mam-mary gland must be studied in more detail, e.g., by comparing levels of virus (viral antigens or viral RNA) in mammary gland cells of C3H compared to C57BL/fC3H and BALB/cfC3H.

Mammary tumors arising in sublines derived from high-cancer strain mice by means of foster-nursing on low-cancer strain females harbor an endogenous low oncogenic virus which has the same morphology as the exogenous milk factor. This is also true for artifi-cially established RIII strain sublines (Charney and Moore, 1972). However, in late-appearing mammary tumors in hybrids of "virus-free" BALB/c mice with the RIII line which has lost its milk factor, no B particles can be found by electron microscopy (Smith et al., 1970). Tumors arising in the hybrids of BALB/c and C3Hf produce such parti-cles abundantly. It seems to us that the genetic mutation which caused the loss of exogenous virus in RIII also inhibits the expression of the endogenous low oncogenic virus in this line.

B. Disappearance of MTV from High Mammary Cancer Strains

As mentioned above, the offspring of certain females of low-cancer strains bearing an early mammary tumor can develop a high incidence of mammary cancer. This can be attributed to either horizontal transmission or, more likely, *de novo* appearance of a virulent MTV. The opposite phenomenon has also been observed in quite a few high-cancer strains.

Burrows (1941) reported on the mammary tumor incidence of five sublines of the DBA strain, one of which had a low mammary cancer incidence. The founding mother of this so-called E subline lived 698 days and did not have a mammary tumor. A mammary cancer appeared in two of her daughters, but the incidence over 10 generations of her offspring was 10%. It could be excluded that this loss in susceptibility to mammary carcinogenesis was due to accidental crossing with a mouse of a low-cancer strain for no aberrations in coat color were observed; this certainly would have been seen, since the DBA strain carries three recessive coat color genes. Murray and Warner (1947) reported that 50 generations of descendants from a female of the 37th inbred generation of the MA strain did not develop mammary tumors. This progeny consisted of 351 breeding females. Sisters of that particular female produced offspring which developed tumors for several generations. The authors speculated that either a mutation had occurred in that female, which made her unreceptive to the virus, or a change in physiology had caused propagation of the virus with varying degrees of potency. Detailed analysis of pedigree charts of the MA strain from its 21st generation of sib-mating indicated great irregularity in the vertical transmission of the virus in this mouse strain, although not as clear-cut as the case mentioned above. Retrospective analysis of studies by Warner *et al.* (1945), in which several MA females were mated with A strain males, indicated that 9 females were derived from a high-cancer line of the MA strain and induced a high incidence of tumors in the F_1 hybrids, 9 came from an intermediate susceptible line giving rise to a moderate incidence in their hybrid offspring and 8 from a low-cancer group resulting in a low percentage of progeny with cancer. Murray and Warner (1947) did not believe the variation among the various sublines to be genetic in nature. They based this opinion on still existing dogmas that, after 20 generations of sib-mating, a mouse strain would be completely homozygous and that mutations would occur infrequently. In our opinion, however, their data support the notion that a recessive mutation which causes resistance to the virus (poor replication of the agent) was segregating in several of the MA lines. Detection of fixation of such a mutation will be delayed by the fact that MTV can be transmitted by homozygous resistant females for some generations (Mühlbock, 1956). Murray and Warner (1947) favored the hypothesis of a change in the virus, but we cannot imagine in the employed experimental set-up a selective mechanism that would favor the replication of the lesser virulent mutant over the highly oncogenic virus. Quite the opposite phenomenon has been observed by Blair (1958, 1960), who noticed the emergence of an extremely virulent variant of MTV in the A strain.

Murray (1963) found that a virus-free MA line was susceptible to the C3H virus. The C57BL strain is resistant to the C3H virus, but quite susceptible to the RIII an GR strain viruses. In the same way, this MA subline might be resistant to the virus present in the initial stock, but susceptible to C3H virus. Another explanation is that, although the subline was derived from a resistant female which had lost the virus, the resistance gene did not become fixed.

Rudali et al. (1956) and Andervont (1959) observed the disappearance of the milk factor from RIII strain mice. In an extensive analysis, Andervont and Dunn (1962) demonstrated that this might be a quite common phenomenon for the various sublines of th RIII strain. Liebelt and Liebelt (1967) had obtained RIII mice from Andervont in 1954. Initially, their RIII line had a high incidence of mammary tumors, but it had changed into a low-cancer strain 6 years later. Andervont and Dunn (1962) foster-nursed RIII mice which had lost their milk agent on virus-carrying C3H females. In the fifth generation of one family, they noticed the rapid disappearance of the C3H virus. Obviously, this line was resistant to both the RIII and C3H virus. Three other related families seemed to have remained susceptible to the C3H agent. A possible explanation for this is that the four families were derived from a cross between a homozygous resistant RIII female which had lost the agent and a heterozygous male, giving rise to one resistant female and three susceptible but virus-free founding females.

Smith (1966) and Blair (1960) noticed that their C3H sublines had lost the milk factor as shown by transmission experiments. Smith (1966) claims that this subline remains susceptible to the virus from other C3H sublines. However, he has not studied the vertical transmission of the newly introduced milk factor in subsequent generations. It is quite possible that the virus will disappear in a few generations, as has been described for the C3H milk factor in the CBA strain by Mühlbock (1956).

The A/He in three different laboratories has changed into a strain with a moderate mammary tumor incidence (Blair, 1960; Heston et al., 1970; W. Van Ebbenhorst-Tengbergen, and P. Bentvelzen, unpublished results). It was suggested by Heston et al. that the genotype of the A strain could hardly maintain a high titer of virus or that there would be some variation in genes controlling virus replication. Since some high mammary cancer A lines are still in existence (e.g., Murray and Little, 1967), the most likely explanation is that a resistance-inducing mutation which has later become fixed in the various laboratories has occurred in the A/He colony. This has not yet led to the complete disappearance of the virus, but certainly to the diminution as becomes evident from immunological assays for MTV (Heston et al., 1970) or foster-nursing experiments (P. Bentvelzen, unpublished results).

Matsuzawa et al. (1970) observed a sudden decline in tumor incidence in the DDD mouse strain. By means of foster-nursing of BALB/c mice on DDD, it was established that the virus was still present. The authors speculated that either a genetic change which conferred resistance to the oncogenic action of the virus had occurred or an increase in leukemia virus occurred, which would interfere with MTV-induce mammary tumorigenesis. A subsequent study (Matsuzawa and Yamamoto, 1972) seems to confirm the latter hypothesis. A similar interference between leukemia virus and mammary tumor virus has been postulated by Squartini et al. (1967).

Reinhard et al. (1955) suggested that the disappearance of MTV from high-cancer strains might have resulted from the inadvertent use of a predominance of first-litter offspring for the propagation of the strains, with a progressive reduction in the amount of virus transmitted from generation to generation. It is known that the amount of virus is rather low in the first lactation period, as detected by several immunological assays (Blair, 1969; Charney et al., 1969; Verstraeten et al., 1975). Andervont (1949) described the gradual disappearance of the virus in the C3H strain when newborn mice were exposed each generation to MTV-containing-milk for less than 40 hours. In less susceptible strains, this might also occur when mice are exposed to virus-containing-milk for the whole nursing period. A peculiar note is that, even in the highly sussceptible BALB/c strain, Andervont (1945a) observed two failures of transmission of the C3H virus to the offspring.

Liebelt and Liebelt (1967) reported that their BALB/c line with MTV reverted to a low-cancer strain.

Felluga et al. (1969) described a subline of BALB/cfC3H which had lost its high mammary tumor incidence, but instead developed a very high incidence of renal adenocarcinomas. These renal carcinomas abundantly produce intracytoplasmic A particles and are positive for MTV antigens (Hilgers et al., 1975). It might be well that the MTV strain in this line has mutated to a kidney-tumor-inducing virus.

It will be apparent that we favor genetic mutations as an important cause for the disappearance of MTV from a high-cancer strain, but we do not exclude the possibility that loss of virus is due to a fortuitous nongenetic event, such as lack of virus in the first lactation. Several lines that have lost their milk factor are still available. The genetic versus the nongenetic hypothesis can be tested under the condition that vertical transmission of the newly introduced virus will be studied for several generations. Such lines may be precious material for a study of role of genetic factors in susceptibility to virus-induced mammary cancer. It would not be surprising if the difference between these lines and their parental high-cancer stocks are caused by mutations of a single locus. In that case, these lines are comparable to "congenic" lines which have been developed intentionally through selection.

C. Inherited Hormonal Influence

The mammary tumor research area has been dominated for several decades by the three-factor-hypothesis (Bittner, 1942b) that mammary cancer in mice would result from the interaction of hormones, a suitable genetic constitution and an extrachromosomal factor (virus). However, indications that mammary cancer can result from excessive hormonal stimulation in the absence of an extrachromosomal factor, even in resistant genotypes, have been obtained by Boot (1969).

One of the mechanisms by which genes might control mammary tumorigenesis is the regulation of the production of those hormones involved in mammary gland growth and differentiation. Since many different hormones from pituitary, ovaries, pancreas, and adrenals are known to act on mammary gland development, it is extremely difficult to sort out which hormone or what combinations are carcinogenic. One might speculate, for instance, that the hormonal combination which induces optimal growth and/or differentiation is also the most tumorigenic. Most recently, Röpcke (1975) demonstrated that not only excessive stimulation by hormones but also subphysiological doses of steroids (estrone and progesterone) in combination with prolactin may cause mammary cancer in some strains or hybrids which are otherwise highly resistant.

The concept of inherited hormonal influence as coined by Bittner *et al.* (1944) is based on the observation that A strain virgins have a low tumor frequency in contrast to breeding females of that strain. Foster-nursing and reciprocal crossing of A and C3H by Heston and Andervont (1944) indicated the genetic nature of this phenomenon. This was confirmed by a series of crosses between the A and several other strains made by Bittner (1952b). From Bittner's work in 1953 it can be concluded that the same gene(s) cause a similar resistance of virgins of the NH strain to mammary cancer. As the (A × C57BL)F_1 hybrid virgins are also resistant (Mühlbock, 1956), it may be assumed that, in view of the recessiveness of this trait in most crosses with the A strain, the C57BL has a similar genetic resistance mechanism.

In the CE strain, the C3H virus causes a very high tumor incidence in breeding mice, but a moderate incidence (26%) in virgins. The virus is retained in the CE strain for at least 10 generations. When infected CE females are mated to C3Hf/Bi males, 81% tumors are found in virgin F_1 offspring. The tumor incidence in the hybrid offspring of CE × A is only 28% (Bittner, 1954). Probably the same loci as in the A strain cause the virgin resistance but to a lesser extent.

Virgins of the A strain have a low incidence of spontaneous pseudopregnancies (Mühlbock and Boot, 1960). Induction of pseudopregnancies by mating with vasectomized males leads to a strong increase in tumor frequency in A females (Law, 1941).

Ovary transplantation into (A × C3H)F_1 hybrids from either parental strain did not reveal great differences in tumor inducing capacity (Huseby and Bittner, 1948). In an extensive review on hormonal aspects in carcinogenesis, Gardner *et al.* (1959) suggested a difference in control at the pituitary level regulating the persistence or function of corpora lutea (prolactin). The evidence for this is rather weak.

Nandi and Bern (1960) and Nandi (1961) were the first to look for a difference in susceptibility of mammary gland growth and differentiation to various protein and steroid hormones. They concluded that the A strain needed larger amounts of growth hormone than other high-cancer strains. They suggested that growth hormone rather than prolactin would be the tumor-inducing principle in virgins. Röpcke (1975), however, postulated that growth hormone might have an anticarcinogenic action on the mammary gland, that is, it would provide protection against the subsequent carcinogenic activity of prolactin and progesterone.

Ben-David *et al.* (1969) found a normal response of the A mammary gland after prolactin release, induced by perphenazine as judged from the appearance of the glands in whole-mount preparations. Singh *et al.* (1970) could not find a correlation between *in vitro* induction of lobuloalveolar development by various hormone combinations and susceptibility to mammary carcinogenesis. However, they found that C57BL and A strain mice required a remarkably long period of *in vivo* pretreatment with estradiol and progesterone to show outgrowth of explants *in vitro*, as compared to the RIII, I, DBA, C3H, and BALB/c strains.

Mammary gland transplantation experiments performed according to the method of Dux and Mühlbock (1966) could establish whether the resistance of A virgins is due to a special endocrine condition of these virgins or that other factors are involved as well.

The GR strain is exceptional with regard to its response to the carcinogenic action of the various mammary gland growth-potentiating hormones. In most mouse strains the pituitary hormone prolactin is thought to be the predominant carcinogenic principle (Boot, 1969). However, mammary tumors can be induced in the GR strain by estrone and progesterone at a very early age (Van Nie and Thung, 1965). The combined estrone–progesterone effect can be mimicked by implantation of pellets of 17-α-ethynyl-19-nortestosterone (Van Nie et al., 1972). Pituitary isografts which grow well in the GR strain do induce mammary tumors, but with a considerably longer latency period than with the steroid treatment (Van Nie and Dux, 1971). Obviously, prolactin released by the isografts is not very efficient in inducing mammary tumors in the GR strain. The rapid induction of tumors by treatment with steroids proved to be a dominant trait, which was associated with expression of MTV (Van Nie et al., 1972). Introduction of GR strain virus into other mouse strains does not lead to early tumors after steroid treatment (Van Nie and Hilgers, 1976). This again emphasizes the importance of host genes for the particular response of the mammary glands to the carcinogenic action of steroid hormones.

In this era of virus research, we regret the neglect of modern endocrinological approaches to the problem of the role of protein versus steroid hormones in mammary tumorigenesis. It is important to pursue strain differences in mammary gland reaction to various hormones, to study its genetic basis in great detail, and to correlate genetic differences in growth and differentiation with those to susceptibility in mammary tumorigenesis.

It is also necessary to study the presence and quantity of receptors for various steroid hormones in mammary glands of different mouse strains. This is important also from the virological point of view, since there exists a relationship between receptors for glucocorticoids and MTV production (Shyamala and Dickson, 1976).

D. COMPLEMENTATION FOR RESISTANCE

In almost all cases we have encountered, resistance to exogenous MTV transmitted by the milk is a recessive trait. This holds true for both resistance due to interference with replication of the virus and resistance of virgins (inherited hormonal influence). When hybrids between resistant strains are also resistant, one may assume that the same genic system is responsible in both strains. In the case of susceptibility of the hybrid between resistant strains, it is obvious that different genes control the resistance in the parental strains. We refer to this as complementation.

Such complementation was discovered by Andervont (1940) for the resistant strains C57BL and I. While foster-nursing of C57BL and I females on C3H mothers leads to a low incidence of breast cancer, foster-nursing of the F_1 hybrid results in an incidence as high as in the C3H foster strain. As mentioned above, the C3H virus replicates poorly in both mouse strains (Bittner, 1952a; Andervont, 1964). The observed susceptibility of the F_1 hybrid must be explained by two separate genetic systems which are both involved in viral replication. Suggestive evidence for this possibility is obtained from the transplantation experiments of Nandi et al. (1966) in which it was found that mammary glands from either C57BL or I could develop nodules and tumors in infected hybrids, but not in infected parental strains. Much more virus is present in the hybrid environment than in the parental milieus, as becomes evident from the finding of Nandi (1974) that blood cells carry much more infectivity. The poor replication of MTV in the I strain seems to be correlated with a strong immunological response (Nandi, 1974). It is not excluded, however, that a similar mechanism, based on another gene, would not play a role in the C57BL strain (see section on H-2 related resistance to exogenous MTV).

Another striking example of complementation was presented by Bittner (1958). NH females with the C3H milk factor will develop only 27% tumors when kept as breeders. The I strain will not develop tumors, even when infected with the virus. The incidence in the F_1 hybrid of these two strains is 76%. Not much information is available on what mechanism might be responsible for the resistance of the NH strain. There is no indication that the C3H virus is poorly replicated in the NH strain. One might think, therefore, of a hormonal resistance factor. The early-appearing reproductive senility of this poorly breeding strain (Snell et al., 1960) may be held responsible for the low tumor incidence. This will be compensated for by the I strain genome which itself is resistant because of poor replication of the virus.

A similar complementation phenomenon of an endocrinological and an antiviral recessive resistance is represented by the $(A \times I)F_1$ virgins which develop 72% mammary cancer (Bittner, 1958). Mühlbock (1956) and Richardson and Hummel (1959) reported that hybrids of some high-cancer strains developed 100% mammary tumors at strikingly earlier ages than did either parent. As mentioned earlier, Andervont (1949) found that the high-cancer strain C3H replicated its milk virus less competently than did BALB/c. It seems that the C3H carries a gene that has some effect on virus replication. It is quite possible that, in F_1 hybrids of so-called high-cancer strains, such genes with minor effect are mutually complemented. One may also apply the same reasoning in the case of the F_1 hybrids of the high-cancer strain A and the resistant strain CBA, especially since breeders were used which excluded the inherited hormonal influence as expressed in virgins (Mühlbock, 1956). F_1 hybrid mice usually have a longer life-span and therefore may have a greater chance to develop a tumor. But we have discussed only those cases where this phenomenon does not play a significant role.

E. Difference in Virulence of MTV Variants

Strain differences in mammary tumor incidence or length of latency period need not only be due to host genetic factors or the absence of exogenous MTV but many reflect genetic variation among the viruses harbored in the different mouse strains.

Bittner (1936b) had already obtained evidence that the milk factor of the A strain would be more virulent than that of the DBA, as there was a significant difference in average tumor age between the reciprocal hybrids of these strains. A similar finding was reported by Murray (1941a) for the DBA strain versus the MA strain which still carried an exogenous MTV. A slight difference in virulence between C3H and A strain milk factor can be deduced from the studies of Heston and Andervont (1944). Tumors in the $(A \times C3H)F_1$ hybrid appear slightly later than in the reciprocal hybrid. In addition, introduction of the C3H milk factor into the A strain leads to a 16% tumor incidence in virgins, in contrast to 0% in control A mice. It is obvious, however, that not the A-strain virus, but predominantly A-strain host genes, control the resistance of the virgins. In contrast to the virus of the C3H line used by Heston and Andervont, that of the Z subline of this mouse strain (C3H/Bi; for subline differences in the C3H, see McLaren and Michie, 1954) proves to be slightly inferior to the A-strain milk factor (Bittner and Huseby, 1946).

A subtlety must be introduced here: introduction of the A virus into C3H/Bi mice leads to a significant delay in tumor development. This indicates that MTV variants must be tested in the same mouse genotype.

Different types of MTV might be called virulent (or high oncogenic) because they have been tested in a mouse strain that is accidentally very susceptible to those MTV types.

Richardson and Hummel (1959) found a striking difference in average tumor age between the reciprocal hybrids of the high-cancer strains C3H and RIII. In the same way a difference has been found between the milk factor from the C3H and CBA high-cancer sublines (Richardson and Hall, 1963).

Dmochowski (1945a,b, 1948) claims strain differences between viruses when tested in the same "virus-free" but susceptible hybrid mice. In our opinion, however, the observed differences are insignificant, probably due to the low numbers of test mice used. Mühlbock (1951) tested tumor extracts from several mouse strains in $(020 \times DBAf)F_1$ hybrid mice. The virus from the C3H proved to be the most potent in this hybrid: tumors appearing at 7 months average age when forced brcd. Tumors induced by agents from the DBA or WLL strains appeared at 11 months and the virus from the RIII strains induced tumors at 13 months average age. The A strain virus proved to be inactive in this hybrid. In a subsequent study, Mühlbock (1956) found that foster-nursing of $(020 \times DBAF)F_1$ newborn mice on A strain females failed to induce an appreciable tumor incidence. It was obvious that the A strain carried an exogenous virulent MTV, because it could be removed by foster-nursing A strain females on C57BL. Furthermore, if A strain mammary tumor extracts were injected into C3Hf mice, mammary tumors developed and the virus could be transmitted to subsequent generations.

Hummel and Little (1959) foster-nursed BALB/c newborns on four different high-cancer strains: C3H, A, RIII, and DBA. In this experiment, the C3H virus also proved to be the most virulent, inducing tumors at 8 months average age in forced-bred test mice. In contrast, A, RIII, and DBA virus induced tumors a few months later. The technique of forced breeding, however, obscures virus differences in the highly susceptible BALB/c strain. Vlahakis (1973) did not find significant differences in tumor incidence and latency periods on breeding BALB/c mice with C3H, A, and DD milk factors. When virgins were compared, the following tumor incidences were found: for C3H virus, 84% at 11 months; A virus, 64% at 15 months; and DD virus, 22% at 19 months.

Blair (1958) noted a decrease in latency period in one branch of the Berkeley breeding colony of the A strain. Reciprocal crossing between mice from that branch with the parental stock indicated a maternal influence on the early appearance of mammary tumors. Foster-nursing experiments showed that this was not due to a genetic mutation in the host, but must have been due to the emergence of a new type of milk factor. Inoculation of cell-free extracts from mammary glands of either A subline into BALB/c mice confirmed the higher virulence of the new variant (Blair, 1960). It has been assumed that the observed alteration in the A strain milk factor was due to a mutation. In our opinion, such a mutation could be detected only if it would have a somewhat higher rate of replication than the original virus. Such a higher rate of replication might explain the earlier appearance of mammary tumors.

Deringer (1970) describes the BL mouse strain in which 10% mammary tumors appear at 15 months average age. Foster-nursing of C3H on this mouse strain leads to 47% incidence of mammary tumors at 18 months in contrast to 2% at 24 months in the controls. It seems that the BL strain harbors a low oncogenic milk factor, which causes only a low incidence of tumors in its host. This in an unique situation, since all milk-factor-containing mouse strains develop a high incidence of tumors at considerable earlier ages, generally before one year. Unfortunately, no further information has become available on this interesting mouse strain, which was developed in the 1920s by Lynch (1925).

Mühlbock (1966) carried out a very extensive study on the relationship between the MTV harbored by various mouse strains and the genotype of the recipient strain. Table II shows the results of cell-free extracts injected i.p. into 4-week-old females of 8 different low cancer strains. He recorded tumor incidence not only in injected animals but also in their offspring. A rather erratic pattern emerges: the virus from the C3H strain is very efficient in C3Hf, DBAf, C57BL, 020, and IF, and the virus from DBA strain is efficient in WLLf, CBA, and 020. The WLL virus seems to be virulent only in the 020 and IF strains and the A strain virus only in C3Hf. It is obvious that a very close relationship between viral and host genotype determines susceptibility to mammary carcinogenesis. So far, no clear-cut pattern emerges as has been found, e.g., for murine leukemia viruses (Lilly and Pincus, 1973).

Dux (1972) found that the milk factor of C3H induced only 14% mammary tumors in the B10 mouse strain, while foster-nursing of C57BL on GR females leads to a 44% incidence in forced-bred mice. In a subsequent study, Mühlbock and Dux (1972) found the C3H virus given with the milk to be superior to that from the GR when tested in four other mouse strains (MAS, LIS, STS, and 020). Only in the C57BL strain did the GR virus prove to be more efficient. Moore et al. (1974) performed a more quantitative study to compare variant MTVs in relation to the host genotype. Instead of using the foster-nursing tech-

TABLE II

DIFFERENCE IN POTENCY OF MAMMARY TUMOR EXTRACTS FROM DIFFERENT
MOUSE STRAINS IN MICE OF FOUR TEST STRAINS AND THEIR PROGENY[a]

| Strain | Tumor incidence: mammary extract from | | | |
	C3H	WLL	DBA	A
C3Hf	0000	000T	00	TTT
% ma-ca in offspring	80%	10%	20%	60%
DBA	TTTT	0000TT	00TT	00
% ma-ca in offspring	75%	21%	—	0%
WLL	000T	TT	00TT	0000
% ma-ca in offspring	16%	—	79%	6%
CBA	000	000	0000	0000
% ma-ca in offspring	4%	3%	35%	0%
C57BL	0000	0000	000	0000
% ma-ca in offspring	50%	0%	6%	0%
020	000T	0000	0000	0000
% ma-ca in offspring	36%	58%	33%	0%
IF	0000	0000	0	00
% ma-ca in offspring	45%	50%	—	—
RIET	00	000	00	0000
% ma-ca in offspring	0%	—	0%	3%

[a] ma-ca, mammary cancer; 0, mouse without mammary tumor; T, mouse with mammary tumor.

nique, where an excess of virus is usually given, he used graded dilutions of virus-containing-milk of the A, RIII, C3H, and BALB/cfC3H strains. A few striking results were the following: RIIIf mice were very resistant to the virus from the isogenic RIII strain, while Af was highly susceptible to the virus from the isogenic A strain. The C57BL was resistant to infection by virus from C3H, BALB/cC3H, and A, but quite susceptible to the virus from RIII. Moore *et al.* (1976) mentions that the RIII strain MTV is still present in the C57BL mice in the fourth generation. There is no indication that this strain would lose the RIII strain virus.

Besides differences in virulence as measured by the tumor incidences and average ages, the viral genome may differ in the type of tumor it causes. Squartini *et al.* (1963) and Heston and Vlahakis (1971) noted that the virus from the RIII and DD strains could induce hormone-dependent tumors arising from so-called plaques in the BALB/c strain. However, host genetic factors also have an important influence on the histological tumor type and its behavior, since introduction of the DD virus into the C3Hf leads to a low incidence of mammary tumors that arise from plaques.

F. HISTOCOMPATIBILITY GENES AND SUSCEPTIBILITY

Important progress has been made in the genetics of cancer through the use of inbred instead of random-bred mouse strains. A more refined genetic analysis, however, requires the development of so-called congenic lines, where one relevant locus is substituted by a series of crosses combined with selection. Such congenic lines have been developed for the study of histocompatibility loci (Snell, 1958). Lilly (1966) noticed an influence of one of these histocompatibility loci (H-2) on susceptibility to leukemogenesis by the Gross leukemia virus. This prompted Mühlbock and Dux (1971) to investigate the influence of histocompatibility genes on mammary carcinogenesis in the presence of MTV, utilizing congenic strains. They found an influence of the H-2 locus only and not of H-1, H-3, H-4, H-7, H-9, H-12, and H-13 in the case of C3H-MTV induced mammary cancer in lines on the C57BL/10 (B10) background.

A comparison of the 020 strain with the congenic OIR line (H-2^q from DBA strain) indicated greater susceptibility of the latter line to the virus of the DBA, but low susceptibility to the virus from C3H; the parental 020 strain is susceptible to the latter virus (Mühlbock and Dux, 1972). In a subsequent analysis of the B10 congenics Mühlbock and Dux (1974) found the H-2^b and H-2^m haplotypes to cause resistance to the milk-borne C3H virus, the H-2^{pa}, H-2^r, and H-2^k to lead to moderate susceptibility, while mice having the H-2^a, H-2^d, H-2^i, and H-2^f are highly susceptible. By the use of a H-2 congenic line [B10.A(5R)], which resulted from a crossover between the K- and D-end of the H-2 complex, it could be established that the genes on the D-end control susceptibility to MTV. This finding seemed to be unexpected, since the gene controlling susceptibility to Gross leukemia virus was located in the K end (Lilly and Pincus, 1973). One gene, which controls the immune response to various synthetic polypeptides (Ir-1), is located near the K end, and it has been assumed that the role of the H-2 locus in murine leukemogenesis is mediated by this gene. The role of the gene in the D end controlling susceptibility to MTV remains unclear. However, an interaction has been recently found between H-2D-coded and MTV-induced membrane antigens at the cell surface (Kusnierczijk and Peknicova, 1975).

The major component of genetic resistance is localized in the mammary gland itself as revealed by mammary gland transplantation (Dux and Mühlbock, 1968), or the production of tetraparental chimeras of high- and low-cancer strains (Mintz and Slemmer, 1969; Mintz, 1970; Mintz *et al.*, 1971). Therefore, it does not seem to be likely that humoral factors, i.e., immunological factors, play a very important role. This might explain why K-end genes have no influence on susceptibility to MTV.

There does not seem to exist such a H-2 controlled restriction with regard to the GR strain virus, as shown by moderate tumor incidences in all congenic B10 lines foster-nursed on GR (Dux, 1972). Since only two haplotypes (H-2^b and H-2^m) confer resistance to the C3H MTV, it is possible that a hitherto unknown haplotype would induce resistance to the GR MTV.

IV. Endogenous Viruses

Already in 1915, Lathrop and Loeb (1915a,b) found an indication for an extrachromosomal influence in the origin of mammary tumors in mice. These findings have been largely ignored because they did not work with sib-mated lines, although their mice might have been inbred to a large extent. The mouse colony "cream" developed only 3% mammary tumors while the stock "English sable" developed 70%. When "cream" females were mated with "English sable" males, no tumors developed in the offspring, but no less than 60% tumors were observed in the reciprocal cross.

The stock "English tan" had a tumor incidence of 73%. When "cream" females were mated with these "English tan" mice, 42% tumors developed in the hybrids. This case, in contrast to the first one, might have been due to genetic transmission of a mammary tumor virus by the "English tan" male, as has been described for the inbred GR mouse (Mühlbock, 1965; Bentvelzen, 1968a).

Korteweg, who contributed to the discovery of the milk factor, was already aware in 1936 (Korteweg, 1936a,b) that mammary tumors could develop in the absence of this factor and would result from the action of genetic factors only. It was several decades before it was realized that these genetic factors may be genetically transmitted viruses.

A. THE C3Hf SYSTEM AND THAT OF OTHER FOSTERED SUBLINES

Soon after Andervont's discovery of the extrachromosomal male transmission of the Bittner virus, Andervont and Dunn (1948b) realized that not all mammary tumors in (BALB/c × C3Hf)F$_1$ mice were caused by this virulent virus. After elimination of this mode of transmission, mammary tumors could still be found in these F_1 hybrids. They stated that apparently, inherited tendencies together with hormonal stimulation were predominant influences in the origin of these tumors.

Heston et al. (1950) did an extensive study on the possible presence of virus in a C3Hf subline which was derived from the high-cancer strain C3H by cesarean section and subsequent foster-nursing on low cancer strain C57BL mice. This line develops a relatively high incidence of mammary tumors (38%), but at a late age (20 months). Cell-free extracts of 24 such late tumors did not induce an appreciable higher incidence when injected into newborn C3Hf mice. However, they reported a statistically significant difference in tumor incidence between females from mothers with tumors as compared to those born from mothers who remained nontumorous. In crosses between C3Hf and C57BL, Heston and Deringer (1952) found no evidence against the possible presence of a virus in the C3Hf strain. This view was confirmed in even more extensive studies with double-foster-nursed sublines of the C3H strain (C3Hff) (Heston, 1958).

However, in the meantime, it was reported that C3Hf mammary tumors contain viruslike particles not distinguishable from those suspected to be the milk factor. Dmochowski, in a series of abstracts (Dmochowski et al., 1954; Dmochowski, 1954), claims to have been the first to see these particles. During the Amsterdam Conference in 1956, both Bernhard et al. (1956) and Dmochowski (1956) reported on the presence of virus particles in C3Hf mammary tumors. Bang et al. (1956) also independently showed such particles. By far, the best pictures were presented by Bernhard's group.

In contrast to the negative bioassays of C3Hf mammary tumor extracts as reported by Heston et al. (1950) and Boot and Mühlbock (1956), Dmochowski and Grey (1957), and Dmochowski et al. (1963) claimed tumorigenic action of such extracts in $(C57B1 \times RIIIf)F_1$ and $(C57BL \times Af)F_1$ test animals. A few mammary tumors appeared at a very early age (6 months) with some extracts in these test mice. The general opinion at that time was against accepting this as proof of the presence of virus in these tumors. We are presently willing to accept this. It would imply that the C3Hf virus, which has been earlier called low oncogenic (Bentvelzen and Daams, 1969), must be regarded as highly oncogenic in certain genotypes. Unfortunately, extensive host-range studies with respect to oncogenicity have not been carried out with the C3Hf virus. High concentrations of virus particles isolated from C3Hf do not induce mammary tumors before 1 year of age in

BALB/c mice (Hageman *et al.*, 1968), but induce a high incidence of late-appearing tumors (Hageman *et al.*, 1972; Hageman, 1973).

Moore *et al.* (1976) recently investigated the infectivity of virus in the milk of C3Hf mice for 4 different mouse strains. Infectivity was assayed by the appearance of an MTV specific antigen in the milk at the third lactation as detected by immunodiffusion. A very high incidence of infected animals was found in the Balb/c strain (more than 90%). The Af strain had a similar susceptibility as the BALB/c strain, but the RIIIf strain proved to be even more susceptible: 46% of the animals produced the MTV antigens when injected with a high dilution of the milk, which does not infect BALB/c or Af mice. Surprisingly, C57BL mice could also be infected with the C3Hf virus, although this strain is considered to be less susceptible. It will be very interesting to determine the oncogenic activity of C3Hf strain MTV in those mouse strains.

In a comprehensive review, Moore (1963) speculated that it was possible that the potential for virus production could be carried in the ova from one generation to the next and thereby likened it to the phenomenon of lysogeny in bacteria.

Pitelka *et al.* (1964) found typical virus particles, by now called B particles (Bernhard and Guérin, 1958), in both hybrids of C3Hf and the "particle-free" BALB/c. Such particles could not be found in mammary hyperplasia of BALB/c mice foster-nursed by C3Hf. They suggested that "the C3Hf particle may represent a second agent (morphologically indistinguishable but biologically distinct from MTV) normally transmitted to offspring by either parent at conception but ordinarily not passed through milk." However, Van Nie and Verstraeten (1975), utilizing the sensitive radioimmunoassay, clearly demonstrated that C3Hf-MTV can be transmitted to BALB/c by the milk, but with a relatively low efficiency, as viral antigens appear at the third lactation in low quantities; while in hybrids of BALB/c × C3Hf, viral antigens can already be detected in relatively large amounts in the first lactation. The C3Hf agent was introduced as the "nodule inducing virus," or NIV, by Nandi and DeOme (1965). DeOme *et al.* (1967), after a complicated procedure, were able to introduce this virus into BALB/c mice. In that strain, virus could be transmitted by the milk only. Obviously, the genotype of the C3Hf mouse controls the gamete-borne transmission.

In analogy to this work on the transmission of a virulent MTV in the GR mouse strain, as will be discussed below, Bentvelzen (1968a) and Bentvelzen and Daams (1969) explained the close relationship between C3Hf genotype and C3Hf virus with regard to gamete-borne transmission by genetic transmission of the virus in the C3Hf mouse strain. Suggestive evidence for this hypothesis was the observation that in F_1 hybrids between C3Hf and (particle-free) 020, no virus particles could be demonstrated, whereas 4 out of 11 tumors originating in the F_2 generation contained many B-type particles (Bentvelzen and Daams, 1969). The logical explanation for this phenomenon was that genetic information for the virus must be present in the F_1 generation, but that its expression is inhibited owing to a dominant genetic factor coming from the 020 strain.

The results of different studies at the Netherlands Cancer Institute on the presence of B particles or MTV antigens in hybrids between various low cancer strains are presented in Table III. No B-type particles have ever been observed in mammary tumors of CBA, 020, or BALB/c strains. Most tumors are also negative for MTV antigens in the immunofluorescence absorption (IAF) test (Hilgers et al., 1972, 1973). However, with more sensitive immunological techniques, such as the radioimmunoassay (RIA), small amounts of viral antigens can be found in tumors of the BALB/c strain (Van Nie and Verstraeten, 1975; P. Bentvelzen, unpublished results).

The majority of tumors in mouse strains which have been derived from high-cancer strains by means of foster-nursing are positive for B particles as well as MTV antigens by IFA. Hybrids both of whose parents produce B-type particles also contain these particles in their tumors. Hybrids of mouse strains in which neither parent has particles or antigens are negative in both tests. In general, hybrids between "particle-free" and particle-positive strains are devoid of particles in their tumors, and the quantity of antigens in the IFA test is very low. As seen by immunofluorescence on trypsinized, acetone-fixed mammary tumor cells of such hybrids, only a small percentage of cells show bright positive staining with an antiserum to MTV (J. Hilgers, unpublished results), while all cells in the C3Hf are positive. Noteworthy exceptions are hybrids of the C3Hf with "particle-free" BALB/c. Tumors produce B particles abundantly, antigen levels are extremely high and all cells are positive by IF.

Van Nie and Verstraeten (1975), utilizing the RIA test to detect MTV antigens in the milk, found that the release of virus of the C3Hf, in crosses with the BALB/c strain, is controlled by a single gene (Mtv-1) located on chromosome 7 (linkage group I), approximately 20 cM from the albino locus. This chromosome also carries Akv-1, the proviral gene of a murine leukemia virus in the AKR mouse (Chattopadhyay et al., 1975).

In the backcross BALB/c $\times$ (BALB/c $\times$ C3H)F_1, the Mtv-1 gene is

TABLE III

B Particles and MTV Antigens in Mammary Tumors of Low Mammary Cancer Strains and Hybrids; Genetic Interference with Endogenous C3Hf-MTV[a]

Strain or hybrid	Electron microscopy		Immunology	
	No. of tumors tested	No. with B particles	No. of tumors tested	No. positive in IF[b] or IFA test
Group I				
CBA[c]	8	0	30	1
020	7	0	29	1
Balb/c/AnDe	15	0	5	0
Group II				
C3Hf[d]	Many	Many	62	57
DBAf	7	5	—	—
AF	5	3	—	—
Group III				
(C3Hf × DBAf)F₁	5	4	—	—
(DBAf × C3Hf)F₁	4	2	—	—
Group IV				
(C57BL × CBA)F₁	14	0	31	0
(020 × IF)F₁	12	0	—	—
(C57BL × TSI)F₁	3	0	—	—
Group V				
(C57BL × Af)F₁	3	0	—	—
(C57BLcC3Hf)F₁[e]	8	0	15	4
(C57BL × DBAf)F₁[f]	—	—	24	6
(020 × DBAF)F₁	9	0	—	—
(020 × C3Hf)F₁	5	0	12	11[g]
(C3Hf × 020)F₁	7	0	—	—
(Balb/c/AnDe × C3Hf)F₁	14	14	14	13[g]
(Balb/c/Crgl × C3Hf)F₁	—	—	20	20[g]

[a] Partly from thesis of Dr. L. Boot (1969), with EM results from, Dr. J. Calafat; partly from thesis of Dr. G. Röpcke (1975) with IFA results from Dr. J. Hilgers; partly from Hilgers et al. (1973); and partly unpublished with IF and IFA results from Dr. J. Hilgers and EM results of Dr. J. Calafat and Dr. P. Bentvelzen.

[b] IF is immunofluorescence on fixed cells (Hilgers et al., 1971, 1972) and IFA is quantitative immunofluorescence absorption.

[c] The one positive tumor was a carcinoma, 26 of 30 tumors were acanthomas.

[d] C3Hf is the C3H/He/fA subline which might be a higher expressor of endogenous MTV than the C3H sublines from Strong and Bittner. The 5 IFA-negative tumors were acanthomas.

[e] Two of 9 carcinomas and 2 of 6 acanthomas were IFA positive.

[f] Five of 18 carcinomas and 1 of 6 acanthomas were IFA positive.

[g] Seven of 11 (020 × C3Hf)F₁ tumors had low titers (1/1–1/4) by IFA; the majority of the (BALB/c × C3Hf)F₁ crosses had high titers (1/32 or higher) by IFA.

associated with the appearance of mammary tumors at a relatively early age of around 12 months. The animals in the backcross which are negative by RIA for MTV antigens in the milk develop tumors at a considerably later age or no tumors at all. This group of negative animals resembles the BALB/c strain with regard to tumor incidence and latency period. Tumors in this group had considerably lower quantities of MTV antigens, like BALB/c mammary tumors.

The inhibition of expression of C3Hf virus in hybrids with C57BL seems to be controlled by a single gene, which is located on a different chromosome than Mtv-1 (P. Bentvelzen, unpublished results). Mintz (1970) produced parental chimeras of C3Hf and C57BL strains. The mammary tumor incidence in the chimeras is 50% at 18 months average age, which is comparable to incidence and tumor age of the C3Hf strain. One out of six tumors proved to be of C57BL origin. These results suggest that susceptibility to the oncogenic action of the C3Hf strain virus is localized at the level of the mammary gland. The inhibitory action of the C57BL genome, as detected in F_1 hybrids, does not show in the chimeras.

A remark should be made here on the histology of mammary tumors in these studies. It is our experience that adenoacanthomas contain lower quantities of MTV antigens than adenocarcinomas and, in general, no B type particles can be detected by means of electron microscopy. For example, the few adenoacanthomas appearing in the C3Hf strain were negative by IFA (see Table III). Spontaneous mammary tumors of the BALB/c are often adenoacanthomas. BALB/c mice infected with the C3Hf virus produce mostly adenoacarcinomas which contain a large amount of B particles and MTV antigens, in contrast to spontaneous BALB/c tumors (P. Hageman, J. Calafat, and J. Hilgers, unpublished results).

B-type particles have been found not only in tumors of the C3Hf substrain, but also in some other foster-nursed lines, such as DBAf and Af (see Table III). Dmochowski et al. (1963) demonstrated B-type particles in the milk of Af mice; these proved to be oncogenic in $(C57BL \times Af)F_1$ hybrid test mice. Comparatively few studies have been carried out with presumed viruses in these foster-nursed sublines, but, recently, Moore et al. (1976) demonstrated the infectivity of Af strain milk in RIII and BALB/c; C57BL proves to be rather resistant to the virus in Af milk. Infectious virus was also found in RIIIf milk. The Af strain is highly susceptible to the virus of this milk, like the BALB/c strain, while C57BL is refractory to the virus of the RIIIf.

Bentvelzen (1974b) has grouped the C3Hf, DBAf, and Af viruses together as MTV-L, as though all these viruses are low oncogenic. Host-range studies are needed, in terms of both infectivity and oncogenicity to determine whether this classification holds true.

Verstraeten *et al.* (1975), using the RIA test, found MTV antigens in the milk of C3Hf and DBAf and Verstraeten *et al.* (1976) additionally reported on the presence of such antigens in the milk of Af and DDf strains, whereas LTSf and RIIIf milk proved to be negative. The MTV negative RIIIf mouse strain kept in Amsterdam could well be different from the MTV-positive RIIf strain of Moore, since isoenzyme patterns of various RIII strains in America and European laboratories differ markedly (J. Hilgers, unpublished observations). Noteworthy in this respect is that the LTS parental line has lost its milk factor (A. A. Verstraeten an R. Van Nie, unpublished results) and that the RIII strain is known to have repeatedly lost its milk factor (see section on disappearance of MTV from high cancer strains).

B. THE GR SYSTEM

According to Mühlbock (1965), it would be desirable to have inbred strains developed in other parts of the world than in the United States in order to expand the gene pool of the laboratory mouse. In that paper, Mühlbock reported on a new albino European mouse strain which had a peculiar characteristic with regard to mammary tumors which had not been reported for other mouse strains and which he thought might, therefore, be of importance for cancer research. This mouse strain, GR, which came from Grumbach in Zürich (Switzerland) and was subsequently inbred in Amsterdam, proved to be a high mammary cancer strain. When GR young were taken out of the uterus and then foster-nursed by a mother of the low-cancer C57BL strain, the high incidence of mammary tumors was retained. It was then thought in Mühlbock's laboratory that this exceptional susceptibility to mammary cancer was a genetic trait. This seemed to be supported by the observation that F_1 hybrids of a C57BL female mated with a GR male had exactly the same high incidence of mammary tumors as did the reciprocal hybrid. However, foster-nursing of so-called virus-free $(020 \times DBAf)F_1$ mice by GR females revealed the presence of a milk-borne mammary tumor virus. In mammary tumors of the GR strain, abundant numbers of B-type particles could be detected by electron microscopy. Mühlbock (1965) concluded that the GR agent is apparently transmitted by the male as effectively as by the female.

Introduction of the GR strain virus into other mouse strains by means of foster-nursing abrogates the effective male transmission (Bentvelzen, 1968a, 1975; Mühlbock and Bentvelzen, 1968). This indicates that male transmission is a genetic pecularity of the GR strain.

Mendelian analysis of this trait proved it to be controlled by a single dominant gene (Bentvelzen, 1968a, 1972a; Mühlbock and Bentvelzen, 1968; Bentvelzen and Daams, 1969; Van Nie et al., 1972; Van Nie and Hilgers, 1976). In the early stage of genetic studies on male transmission, results were mainly based on incidences of palpable mammary tumors arising early in life, and in a few cases on the presence of virulent virus in the milk, which can be effectively transmitted by foster-nursing. In subsequent studies, virus was also determined by immunological means such as immunofluorescence on acetone-fixed mammary gland cell preparations, cytotoxicity absorption tests on mammary gland extracts, and immunodiffusion tests with milk (Van Nie et al. 1972; Van Nie and Hilgers, 1976). Mammary tumor induction was standardized, in that ovariectomized mice were treated with progesterone and estrone or the hormonal compound 17-ethynyl-19-nortestosterone, leading to early stages of mammary tumors in a few weeks (Van Nie et al., 1972; Van Nie and Hilgers, 1976).

The intimate relationship between the GR host genome and the GR strain MTV with regard to the male transmission has led to the hypothesis that the virus is genetically transmitted by the GR male (Bentvelzen, 1968a; Mühlbock and Bentvelzen, 1968; Bentvelzen and Daams, 1969; Bentvelzen et al., 1970). This concept of genetic transmission was supported by the observation that blastocysts of the genotype $(GR \times C57BL)F_1$ and pronuclear ova of the genotype $(GR \times BALB/c)F_1$ gave rise to tumorous mice despite transfer to low-cancer strain mice uteri. In the control experiment in which "virus-free" blastocysts or pronuclear eggs were transferred to GR mice uteri, no sign of virus infection was observed (Zeilmaker, 1969). These experiments indicate that the GR strain virus is not transmitted through the placenta, but that genetic information for the virus is present in the ovum. Bentvelzen (1968a) found some indications that this mode of transmission in the GR females is controlled by a single gene, which seems to be identical with the gene controlling male transmission.

A detailed discussion of the genetical crosses involved in these experiments has been presented by Bentvelzen (1972a).

An alternative for the hypothesis of "genomic transmission" of the GR strain MTV was presented by Nandi (1972) and Nandi and McGrath (1973). This hypothesis suggests that in the GR, there would be a gene for extreme susceptibility of embryos to the GR strain virus, called MTV-P (Bentvelzen and Daams, 1969). The C3Hf embryos would be susceptible only to C3Hf-MTV, but refractory to the milk-borne virulence of C3H-MTV. It must then also be assumed that the C3Hf embryos would be resistant to the GR strain virus. However, newborn mice of C3Hf as well as various other strains would be susceptible to the milk-borne viruses, in contrast to the embryos. This hypothesis had been earlier discussed by Bentvelzen (1968a, 1972a) in which he also admitted that it could not be completely excluded for the GR strain, but he regarded this as very untenable for the C3Hf situation. For that reason, he assumed that the virus would also be genetically transmitted in the case of the GR. Molecular hybridization studies, as will be discussed below (Varmus et $al.$, 1972, 1975; Michalides and Schlom, 1975) definitely proved the correctness of the "genomic transmission" hypothesis.

The conclusion of the Dutch investigators that gamete-borne transmission of an MTV in the GR strain is controlled by a single dominant gene has been disputed by Nandi and Helmich (1974) and Heston and Parks (1975).

In our opinion, analysis of the data presented by Nandi and Helmich (1974) does not reveal that two independent dominant genes are associated with gamete-borne transmission of an MTV. F_1 hybrids of BALB/c and GR develop 100% tumors by 7 months of age. In the F_2 generation, 75% mammary tumors are found at that age. In the case of the single-gene hypothesis approximately 75% is expected; for the two-gene hypothesis, this incidence must be around 94%. In the backcross to BALB/c, the authors found a 53% incidence at 7 months, which is in accordance with the single-gene hypothesis, while in the case of the two gene hypothesis, 75% would be anticipated. The incidence in the backcross to GR is 95%. For both hypotheses, 100% is expected. It is obvious that a single gene is responsible for the early appearance of mammary tumors in the GR strain as found earlier by Bentvelzen (1968a) and Van Nie et $al.$ (1972). In the F_2 generation, the higher incidence of mammary lesions (mammary tumors or hyperplastic alveolar nodules) at 12 months of age, may be partly due to extrachromosomal male transmission by the F_1 parent. The effect of this on mammary lesions becomes evident considerably later than in the case of genetic transmission. This phenomenon cannot play any role in the case of the backcross to the BALB/c, and it can therefore not be excluded that a second gene associated with release of a less oncogenic virus than MTV-P is involved (Bentvelzen, 1974b; Van Nie and Hilgers, 1976).

Van Nie and Verstraeten (1976) performed exactly the same backcross to BALB/c experiment. They found large amounts of MTV antigens, detectable by immunodiffusion (ID), in 40 out of 91 mice. In the positive animals, mammary tumors appeared at the mean age of 7.3 months. Twenty-six ID-negative animals were killed on the day a litter was born (3rd to 8th litter). No tumors were present in the mammary glands of these mice. The remainder of the negative animals continued to be tumor-free for more than 1 year.

The GR gene for release of MTV-P and early development of mammary tumors has been called Mtv-2 by Van Nie and Verstraeten (1975). This gene is not allelic to Mtv-1 because it is not linked to the c locus (albino). Van Nie and Hilgers (1976) have tested 18 genetic markers, representing approximately 40% of the mouse genome, for possible linkage with Mtv-2. The results were negative.

Van Nie and Verstraeten (1976) have developed a congenic GR line that lacks the gene for the appearance of early mammary tumors, Mtv-2. No MTV antigens were detectable with the ID test in the milk of this subline, but small amounts of MTV antigens can be discovered with the radioimmunoassays (R. Van Nie and A. A. Verstraeten, personal communication). This is probably due to a gene associated with another MTV strain endogenous to the GR.

Heston and Parks (1975) presented some preliminary results on the presence of MTV antigens in the milk of a series of crosses and backcrosses of GR to C57BL as determined by RIA with antisera to purified MTV proteins (Parks et al., 1974; Noon et al., 1975). When only incidences of antigen-positive animals are taken into account, the results might seem to be in conflict with results obtained by the Dutch investigators. However, low levels of antigens can be due to milk transmission as well as extrachromosomal male transmission and to a second gene associated with the release of a less productive virus, as postulated above. If these experiments had been controlled for both milk and extrachromosomal male transmission and if levels of MTV antigens are taken into account, a pattern of a single gene controlling large amounts of virus release which is associated with the early pregnancy-dependent tumorigenesis would most likely emerge.

Genetic factors with a minor effect on tumor development by MTV-P from the GR strains have recently been described by Van Nie and Hilgers (1976). Two types of resistance phenomena were observed. Neither type could prevent the early development of tumors after hormone treatment, however, they could delay it. One resistance factor was noticeable and dominant in reciprocal hybrids of GR and DBAf strains, whereas another factor was detected in the backcross population only (i.e., in the C57BL × (C57BL × GR) backcross), but not in hybrids. Therefore this factor is recessive.

C. Endogenous MTV in Low Mammary Cancer Strains

The *de novo* appearance of MTV in several low-mammary cancer strains might be regarded as an indication of the existence of genetic information for MTVs in such strains (see section on *de novo* appearance in this review). Appearance of a virulent MTV has been reported for the Af, C3Hf/Bi, NLC, CBA, C57BL, RIIIf, AKR, and BALB/c strains. The expression of this information is usually strongly inhibited, but virus might be accidentally released and subsequently transmitted as a milk factor, transforming the low cancer strains into high-mammary tumor lines. According to Bentvelzen (1968a), when the genetic transmission and spontaneous release of MTV in the C3Hf and GR mouse strains is compared with the phenomenon of lysogeny in bacteria, the spontaneous virus release would be a feature that does not fit into the accepted scheme. It is conceivable that the GR and C3Hf strains contain mutations in the genetic system which would normally repress the release of virus so that MTV could become expressed. Strains without any detectable MTV, such as BALB/c, C57BL, and 020, on the other hand, might possess a normal chromosomal form of MTV which does not become released spontaneously.

Timmermans *et al.* (1969) treated 020 mice with whole-body irradiation (200 rad) and 0.05% urethane in the drinking water. Four out of 7 animals developed mammary tumors before 1 year of age, while no tumors developed before that age in the controls. One of these tumors contained B particles. Cell-free filtrates of two other tumors induced mammary tumors in BALB/c mice (a total of 12 out of 20 animals developed mammary tumors before 1 year of age). It must be noted here that occasionally 020 females release MTV antigens into their milk (R. Nowinski, personal communication; Verstraeten *et al.*, 1976).

Boot *et al.* (1971) reported that injection of blood from previously irradiated C57BL male mice induces some mammary tumors before 1 year of age in (C57BL × C3Hf)F₁ and (020 × DBAF)F₁ mice which were forced-bred. No tumors are observed in control forced-bred mice of these hybrids.

Bentvelzen (1972a) reported on the appearance of MTV antigens as detected by immunofluorescence in organs of irradiated C57BL mice. Gillette *et al.* (1974) found MTV antigens on the membranes of lymphoid cells of low cancer strains such as BALB/c, NIH C57BL. However, one must be aware that antisera to purified MTV antigens generally contain high levels of antibodies to nonviral antigens and that rigorous absorption procedures are needed to remove such antibodies (Hilgers *et al.*, 1972). The same criticism holds for the application of the hemagglutination assay of Gillette and Junker (1973) or complement fixation (Parks *et al.*, 1972) for the detection of MTV antigens in the milk of low cancer strains (Gillette *et al.*, 1973).

With the much more sensitive radioimmunoassay, Verstraeten *et al.* (1976) found only MTV-antigen positives in the milk of the low cancer strains 020 and TSI, while C57BL, BALB/c, CBA, and MAS were negative. On the other hand, J. Haayman (unpublished results), utilizing the highly sensitive Sepharose bead immunofluorescence assay found that, at high parities, C57BL mice release small amounts of viral antigens (a few nanograms per milliliter) into their milk.

After incidental observations of MTV-like activity in a spontaneous BALB/c leukemia and the finding of some B particles in mammary gland extracts, Hageman *et al.* (1972) made a systematic study of the presence of an MTV in mammary glands of old BALB/c females. Inoculation of preparations from glands of retired breeding females induce a very high mammary tumor incidence at an early age (6–7 months) in forced-bred BALB/c females. These mammary tumors contain large quantities of B particles. It is quite possible, in view of the extreme susceptibility of BALB/c mice to exogenous MTV, that the appearance of virus in old BALB/c mice is due to horizontal transmission. Daams and Hageman (1972) claim that the virus isolated from old BALB/c mice and passaged in this strain is antigenically different from three other MTV strains (C3Hf-MTV, C3H-MTV, and GR-MTV) maintained in mice of the Netherlands Cancer Institute. Bentvelzen (1975) isolated a virulent MTV from germfree retired BALB/c breeders. He found that 4 out of 41 spontaneous mammary tumors of this strain had a high mammary tumor inducing activity.

Kimball *et al.* (1976a,b) reported that two spontaneous mammary tumors of the BALB/c produce significant amounts of MTV antigens and particles in tissue culture.

Links *et al.* (1972) transformed BALB/c kidney cells *in vitro* with methylcholanthrene. The resulting cell line produces MTV antigens and B-type particles (Calafat *et al.*, 1974). The virus is highly oncogenic (Links *et al.*, 1974). A similar procedure can induce MTV antigens in other low-cancer strains, such as the C57BL (J. Links and J. Calafat, personal communication).

V. Molecular Biological Studies

Despite the use of an inferior MTV-cDNA probe, which represented only a small portion of the viral genome, it is generally accepted that Varmus *et al.* (1972) are the first to have shown the presence of DNA homologous to MTV-RNA in normal cellular DNA of the mouse. This study can be regarded as the beginning of the molecular era in MTV research.

Varmus *et al.* (1972) found the same high copy number (90) of viral sequences per diploid cell in the GR as well as in the C57BL. The immediate impact of this observation was that it confirmed the hypothesis of genetic transmission of MTV in the GR (Bentvelzen, 1968a); it also provided evidence that low-cancer strains would contain information for such a virus. The fact that Varmus and co-workers were unable to detect any genotypic differences between these phenotypically dissimilar strains indicated to them that the inherited difference between them would reside in regulatory genes that govern the expression of viral information, as was postulated earlier by Bentvelzen (1968a) from his Mendelian analysis.

In a subsequent study Varmus *et al.* (1975), using more representative reagents (a single-stranded cDNA instead of a double-stranded polymerase product used in the earlier study), found a considerably lower copy number per cell (16–22) in 5 different mouse strains. Only the GR had in this study a remarkably high number of viral DNA copies per cell, 56.

Scolnick *et al.* (1974) found the same amount of MTV-specific DNA in a great variety of mouse cell lines including one derived from a wild mouse. The GR mouse strain was not included in this study.

Michalides and Schlom (1975) found 14–18 copies per mammary tumor cell of the RIII and C3H strains and 36 for GR tumor cells.

In a subsequent study Michalides *et al.* (1976) reported for the DNA of livers of RIII, C3H, and BALB/c, fewer than 10 copies; 32 copies were found in the DNA of GR livers. In mammary tumors induced by milk-borne (exogenous) MTV in RIII and C3H, a slightly higher copy number was found than in the liver. There seemed also to be qualitative differences in nucleotide sequences between the exogenous MTV and the endogenous ones, as was concluded earlier (Michalides and Schlom, 1975) from competition hybridization experiments.

No differences were found in the number and nature of MTV-DNA copies in livers and mammary tumors of the GR strain (R. Michalides, personal communication). This proves once more that mammary tumors in the GR strain are caused by a genetically transmitted (germinal) provirus.

In the molecular competition hybridization experiments of Michalides and Schlom (1975), no differences were detected among the RNAs of the MTVs from GR, RIII, A, and C3H, but they found a 25% difference between these viruses and the endogenous MTV-L of the C3Hf strain. This is in contrast with results from comparable studies by Ringold *et al.* (1976). The latter authors found no difference among the RNAs from GR strain virus (MTV-P), MTV-S, and MTV-L from the C3H and C3Hf strains, respectively. They also did not find a difference in the so-called MTV-S strains from C3H, DBA, and A and MTV from wild mice passaged in the BALB/c strain.

Varmus *et al.* (1973), using a single-stranded probe synthesized in the presence of antinomycin D, found a strain-dependent variation in the amount of MTV-RNA in lactating mammary glands. High levels of such RNA were found in the glands of high-cancer strains such as GR and C3H, and considerably lower numbers of genome equivalents per cell were found in glands from C57BL or BALB/c. The implication of this study for the presence of MTV-RNA is that the occasional mammary tumor arising in such low-cancer strains is associated with the (partial) switching-on of genetic information of an endogenous MTV.

Another consequence of these studies is that the phenotypic difference between high- and low-cancer strains is due to a quantitative control at the transcriptional level.

Very interesting was the observed correlation between virus production and the amount of MTV-RNA in the progeny of backcrosses between GR and C57BL strains. However, Spiegelman *et al.* (1972) failed to detect MTV-RNA in lactating glands of the C57BL. A possible explanation was that their MTV-DNA probe did not reflect a large enough portion of the MTV genome in order to detect small amounts of viral RNA. Schlom *et al.* (1973) found, however, that various tissues of aging or carcinogen-treated low-cancer strain mice contain significant amounts of MTV-specific RNA. This would imply that aging or treatment with nonviral carcinogens abrogates the transcriptional control of the MTV germinal provirus.

VI. Speculative Considerations and Concluding Remarks

A clear distinction must be made between somatic and germinal proviruses in oncorna virology (Bentvelzen and Daams, 1972). The first category, the existence of which was postulated by Temin (1964), made acceptable by the discovery of reverse transcriptase (Temin and

Mizutani, 1970; Baltimore, 1970) and definitely proved by transfection experiments (Hill and Hillova, 1972), concerns the DNA copy of infecting, exogenous virus. The second category, first postulated by Bentvelzen (1968a) on the basis of his studies on the genetic transmission of MTV and definitely proved for the mouse leukemia virus (Chattopadhyay et al., 1974), refers to the integrated DNA copy of endogenous virus.

In contrast to the somatic provirus, the germinal provirus is present in all cells of the organism and is transmitted via the germ cells to the offspring. The somatic provirus can be present only in those cell species that have a receptor for the exogenous virus. Besides the target organ for tumorigenesis, many other tissues must have such receptors. It is known that MTV has a relatively wide organ distribution (Nandi and McGrath, 1973, for review), but so far, the mammary gland seems to be the only tissue that can be transformed by MTV. However, in the molecular biological studies of Michalides et al. (1976), MTV-S specific nucleotide sequences of the exogenous virus could not be detected in the liver but were present in the mammary tumor.

So far, a complete B-type particle has not been isolated from every mouse strain. Molecular biological studies failed to prove definitely that every mouse strain contains genetic information for an MTV. It is possible that some strains, like C57BL, carry only a fragment of a germinal provirus. In that case, it would be more appropriate to use the term protovirus (Temin, 1972). De novo appearance of MTV in certain low-cancer strains might be due to the ontogenetic evolution of such a protovirus.

A very important aspect of endogenous mammary tumor viruses in mice is their oncogenicity for the natural host. This remains to be established for the endogenous C-type viruses in many vertebrate species. The few cases with established oncogenicity for endogenous viruses have been demonstrated only by using the endogenous virus as an exogenous virus, i.e., by passage of cell-free material (for review, see Gross, 1970). If, however, the C-type viral induction genes Akv-1 and/or Akv-2 (Rowe, 1972; Rowe and Hartley, 1972) are demonstrated to be associated with spontaneous leukemogenesis, the final proof for natural oncogenicity of C-type viruses may be regarded as provided. This has already been accomplished for endogenous mammary tumor viruses.

Endogenous mammary tumor viruses are good tools for understanding neoplastic transformation, because various bottlenecks encountered with exogenous viruses such as inability to penetrate the target cell due to the absence of receptors are circumvented. Formal genetic analysis might make it possible to localize on the chromosome that gene of the germinal provirus which codes for the neoplastic transformation of the mammary gland, which we propose to call the "mam" gene in analogy to the "sarc" gene of sarcoma viruses (Stehelin et al., 1976). The Mendelian approach (crossing-over studies, development of congenic lines) would be comparable with the molecular approach of analyzing the genome of DNA viruses with restriction enzymes (Graham et al., 1975).

There is a discrepancy in the number of MTV DNA copies in normal cellular DNA between Varmus et al. (1972), on the one hand, and Michalides et al. (1976) on the other hand. This difference might be due not only to differences in technique, but also in the cDNA probes, that of Varmus et al. (1972) representing a considerably smaller portion of the viral genome. Since Varmus and co-workers reported 45 copies per haploid genome in two mouse strains and the other 2–16 in various mouse strains, it is possible that the segment detected by the probe prepared by Varmus is present in a much higher number than the complete germinal proviruses.

It has been reported for DNA tumor viruses (Sambrook et al., 1975) that more copies of certain portions of the viral genome are integrated into the transformed cells. These reiterated segments seem to contain the transforming genes, as detected by transformation experiments with DNA fragments prepared with restriction enzymes (Graham et al., 1975). The reiterated sequences detected by Varmus and co-workers might represent the "mam" gene.

Speculating further, it might be assumed that the multiple "mam" genes play a role in the normal functioning of the mammary gland, as has been proposed for the "sarc" gene detected in normal avian DNA (Stehelin et al., 1976). The detection of MTV-RNA in the lactating mammary glands of low-mammary cancer strains (Varmus et al., 1973) may be explained as functional expression of such "mam" genes instead of expression of the germinal provirus. Continuous expression of such genes, as is the case, for instance, when endogenous virus is continuously released, leads to neoplastic transformation. It is possible that mammary tumors result from unregulated expression of cellular "mam" genes in the absence of endogenous virus production. This "unitarian" hypothesis of mammary carcinogenesis attempting to explain viral, hormonal, chemical, and radiation-induced carcinogenesis on the basis of expression of the "mam" gene can be tested with the new molecular and immunological techniques available.

This hypothesis bears a great resemblance to the "oncogene" hypothesis of Huebner and Todaro (1969). The important difference is the assumption of a tissue-specific gene for conversion of the mammary gland in contrast to the "omnipotent" oncogene operative in all cases of carcinogenesis.

Lymphoid leukemias occasionally occur in the GR mouse strain without expression of C-type virus. These leukemias always exhibit MTV antigens in the cytoplasm and at the cell surface (Calafat *et al.*, 1974; Hilgers *et al.*, 1975). The hypothesis that these leukemias would be induced by endogenous MTV-P is presently being tested by comparing leukemia incidences between the parental GR strain and a congenic strain in which the gene for MTV-P (Mtv-2) has been removed. If this hypothesis holds true, the "mam" gene hypothesis should be considerably modified, as that the "mam" gene does not have such a narrow tissue specificity.

Although Michalides *et al.* (1976) found considerably fewer DNA copies of MTV in the normal cellular DNA of the GR strain than did Varmus *et al.* (1972), the reported number for this strain is remarkably higher (16) than for the other strains—BALB/c (2), C3H and RIII (3–4) per haploid genome. This high number in the GR strain seems to be in conflict with the single gene (Mtv-2) reported to be associated with MTV-P. It is possible that multiple copies of the MTV genome are randomly distributed throughout the cellular genome with a considerably reduced rate of expression than that of MTV-P. It is more likely, however, that 12 copies of MTV-P proviral genome are located in tandem in a single chromosome, as has been postulated for RD-114 and the protovirus of feline leukemia virus in the domestic cat (Beneveniste and Todaro, 1975b). This hypothesis can be proved when a congenic line of GR lacking Mtv-2 has 4 or fewer copies, and reciprocally when a congenic line of C57BL with Mtv-2 has 16 copies.

In F_1 hybrids of GR with any other mouse strain, such as BALB/c, one may imagine a loop consisting of a string of MTV proviruses (see Fig. 2). The existence of this loop would explain the very high rate of virus production in the GR strain (Souissi *et al.*, 1974; Verstraeten *et al.*, 1975; Noon *et al.*, 1975) as compared to other high-cancer strains. The loop on the Mtv-2 locus is not allelic with the Mtv-1 locus controlling the release of MTV-L in the C3H strain. It is possible that the large number of MTV copies are integrated at a site where in other mouse strains a germinal provirus of MTV is also located, e.g., with one of the two possible proviruses present in the BALB/c.

In our opinion, the GR strain has acquired this string of proviruses relatively recently, because mouse strains that are genetically closely related to the GR strain, as determined by their isoenzyme pattern and their H-2 determinants (J. Hilgers, unpublished results; A. Dux and O.

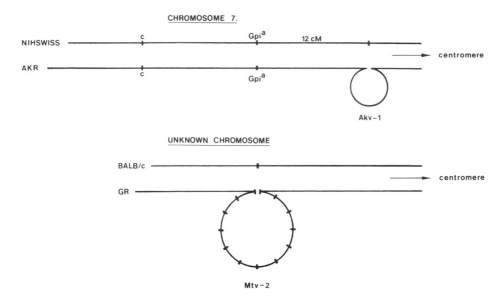

FIG. 2. Chromosomal localization of acquired germinal proviruses in hybrid mice.

Mühlbock, personal communication), are lacking the Mtv-2 gene. Surprisingly, this trait was not selected for, in contrast to spontaneous leukemia in the AKR strain (Cole and Furth, 1941).

Similarly, one can speculate about the Mtv-1 gene of the C3Hf, which is presumably also present in RIIIf. These strains have 1 or 2 more copies of MTV-DNA than does the BALB/c. The BALB/c strain might be regarded as the strain with the "primordial" MTV proviruses only. At least one of these seems to be highly oncogenic upon passage in an exogenous form. The *de novo* appearance of virulent agents in the C3Hf and other strains suggests that many if not all laboratory mouse strains carry a primordial provirus coding for a virulent MTV.

Somatic cell hybridization, as has been employed by Strand *et al.* (1976) for the localization of germinal proviruses of murine leukemia viruses in mouse–human cell hybrids, can also be applied for the localization of Mtv-2 and other germinal proviruses of endogenous MTVs. This method can also be used for detecting the chromosome(s) that harbor somatic proviruses.

MTV-specific sequences have been found in the DNA of commensal and feral *Mus musculus,* in *Mus caroli* and *Mus cervicolor,* but not in other rodent genera, such as *Rattus, Cricetulus, Microtus,* and *Peromyscus* (Ringold *et al.,* 1976). It seems very likely that MTV sequences were acquired by the genus *Mus* 10–15 millions of years ago in a similar way to that suggested for the acquisition of baboon-type virus by the ancestor of the domestic cat some 3–10 million years ago and the acquisition of the protovirus for feline leukemia virus from a primitive rodent by the pig and some cats (Benveniste and Todaro, 1974, 1975a; Benveniste *et al.*, 1975).

The crucial experiment in which acquisition of a provirus by the germ line has been accomplished in the laboratory was performed by Jaenisch *et al.* (1975), who inoculated blastocysts with Moloney leukemia virus, resulting in occasional Mendelian transmission of this virus. Zeilmaker attempted to do this in the mid-1960s with MTV, but failed (Nandi, 1972). His failure is probably due to a difference in the infection procedure, in that he injected virus into the blastocysts, making the proper processing of the virus difficult.

It seems to be the consensus at present that differences between high- and low-cancer strains can be due to differences in the regulation of the expression of endogenous MTV (excluding those cases in which an exogenous milk factor is involved). However, relatively little is known about the nature of regulation. In the BALB/c mouse strain, there is considerable inhibition of the expression of endogenous MTV. When this virus after occasional retrieval is passaged in the BALB/c, no obvious inhibition is encountered. The BALB/c genome also does not inhibit the release of MTV-L from the C3Hf strain in F_1 hybrids. The BALB/c mouse strain seems to provide even a promoting factor as far as MTV-L is concerned, because (1) the amount of virus in the milk is considerably higher than in the C3Hf strain and (2) mammary tumors appear at a higher incidence and earlier (Bentvelzen and Daams, 1969; Van Nie and Verstraeten, 1975). In this mouse strain, exogenous MTV-S and MTV-P are also extremely well replicated, and tumors can be induced with these viruses at high frequency.

The inhibition of spontaneous release of the endogenous virus has been explained by the existence of a regulatory gene that is closely linked to the germinal provirus and represses its transcription. Its action would be limited to only that provirus with which it is closely linked, but not to other proviruses, either germinal or somatic. If the somatic provirus is integrated close to an endogenous virus, as has been postulated for exogenous avian tumor viruses by Shoyab *et al.* (1976), the range of the repressor is truly limited. The high rate of release of MTV-P in the GR strain is probably due to the lack of such a closely linked inhibitory gene.

In contrast to hybrids of C3Hf and BALB/c, hybrids of C3Hf with C57BL or 020 have limited expression of endogenous MTV-L being associated with a lower tumor incidence and a prolonged latency period. There seems to be an inhibitory gene in these strains which does not display the position effect postulated for the BALB/c strain. This gene might be comparable to the Fv-1 gene limiting C-type virus replication in mice (Lilly and Pincus, 1973), according to Hilgers and Galesloot (1973). In contrast to the gene that has a short-range action, the latter gene has only a quantitative effect on the expression of endogenous virus. There is no complete inhibition in the production of MTV antigens.

A noteworthy exception to the correlation between low quantities of endogenous MTV-L and delayed tumor appearance in hybrids of C3Hf with low cancer strains is the hybrid $(TSI \times C3Hf)F_1$. There is good virus expression in tumors arising at a very late age (J. Hilgers and L. M. Boot, unpublished results). This situation resembles the observed delayed leukemogenesis in AKR hybrids of the $Fv-1^{nn}$ type, for example with CBA, where levels of endogenous virus are as high as in the high-leukemia strain (Barnes, 1976).

The release of MTV-P does not seem to be hampered in the GR strain by the presence of a repressor. Epigenetic factors may control transcription of the provirus, since only a few viral RNA molecules are found in GR liver cells (Varmus et al., 1973). It can be envisaged that initiating factors which can be provided by only certain cell species are needed for transcription. In other words, its expression is dependent on the differentiation process.

It has been a rewarding experience for us to review several old papers on the transmission of and susceptibility to mouse mammary tumor virus. Various phenomena that were poorly understood in the 1940s and the 1950s can now be interpreted with our present knowledge of proviruses, either germinal or somatic. MTV research has entered its molecular era. Certain hypotheses have been affirmed by the use of molecular biological methods. Several postulates brought forward in this review can be readily tested with these techniques. However, it is obvious to us that "old-fashioned" biological studies, e.g., host range studies or Mendelian analysis in which tumor incidences are also taken into account, remain essential and will be complementary to the molecular and immunological studies.

Acknowledgment

This work was supported in part by contracts with the National Cancer Institute (United States), contract numbers NO1-CP-33368 (J. H.) and NOI-CP-43328 (P. B.). We are grateful to Professor Dr. O. Mühlbock for critical reading of the manuscript.

References

Andervont, H. B. (1940). *J. Natl. Cancer Inst.* 1, 147–153.
Andervont, H. B. (1945a). *J. Natl. Cancer Inst.* 5, 383–390.
Andervont, H. B. (1945b). *J. Natl. Cancer Inst.* 5, 391–395.
Andervont, H. B. (1949). *J. Natl. Cancer Inst.* 10, 201–204.
Andervont, H. B. (1950). *J. Natl. Cancer Inst.* 11, 545–553.
Andervont, H. B. (1952). *Ann. N.Y. Acad. Sci.* 54, 1004–1011.
Andervont, H. B. (1959). *Acta Unio Int. Cancrum* 15, 124–127.
Andervont, H. B. (1963). *J. Natl. Cancer Inst.* 31, 261–272.
Andervont, H. B. (1964). *J. Natl. Cancer Inst.* 32, 1189–1198.
Andervont, H. B., and Dunn, T. B. (1948a). *J. Natl. Cancer Inst.* 8, 227–233.
Andervont, H. B., and Dunn, T. B. (1948b). *J. Natl. Cancer Inst.* 9, 89–104.
Andervont, H. B., and Dunn, T. B. (1953). *J. Natl. Cancer Inst.* 14, 317–327.
Andervont, H. B., and Dunn, T. B. (1962). *J. Natl. Cancer Inst.* 28, 159–185.
Andervont, H. B., and McEleney, W. J. (1938). *Public Health Rep.* 53, 777–783.
Andervont, H. B., Shimkiu, M. B., and Bryan, W. R. (1942). *J. Natl. Cancer Inst.* 3, 309–318.
Baltimore, D. (1970). *Nature (London)* 226, 1209–1211.
Bang, F. B., Andervont, H. B., and Vellisto, I. (1956). *Bull. Johns Hopkins Hosp.* 98, 287–306.
Barnes, R. D. (1976). *Eur. J. Cancer* 12, 283–290.
Ben-David, M., Heston, W. E., and Rodbard, D. (1969). *J. Natl. Cancer Inst.* 42, 207–218.
Bentvelzen, P. (1968a). Ph.D. Thesis, University of Leiden, Hollandia, Amsterdam.
Bentvelzen, P. (1968b). *J. Natl. Cancer Inst.* 41, 757–765.
Bentvelzen, P. (1972a). In "RNA Viruses and Host Genome in Oncogenesis" (P. Emmelot and P. Bentvelzen, eds.), pp. 309–337. North-Holland Publ., Amsterdam.
Bentvelzen, P. (1972b). *Int. Rev. Exp. Pathol.* 11, 259–297.
Bentvelzen, P. (1974a). *Biochim. Biophys. Acta* 355, 236–259.
Bentvelzen, P. (1947b). In "Viruses, Evolution and Cancer" (E. Kurstak and K. Maramorosch, eds.), pp. 279–367. Academic Press, New York.
Bentvelzen, P. (1975). *Cold Spring Harbor Symp. Quant. Biol.* 39, 1145–1150.
Bentvelzen, P., and Daams, J. H. (1969). *J. Natl. Cancer Inst.* 43, 1025–1035.
Bentvelzen, P., and Daams, J. H. (1972). *Eur. J. Clin. Biol. Res.* 13, 245–248.
Bentvelzen, P., Daams, J. H., Hageman, P., and Calafat, J. (1970). *Proc. Natl. Acad. Sci. U.S.A.* 67, 377–384.
Benveniste, R. E., and Todaro, G. L. (1974). *Nature (London)* 252, 456–459.
Benveniste, R. E., and Todaro, G. J. (1975a). *Proc. Natl. Acad. Sci. U.S.A.* 72, 4090–4094.
Benveniste, R. E., and Todaro, G. L. (1975b). *Nature (London)* 257, 506–508.
Benveniste, R. E., Sherr, C. J., and Todaro, G. J. (1975). *Science* 190, 886–888.
Bernard, W., and Guérin, M. (1958). *C. R. Hebd. Seances Acad. Sci., Ser. D* 247, 1802–1805.
Bernhard, W., Guérin, M., and Oberling, C. (1956). *Acta Unio Int. Cancrum* 12, 545–554.
Biancifori, C., Lotti, G., and Martinez, C. (1958). *Int. Symp. Mammary Cancer, Proc., 2nd, 1957* pp. 419–422.
Bittner, J. J. (1936a). *Science* 84, 162.
Bittner, J. J. (1936b). *Proc. Soc. Exp. Biol. Med.* 34, 42–48.
Bittner, J. J. (1940). *J. Natl. Cancer Inst.* 1, 155–168.

Bittner, J. J. (1941). *Cancer Res.* **1**, 113–114.
Bittner, J. J. (1942a). *Cancer Res.* **2**, 540–545.
Bittner, J. J. (1942b). *Cancer Res.* **2**, 710–721.
Bittner, J. J. (1943). *Cancer Res.* **3**, 441–447.
Bittner, J. J. (1944a). *Cancer Res.* **4**, 159–167.
Bittner, J. J. (1944b). *Cancer Res.* **4**, 779–784.
Bittner, J. J. (1945). *Proc. Soc. Exp. Biol. Med.* **59**, 43–44.
Bittner, J. J. (1952a). *Cancer Res.* **12**, 387–398.
Bittner, J. J. (1952b). *Cancer Res.* **12**, 594–601.
Bittner, J. J. (1953). *Cancer Res.* **13**, 672–676.
Bittner, J. J. (1954). *Cancer Res.* **14**, 783–789.
Bittner, J. J. (1956). *J. Natl. Cancer Inst.* **16**, 1263–1286.
Bittner, J. J. (1957). *Ann. N.Y. Acad. Sci.* **68**, 636–648.
Bittner, J. J. (1958). *Ann. N.Y. Acad. Sci.* **71**, 943–975.
Bittner, J. J., and Frantz, M. J. (1954). *Proc. Soc. Exp. Biol. Med.* **86**, 698–701.
Bittner, J. J., and Huseby, R. A. (1946). *Cancer Res.* **6**, 235–239.
Bittner, J. J., Huseby, R. A., Visscher, M. B., Ball, Z. B., and Smith, F. (1944). *Science* **99**, 83–85.
Blair, P. B. (1958). *Science* **127**, 518.
Blair, P. B. (1960). *Cancer Res.* **20**, 635–642.
Blair, P. B. (1968). *Curr. Top. Microbiol. Immunol.* **45**, 1–69.
Blair, P. B. (1969). *Cancer Res.* **29**, 745–748.
Blair, P. B., and Lane, M. A. (1974a). *J. Immunol.* **112**, 439–443.
Blair, P. B., and Lane, M. A. (1974b). *J. Immunol.* **113**, 1446–1449.
Blair, P. B., and Lane, M. A. (1975). *J. Immunol.* **114**, 17–23.
Blair, P. B., Lane, M. A., and Yagi, M. J. (1974). *J. Immunol.* **112**, 693–705.
Boot, L. M. (1969). Ph.D. Thesis, University of Amsterdam, Noord-Hollandse Uitgevers Maatschappij N.V., Amsterdam.
Boot, L. M., and Mühlbock, O. (1956). *Acta Unio Int. Cancrum* **12**, 569–581.
Boot, L. M., Bentvelzen, P., Calafat, J., Röpcke, G., and Timmermans, A. (1971). *Proc. Int. Cancer Congr., 10th, 1970* Vol. 1, pp. 434–440.
Bryan, W. R., Kahler, H., Shimkin, M. B., and Andervont, H. B. (1942). *J. Natl. Cancer Inst.* **12**, 451–455.
Bucciarelli, E., Bolis, G. B., and Squantini, F. (1970). *Lav. Ist. Anat. Istol. Patol. Univ. Studi Perugia* **30**, 57–72.
Burrows, H. (1941). *Cancer Res.* **1**, 121–122.
Calafat, J., Buijs, F., Hageman, P. C., Links, J., Hilgers, J., and Hekman, A. (1974). *J. Natl. Cancer Inst.* **53**, 977–991.
Charney, J., and Moore, D. H. (1972). *J. Natl. Cancer Inst.* **48**, 1125–1129.
Charney, J., Pullinger, B. D., and Moore, D. H. (1969). *J. Natl. Cancer Inst.* **43**, 1289–1296.
Chattopadhyay, S. K., Rowe, W. P., Teich, N. M., and Lowy, D. R. (1975). *Proc. Natl. Acad. Sci. U.S.A.* **72**, 906–910.
Cole, R. K., and Furth, J. (1941). *Cancer Res.* **1**, 957–965.
Daams, J. H., and Hageman, P. C. (1972). *In* "Fundamental Research on Mammary Cancer" (J. Mouriquand, ed.), pp. 97–100. Inserm, Paris.
DeOme, K. B., Young, L., and Nandi, S. (1967). *Proc. Am. Assoc. Cancer Res.* **8**, 13 (abstr.).
Deringer, M. K. (1959). *J. Natl. Cancer Inst.* **22**, 995–1002.
Deringer, M. K. (1962). *J. Natl. Cancer Inst.* **28**, 203–210.
Deringer, M. K. (1970). *J. Natl. Cancer Inst.* **45**, 215–218.

Dmochowski, L. (1945a). *Br. J. Exp. Pathol.* **26**, 192–197.

Dmochowski, L. (1945b). *Br. J. Exp. Pathol.* **26**, 267–269.

Dmochowski, L. (1948). *Br. J. Cancer* **2**, 94–102.

Dmochowski, L. (1953a). *Adv. Cancer Res.* **1**, 104–172.

Dmochowski, L. (1953b). *Br. J. Cancer* **7**, 73–119.

Dmochowski, L. (1954). *Proc. Am. Assoc. Cancer Res.* **1**, 11–12 (abstr.).

Dmochowski, L. (1956). *Acta Unio Int. Cancrum* **12**, 582–618.

Dmochowski, L. (1971). *Tex. Rep. Biol. Med.* **29**, 370.

Dmochowski, L., and Grey, C. E. (1957). *Ann. N.Y. Acad. Sci.* **68**, 559–615.

Dmochowski, L., Haagensen, C. D., and Moore, D. H. (1954). *Proc. Am. Assoc. Cancer Res.* **1**, 12 (abstr.).

Dmochowski, L., Grey, C. E., and Sykes, J. A. (1963). *Acta Unio Int. Cancrum* **19**, 276–279.

Dmochowski, L., Langford, P. L., Williams, W. C., Liebelt, A. G., and Liebelt, R. A. (1968). *J. Natl. Cancer Inst.* **40**, 1339–1358.

Dux, A. (1972). *In* "RNA Viruses and Host Genome in Oncogenesis" (P. Emmelot and P. Bentvelzen, eds.), pp. 301–308. North-Holland Publ., Amsterdam.

Dux, A., and Mühlbock, O. (1966). *Int. J. Cancer* **1**, 5–17.

Dux, A., and Mühlbock, O. (1968). *J. Natl. Cancer Inst.* **40**, 1259–1265.

Fekete, E., and Little, C. C. (1942). *Cancer Res.* **2**, 525–530.

Felluga, B., Claude, A., and Mrena, E. (1969). *J. Natl. Cancer Inst.* **43**, 319–330.

Fieldsteel, A. H., Dawson, P. J., Kurahara, C., and Brooks, R. E. (1975). *Br. J. Cancer* **32**, 741–744.

Foulds, L. (1949). *Br. J. Cancer* **3**, 230–239.

Gardner, W. U. (1941). *Cancer Res.* **1**, 345–348.

Gardner, W. U., Pfeiffer, C. A., and Trentin, J. J. (1959). *In* "The Physiopathology of Cancer" (F. Hamburger, ed.), pp. 152–237. Harper (Hoeber), New York.

Gillette, R. W., and Junker, D. (1973). *Appl. Microbiol.* **26**, 63–65.

Gillette, R. W., Sorio, M., and Parks, W. P. (1973). *8th Meet. Mammary Cancer Exp. Anim. Man* Abstr., p. 37.

Gillette, R. W., Robertson, S., Brown, R., and Blackman, K. E. (1974). *J. Natl. Cancer Inst.* **53**, 499–505.

Graham, F. L., Abrahams, P. J., Mulder, C., Heyneker, H. L., Warnaer, S. D., De Vries, F. A. J., Fiers, W., and Van der Eb, A. J. (1975). *Cold Spring Harbor Symp. Quant. Biol.* **39**, 637–650.

Gross, L. (1951). *Proc. Soc. Exp. Biol. Med.* **76**, 27–32.

Gross, L. (1970). "Oncogenic Viruses." Pergamon, Oxford.

Hageman, P. (1973). *8th Meet. Mammary Cancer Exp. Anim. Man* Abstr., p. 46.

Hageman, P. C., Links, J., and Bentvelzen, P. (1968). *J. Natl. Cancer Inst.* **40**, 1319–1324.

Hageman, P. C., Calafat, J., and Daams, J. H. (1972). *In* "RNA Viruses and Host Genome in Oncogenesis" (P. Emmelot and P. Bentvelzen, eds.), pp. 283–300. North-Holland Publ., Amsterdam.

Heston, W. E. (1958). *Ann. N.Y. Acad. Sci.* **71**, 931–942.

Heston, W. E. (1972). *In* "RNA Viruses and Host Genome in Oncogenesis" (P. Emmelot and P. Bentvelzen, eds.), pp. 13–24. North-Holland Publ., Amsterdam.

Heston, W. E. (1976). *Adv. Cancer Res.* **23**, 1–21.

Heston, W. E., and Andervont, H. B. (1944). *J. Natl. Cancer Inst.* **4**, 403–407.

Heston, W. E., and Deringer, M. K. (1952). *J. Natl. Cancer Inst.* **13**, 167–175.

Heston, W. E., and Parks, W. P. (1975). *Can. J. Genet. Cytol.* **17**, 493–503.

Heston, W. E., and Vlahakis, G. (1967). *Collect. Pap. Annu. Symp. Fundam. Cancer Res.* **12**, 347–363.

Heston, W. E., and Vlahakis, G. (1971). *Int. J. Cancer* **7**, 141–148.

Heston, W. E., Deringer, M. K., and Andervont, H. B. (1945). *J. Natl. Cancer Inst.* **5**, 289–307.

Heston, W. E., Deringer, M. K., Dunn, T. B., and Levillian, W. D. (1950). *J. Natl. Cancer Inst.* **10**, 1139–1155.

Heston, W. E., Deringer, M. K., and Dunn, T. B. (1956). *J. Natl. Cancer Inst.* **16**, 1309–1334.

Heston, W. E., Vlahakis, G., and Deringer, M. K. (1960). *J. Natl. Cancer Inst.* **24**, 721–731.

Heston, W. E., Hall, W. T., Vlahakis, G., Charney, J., and Moore, D. H. (1970). *J. Natl. Cancer Inst.* **45**, 937–940.

Hilgers, J., and Galesloot, J. (1973). *Int. J. Cancer* **11**, 780–793.

Hilgers, J., Williams, W. C., Myers, B., and Dmochowski, L. (1971). *Virology* **45**, 470–483.

Hilgers, J., Nowinski, R. C., Geering, G., and Hardy, W. (1972). *Cancer Res.* **32**, 98–106.

Hilgers, J., Theuns, G., and Van Nie, R. (1973). *Int. J. Cancer* **12**, 568–576.

Hilgers, J., Haverman, J., Nusse, R., Van Blitterswijk, W. J., Cleton, F. J., Hageman, P. C., Van Nie, R., and Calafat, J. (1975). *J. Natl. Cancer Inst.* **54**, 1323–1333.

Hill, M., and Hillova, J. (1972). *Virology* **49**, 309–313.

Huebner, R. J., and Todaro, G. J. (1969). *Proc. Natl. Acad. Sci. U.S.A.* **64**, 1087–1094.

Hummel, K. P., and Little, C. C. (1959). *J. Natl. Cancer Inst.* **23**, 813–821.

Huseby, R. A., and Bittner, J. J. (1948). *Acta Unio Int. Cancrum* **6**, 197–205.

Jackson Laboratory Staff. (1933). *Science* **78**, 465–466.

Jaenisch, R., Fan, H., and Croker, B. (1975). *Proc. Natl. Acad. Sci. U.S.A.* **10**, 4008–4012.

Kimball, P. C., Boehm-Truitt, M., Schochetman, G., and Schlom, J. (1976a). *J. Natl. Cancer Inst.* **56**, 111–117.

Kimball, P. C., Michalides, R., Colcher, D., and Schlom, J. (1976b). *J. Natl. Cancer Inst.* **56**, 119–124.

Korteweg, R. (1934). *Ned. Tijdschr. Geneeskd.* **78**, 240–245.

Korteweg, R. (1935a). *Ned. Tijdschr. Geneeskd.* **79**, 1463–1505.

Korteweg, R. (1935b). *Verh. Conf. Leeuwenhoekvereeniging, 4th*, pp. 57–62.

Korteweg, R. (1936a). *Genetica (The Hague)* **18**, 350–371.

Korteweg, R. (1936b). *Mitt. Int. Kongr. Krebsforsch., 2nd*, pp. 151–153.

Kusnierczijk, P., and Pèknicova, J. (1975). *Folia Biol. (Prague)* **21**, 435 (abstr.).

Lane, M. A., Roubinian, J., Slomick, M., Trefts, P., and Blair, P. (1975). *J. Immunol.* **114**, 24–29.

Lathrop, A. E. C., and Loeb, L. (1913). *Proc. Soc. Exp. Biol. Med.* **11**, 34–38.

Lathrop, A. F. C., and Loeb, L. (1915a). *J. Exp. Med.* **22**, 646–673.

Lathrop, A. E. C., and Loeb, L. (1915b). *J. Exp. Med.* **22**, 713–731.

Law, L. W. (1941). *Proc. Soc. Exp. Biol. Med.* **48**, 486–487.

Liebelt, A. G., and Liebelt, R. A. (1967). *In* "Carcinogenesis, A Broad Critique," pp. 315–340. Williams & Wilkins, Baltimore, Maryland.

Lilly, F. (1966). *Natl. Cancer Inst., Monogr.* **22**, 631–642.

Lilly, F., and Pincus, T. (1973). *Adv. Cancer Res.* **17**, 231–277.

Links, J., Buys, F., and Tol, O. (1972). *In* "Fundamental Research on Mammary Cancer" (J. Mouriquand, ed.), pp. 263–268. Inserm, Paris.

Links, J., Buys, F., Calafat, J., and Tol, O. (1974). *9th Meet. Mammary Cancer Exp. Anim. Man* Abstr. No. 38, p. 53.

Lopez, D. M., Ortis-Muniz, G., and Sigel, M. M. (1976). *Proc. Soc. Exp. Biol. Med.* **151**, 225–230.

Luria, S. E. (1958). *Ann. N.Y. Acad. Sci.* **71**, 1085–1091.

Lynch, C. J. (1925). *J. Exp. Med.* **42**, 829–840.

MacDowell, E. C., Potter, J. S., and Taylor, M. J. (1945). *Cancer Res.* **5**, 65–83.

McLaren, A., and Michie, D. (1954). *J. Embryol. Exp. Morphol.* **2**, 149–161.

Matsuzawa, A., and Yamamoto, T. (1972). *Exp. Leukemogenesis, Pop. Jpn. Cancer Assoc. Symp. Exp. Lenk. Res. Jpn., 1970* Gann Monogr. Cancer Res. No. 12, pp. 119–130.

Matsuzawa, A., Yamamoto, T., and Suzuki, K. (1970). *Jpn. J. Exp. Med.* **40**, 159–181.

Michalides, R., and Schlom, J. (1975). *Proc. Natl. Acad. Sci. U.S.A.* **72**, 4635–4639.

Michalides, R., Vlahakis, G., and Schlom, J. (1976). *Int. J. Cancer* **18**, 105–115.

Miller, E. W., and Pybus, F. C. (1944). *Cancer Res.* **4**, 84–93.

Mintz, B. (1970). *Collect. Pap. Annu. Symp. Fundam. Cancer Res.* **23**, 477–520.

Mintz, B., and Slemmer, G. (1969). *J. Natl. Cancer Inst.* **43**, 87–95.

Mintz, B., Custer, R. P., and Donelly, J. (1971). *Int. Rev. Exp. Pathol.* **10**, 143–179.

Moore, D. H. (1963). *Nature (London)* **198**, 429–433.

Moore, D. H., Charney, J., and Holben, J. A. (1974). *J. Natl. Cancer Inst.* **52**, 1757–1762.

Moore, D. H., Holben, J. A., and Charney, J. (1976). *J. Natl. Cancer Inst.* (in press).

Mühlbock, O. (1950a). *J. Natl. Cancer Inst.* **10**, 861–864.

Mühlbock, O. (1950b). *Acta Physiol. Pharmacol. Neerl.* **1**, 645–650.

Mühlbock, O. (1951). *Proc. K. Ned. Akad. Wet.* **54**, 386–390.

Mühlbock, O. (1952). *J. Natl. Cancer Inst.* **12**, 819–837.

Mühlbock, O. (1956). *Acta Unio Int. Cancrum* **12**, 665–681.

Mühlbock, O. (1965). *Eur. J. Cancer* **1**, 123–124.

Mühlbock, O. (1966). *Jaarb. Kankeronder. Kankerbestr.* **16**, 9–16.

Mühlbock, O. (1972). *In* "RNA Viruses and Host Genome in Oncogenesis" (P. Emmelot and P. Bentvelzen, eds.), pp. 339–349. North-Holland Publ., Amsterdam.

Mühlbock, O., and Bentvelzen, P. (1968). *Perspect. Virol.* **6**, 75–87.

Mühlbock, O., and Boot, L. M. (1960). *Natl. Cancer Inst., Monogr.* **4**, 129–137.

Mühlbock, O., and Dux, A. (1971). *Transplant. Proc.* **3**, 1247–1250.

Mühlbock, O., and Dux, A. (1972). *In* "Fundamental Research on Mammary Cancer" (J. Mouriquand, ed.), pp. 11–19. Inserm, Paris.

Mühlbock, O., and Dux, A. (1974). *J. Natl. Cancer Inst.* **53**, 993–996.

Mühlbock, O., and van Rijssel, T. G. (1954). *J. Natl. Cancer Inst.* **15**, 73–97.

Mühlbock, O., van Ebbenhorst Tengbergen, W., and van Rijssel, T. G. (1952). *J. Natl. Cancer Inst.* **18**, 505–531.

Müller, M., and Zotter, S. (1973). *J. Natl. Cancer Inst.* **50**, 713–718.

Murray, W. S. (1941a). *Cancer Res.* **1**, 123–129.

Murray, W. S. (1941b). *Cancer Res.* **1**, 790–792.

Murray, W. S. (1963). *J. Natl. Cancer Inst.* **30**, 605–610.

Murray, W. S., and Little, C. C. (1935). *Genetics* **20**, 466–496.

Murray, W. S., and Little, C. C. (1936). *Amer. J. Cancer* **27**, 516–518.

Murray, W. S., and Little, C. C. (1939). *Am. J. Cancer* **37**, 536–552.

Murray, W. S., and Little, C. C. (1967). *J. Natl. Cancer Inst.* **38**, 639–656.

Murray, W. S., and Warner, S. G. (1947). *J. Natl. Cancer Inst.* **7**, 183–188.

Nandi, S. (1961). *Proc. Soc. Exp. Biol. Med.* **108**, 1–3.

Nandi, S. (1972). *In* "Fundamental Research on Mammary Cancer" (J. Mouriquand, ed.), pp. 189–192. Inserm, Paris.

Nandi, S. (1974). *J. Natl. Cancer Inst.* **52**, 1797–1804.

Nandi, S., and Bern, H. A. (1960). *J. Natl. Cancer Inst.* **24**, 907–931.

Nandi, S., and DeOme, K. B. (1965). *J. Natl. Cancer Inst.* **35**, 299–308.

Nandi, S., and Helmich, C. (1974). *J. Natl. Cancer Inst.* **52**, 1285–1290.

Nandi, S., and McGrath, C. M. (1973). *Adv. Cancer Res.* **17**, 353–414.

Nandi, S., Handin, M., Robinson, A., Pitelka, D. R., and Webber, L. E. (1966). *J. Natl. Cancer Inst.* **36**, 783–801.

Noon, M. C., Wolford, R. G., and Parks, W. (1975). *J. Immunol.* **115**, 653–658.

Parks, W., Gillette, R. W., Blackman, K., Verna, J. E., and Sibal, L. R. (1972). *In* "Fundamental Research on Mammary Cancer" (J. Mouriquand, ed.), pp. 77–90. Inserm, Paris.

Parks, W. P., Howk, R. S., Scolnick, E. M., Oroszlan, S., and Gilden, R. V. (1974). *J. Virol.* **13**, 1200–1210.

Peacock, A. (1953). *Br. J. Cancer* **7**, 352–357.

Peacock, A. (1956). *Br. J. Cancer* **10**, 715–718.

Peacock, A. (1963). *Br. J. Cancer* **17**, 252–254.

Pitelka, D. R., Bern, H. A., Nandi, S., and DeOme, K. B. (1964). *J. Natl. Cancer Inst.* **33**, 867–885.

Pogossiantz, H. (1956). *Acta Unio Int. Cancrum* **12**, 690–700.

Reinhard, M. C., Goltz, H. L., and Mirand, E. A. (1955). *Exp. Med. Surg.* **13**, 135–142.

Richardson, F. L., and Hall, G. (1963). *J. Natl. Cancer Inst.* **31**, 529–539.

Richardson, F. L., and Hummel, K. P. (1959). *J. Natl. Cancer Inst.* **23**, 91–107.

Ringold, G. M., Blair, P. B., Bishop, J. M., and Varmus, H. E. (1976). *Virology* **70**, 550–553.

Rongey, R. W., Abtin, A. H., Estes, J. D., and Gardner, M. B. (1975). *J. Natl. Cancer Inst.* **54**, 1149–1156.

Röpcke, G. (1975). Ph.D. Thesis, University of Amsterdam, Mondeel, Amsterdam.

Rowe, W. P. (1972). *J. Exp. Med.* **136**, 1272–1285.

Rowe, W. P., and Hartley, J. W. (1972). *J. Exp. Med.* **136**, 1286–1301.

Rudali, G. (1958). *Int. Symp. Mammary Cancer, Proc., 2nd, 1957* pp. 461–469.

Rudali, G., Yourkovski, N., Juliard, N., and Fautrel, M. (1956). *Bull. Cancer* **43**, 364–383.

Sambrook, J., Botchan, M., Gallimore, P., Ozanne, B., Petterson, U., Williams, J., and Sharp, P. A. (1975). *Cold Spring Harbor Symp. Quant. Biol.* **39**, 615–632.

Schlom, J., Michalides, R., Hehlmann, R., Spiegelman, S., Bentvelzen, P., and Hageman, P. (1973). *J. Natl. Cancer Inst.* **51**, 541–551.

Scolnick, E. M., Parks, W., Kawakami, T., Kohne, D., Okabe, H., Gilden, R., and Hatanaka, M. (1974). *J. Virol.* **13**, 363–369.

Severi, L., Biancifori, C., Olivi, M., and Squartini, F. (1958). *In* Endocrin Aspects of Breast Cancer" (A. R. Currie, ed.), pp. 283–290. Livingstone, London.

Shannon, J. M., Aidells, B. D., and Daniel, C. W. (1974). *J. Natl. Cancer Inst.* **52**, 1157–1160.

Shoyab, M., Dastoor, M. M., and Baluda, M. A. (1976). *Proc. Natl. Acad. Sci. U.S.A.* **73**, 1749–1753.

Shyamala, G., and Dickson, C. (1976). *Nature (London)* **262**, 107–112.

Singh, D. V., DeOme, K. B., and Bern, H. A. (1970). *J. Natl. Cancer Inst.* **45**, 647–675.

Smith, G. H. (1966). *J. Natl. Cancer Inst.* **36**, 685–701.

Smith, G. H., Andervont, H. B., and Dunn, T. B. (1970). *J. Natl. Cancer Inst.* **44**, 657–671.

Snell, G. D. (1958). *J. Natl. Cancer Inst.* **21**, 843–877.

Snell, G. D., Staats, J., Lyou, M. F., Dunn, L. C., Grüneberg, H., Hertwig, P., and Heston, W. E. (1960). *Cancer Res.* **20**, 145–169.

Souissi, T., Hilgers, J., Verstraeten, A., Kwa, H., and Van Nie, R. (1974). *9th Meet. Mammary Cancer Exp. Anim. Man* Abstr., p. 65.

Spiegelman, S., Axel, R., and Schlom, J. (1972). *J. Natl. Cancer Inst.* **48**, 1205–1211.

Squartini, F., and Biancifori, C. (1958). *Lav. Ist. Anat. Istol. Patol. Univ. Studi Perugia* **18**, 119–123.

Squartini, F., Rossi, G., and Paoletti, I. (1963). *Nature (London)* **197**, 505–506.

Squartini, F., Olivi, M., Bolis, G. B., Ribacchi, R., and Giraldo, G. (1967). *Nature (London)* **214**, 730–732.

Stehelin, D., Varmus, H. E., Bishop, J. M., and Vogt, P. K. (1976). *Nature (London)* **260**, 170–173.

Strand, M., August, J. T., and Croce, C. M. (1976). *Virology* **70**, 545–549.

Strong, L. C. (1943). *Proc. Soc. Exp. Biol. Med.* **53**, 257–258.

Temin, H. M. (1964). *Natl. Cancer Inst., Monogr.* **17**, 557–570.

Temin, H. M. (1972). *In* "RNA Viruses and Host Genome in Oncogenesis" (P. Emmelot and P. Bentvelzen, eds.), 350–363. North-Holland Publ., Amsterdam.

Temin, H. M., and Mizutani, S. (1970). *Nature (London)* **226**, 1211–1213.

Timmermans, A., Bentvelzen, P., Hageman, P. C., and Calafat, J. (1969). *J. Gen. Virol.* **4**, 619–621.

Van Gulik, P. J., and Korteweg, R. (1940). *Proc. K. Ned. Akad. Wet., Ser. C* **43**, 891–900.

Van Nie, R., and Dux, A. (1971). *J. Natl. Cancer Inst.* **46**, 885–897.

Van Nie, R., and Hilgers, J. (1976). *J. Natl. Cancer Inst.* **56**, 27–32.

Van Nie, R., and Thung, P. J. (1965). *Eur. J. Cancer* **1**, 41–50.

Van Nie, R., and Verstraeten, A. A. (1975). *Int. J. Cancer* **16**, 922–931.

Van Nie, R., and Verstraeten, A. A. (1976). *10th Meet. Mammary Cancer Exp. Anim. Man* Abstr. No. 35, p. 51.

Van Nie, R., Hilgers, J., and Lenselink, M. (1972). *In* "Fundamental Research on Mammary Cancer" (J. Mouriquand, ed.), pp. 21–29. Inserm, Paris.

Varmus, H. E., Bishop, J. M., Nowinski, R. C., and Sarkar, N. H. (1972). *Nature (London), New Biol.* **238**, 189–190.

Varmus, H. E., Quintrell, N., Medeiros, E., Bishop, J. M., Nowinski, R. C., and Sarkar, N. H. (1973). *J. Mol. Biol.* **79**, 663–679.

Varmus, H. E., Stavnezer, J., Medeiros, E., and Bishop, J. M. (1975). *Bibl. Haematol. (Basel)* 451–461.

Verstraeten, A. A., Van Nie, R., Kwa, H. G., and Hageman, P. C. (1975). *Int. J. Cancer* **15**, 270–281.

Verstraeten, A. A., van der Valk, M. A., and Van Nie, R. (1976). *10th Meet. Mammary Cancer Exp. Anim. Man* Abstr. No. 50, p. 66.

Visscher, M. B., Green, R. G., and Bittner, J. J. (1942). *Proc. Soc. Exp. Biol. Med.* **49**, 94–96.

Vlahakis, G. (1973). *J. Natl. Cancer Inst.* **51**, 1711–1712.

Warner, S. G., Reinhard, M. C., and Goltz, H. L. (1945). *Cancer Res.* **5**, 584–586.

Woolley, G. W., Law, L. W., and Little, C. C. (1941). *Cancer Res.* **1**, 955–956.

Zeilmaker, G. H. (1969). *Int. J. Cancer* **4**, 261–266.

INHIBITORS OF CHEMICAL CARCINOGENESIS

Lee W. Wattenberg

Department of Laboratory Medicine and Pathology, University of Minnesota, Minneapolis, Minnesota

I. Introduction

Current data suggest that chemical carcinogens play a very significant role in the etiology of cancer in man. In this review, information will be presented concerning a substantial number of compounds that have the capacity to inhibit the neoplastic effects of chemical carcinogens when administered either prior to exposure to the carcinogen or at the same time. Most of the inhibitors currently known are synthetic compounds. However, some are constituents of natural products including vegetables consumed by man. The inhibitors identified thus far show a great diversity of chemical structures making it likely that we have only a limited knowledge of the total spectrum of compounds having this property. Thus the question arises whether inhibitors present in the environment have or could have an impact on the response of humans to chemical carcinogens. Geographic differences in the incidence of cancer of a particular organ as well as variations in incidence over a period of time are generally attributed to changes in the magnitude of exposure to cancer-producing compounds. However, it is possible that in some instances the observed differences may be due, at least in part, to alterations in the level of protection against carcinogenic agents.

Experiments on inhibition of chemical carcinogenesis date back to 1929. At that time it was shown that dichloroethyl sulfide inhibits skin tumor formation resulting from repeated painting of mouse skin with carcinogenic tar (Berenblum, 1929). Subsequently, a number of other compounds were found to have similar effects on epidermal neoplasia in mice. These include: hydrolyzable halogen compounds, such as valeryl chloride or benzene sulfochloride (Crabtree, 1941); compounds that are metabolized to mercapturates, such as bromobenzene (Crabtree, 1944); and anhydrides of α,β-unsaturated dicarboxylic acids such as maleic anhydride and citraconic anhydride (Crabtree, 1945; Klein, 1965); and several low-molecular-weight aromatic hydrocarbons, such as naphthalene, anthracene, and phenanthrene (Crabtree, 1946). In experiments with these compounds it was possible to retard, and in some instances prevent, the appearance of carcinogen-induced neoplastic lesions in the mouse.

Suppression of epidermal neoplasia is an unusual situation in allowing for high local concentrations of inhibitors. In addition, toxicity problems are generally less as compared to systemic administrations, thus allowing for the use of compounds that could not be employed in inhibiting neoplasia at other sites. These early studies of inhibition of chemical carcinogenesis have previously been reviewed (Wattenberg, 1966). They were followed by a more diverse group of experiments based on an increasing amount of information concerning the chemistry and metabolism of chemical carcinogens and biochemistry in general. Of importance were the data indicating that carcinogens have a common reactive form; namely, a positively charged electrophilic species which binds to macromolecules. Many carcinogens are metabolized to this active form via the microsomal mixed function oxidase system, some by other metabolic pathways, and a significant group requires no enzyme activation (Miller and Miller, 1973).

In the present review major emphasis will be placed on two groups of inhibitors that have relatively low toxicity. The mechanism of inhibition generally is not known so that the division of the compounds into the two groups designated is somewhat arbitrary. The first group are antioxidants and some related compounds. These were initially chosen for investigation because of the possibility that they might have a scavenging effect on reactive carcinogenic species. One of the properties of this group of inhibitors is that they can exert an inhibitory effect when administered shortly before the carcinogen, i.e., 2–4 hours. The second group are compounds that have as a common property the capacity to alter the activity of the microsomal mixed-function oxidase system. Most of these compounds induce an increase in mixed-function oxidase activity and have a maximum effectiveness when administered 24–48 hours prior to challenge by the carcinogen. This classification is primitive and will almost assuredly be revised when more data on mechanisms are known. However, for the present it allows for a somewhat orderly presentation of many known inhibitors.

In addition to the inhibitors that are included in the above two groups, others exist as well. One of these are compounds structurally related to specific carcinogens. These have been employed in efforts to obtain competitive inhibition. Experiments of this nature have previously been summarized (Falk *et al.*, 1964; Wattenberg, 1966). A second group of inhibitors have as a common property the ability to inhibit proteases (Troll *et al.*, 1971; Hozumi *et al.*, 1972). A method of inhibiting chemical carcinogenesis having unique features has as its objective preventing the formation of the carcinogen. Work of this type has been directed toward suppressing the formation of nitrosamines. In animals given a prerequisite amine and nitrite, nitrosamines have been shown to be formed in the stomach. This nitrosamine formation can be inhibited by sodium ascorbate and also by gallic acid (Mirvish, 1975; Mirvish *et al.*, 1975). An additional area of exploration for means of inhibiting carcinogenesis differing from all of the above is aimed at reversing the early phases of neoplasia. The major emphasis has been on retinoids. This approach is exceedingly interesting and has recently been reviewed by Sporn *et al.* (1976). It is quite distinctive; however, in that the objective is to reverse biological properties of cells which have already been subjected to the effects of chemical carcinogens rather than toward the earlier event of protecting cells from carcinogens. It will not be dealt with in this review, which focuses primarily on inhibitors that alter the manner in which the carcinogen is handled by the organism prior to the time it reacts with critical target sites. Before proceeding to a description of these inhibitors, test systems used for their study will be discussed.

II. Animal Test Systems for the Study of Inhibitors of Chemical Carcinogenesis

Test systems for detecting inhibitors of chemical carcinogenesis have characteristics which are quite distinctive from the more familiar reverse pursuit of determining whether or not a particular compound is a carcinogen. In the latter case, high doses of the test material are generally used. For studies aimed at evaluating the carcinogen-inhibiting capacity of a particular compound, the dose or doses of the carcinogen employed in the test system must be on a portion of the dose-response curve sensitive to alterations in the dose of the carcinogen. Inhibitors of carcinogens, in general, produce the same effect as if a lower dose of the carcinogen was administered than that actually given. Thus they may not be detected if excessive amounts of carcinogen are administered. Let us suppose that a dose of carcinogen is being employed such that a reduction of the concentration of the carcinogen of 50% produces a decrease in tumor incidence of only 5 or 10%. Under these conditions, an inhibitor producing an effective reduction of carcinogen dose of 50% could easily be missed. On the other hand, the inhibitor would be readily detected if the dose of carcinogen employed were on a linear portion of the dose-response curve so that a reduction of the effective carcinogen dose of 50% would produce a 50% decrease in tumor incidence.

In addition to the importance of the biological response being sensitive to changes in carcinogen dose, the absolute amount of the carcinogen administered at one time may be critical. If the inhibitor is operating through a mechanism which has a defined upper limit as to the absolute quantity of carcinogen that can be inactivated, a high dose of carcinogen may overwhelm the system. The microsomal mixed-function oxidase system of the skin is a case in point. With a limited capacity to inactivate chemical carcinogens, it can be effective when low doses of carcinogens are administered but not with high doses.

A desirable attribute of an animal testing system for studying inhibitors is that the duration be as short as possible. In a number of models, an evaluation can be made within a period of 6 months. These entail the use of experimental animals in which one or more tissues are highly sensitive to a particular chemical carcinogen. Even with such high sensitivity, the quest for a short testing period usually results in substantial doses of carcinogen being employed. The systems can be made more sensitive to inhibitors by reducing the dose of carcinogen and prolonging the period that the experimental animals are allowed to survive. This may be warranted when an inhibitor is showing uncertain results or where it is desirable to use low doses of the inhibitor. Human exposures to carcinogen and inhibitor are of low dose and long duration. Animal systems that reflect these conditions are indicated in later stages of inhibitor studies in which evaluations are being made of conditions under which inhibitors will exert their effects.

A considerable number of experimental procedures have been employed to evaluate the carcinogen-inhibiting capacities of test compounds as will be noted from Tables I, IV, and VII. Of these, several have the desirable attributes discussed above and will be described briefly. A very simple test system entails the use of strains of mice that are highly sensitive to carcinogen-induced pulmonary adenoma formation. Pulmonary adenomas are produced by a wide variety of carcinogens, and the dose-response relationships have been extensively studied by Shimkin (1955). The usefulness of this system for studying inhibitors of a number of carcinogens has been demonstrated by several investigators as will be noted in Tables I and VII. A typical testing procedure is to administer 2 or 3 doses of a polycyclic aromatic hydrocarbon carcinogen such as benzo[a]pyrene (BP) or 7,12-dimethylbenz[a]anthracene (DMBA) with an interval of 2 weeks between the administrations. The substance being tested for its inhibitory capacities can be given either in the diet or as discrete single administrations at some specific time interval prior to carcinogen administration (see Table III). About 24 weeks after the initial administration of carcinogen, the animals are sacrificed and pulmonary adenomas are counted. A comparable procedure can be used for urethane, uracil mustard, diethylnitrosamine, and a number of other carcinogens (Wattenberg, 1973). The precise dose level and number of doses varies with the particular carcinogen employed. In some instances, as with urethane, only a single administration is required to give a large enough number of pulmonary adenomas for valid testing. For carcinogens that are less potent in terms of their effects on the mouse lung, a sizable number of administrations may be required.

The forestomach of the mouse is sensitive to a number of carcinogens (Berenblum and Haran, 1955; Neal and Rigdon, 1967). This experimental model has been found to be useful for the study of inhibitors of chemical carcinogens. A typical protocol entails the administration of eight doses of BP by oral intubation. Two doses of the carcinogen are given per week for 4 weeks. Approximately 20 weeks after the initial dose of carcinogen, the experiment is terminated and the number of neoplasms of the forestomach recorded. The substance being tested for its inhibitory capacities can be added to the diet or can be given in the form of discrete administrations at a precise period prior to the carcinogen. Another way in which this model can be employed is to add both the inhibitor and carcinogen to the diet, as is done in the experiments in Table II. A number of variations are possible including the use of very low doses of both carcinogen and inhibitor. An additional positive attribute of the model is that the carcinogen and inhibitor both come into direct contact with the target tissue rather than acting at a remote site.

DMBA-induced mammary tumor formation in the female rat is another experimental system that is readily employed to evaluate potential inhibitors of chemical carcinogenesis. This model has been extensively developed by Huggins *et al.* (1961, 1964). It is very simple in that a single oral administration of DMBA will induce mammary tumors in a large percentage of animals within a period of 3 to 6 months depending upon the particular strain of Sprague-Dawley rat or other sensitive strain of rat employed. A single dose of DMBA is usually given. The system can be made more sensitive to inhibitors by using several smaller doses of carcinogen. Compounds being studied for carcinogen-inhibiting properties can be administered, either as discrete administrations, as shown in Table VI, or added to the diet of animals subsequently subjected to carcinogen challenge. There are some limitations to this particular test system. One of these is that it is almost entirely limited to studies of inhibition of one carcinogen; namely, DMBA. Although other carcinogens can produce mammary tumors in rats, either repeated large doses are required or the time interval necessary for the neoplasms to develop is long. A second limitation of the system is that the hormonal status of the animal affects the tumor incidence. If an investigation is directed toward inhibitors that act by virtue of alteration of detoxification mechanisms or some direct interaction with carcinogen metabolites, then inadvertent changes produced in the hormonal balance might give spurious results.

During the past several years 1,2-dimethylhydrazine (DMH) and some related compounds have been found to be highly effective in inducing neoplasia of the large bowel in a number of rodent species. The morphology and biology of these neoplasms closely resembles their human counterpart. Since cancer of the large bowel is an important neoplasm in man, an experimental model simulating that of the human disease is of considerable interest. A simple procedure for obtaining large-bowel neoplasms has been worked out in the mouse. This entails subcutaneous administration of DMH given at weekly intervals (Thurnherr *et al.*, 1973; Wattenberg, 1975). In studies of inhibitors of DMH-induced large-bowel neoplasia, the compound under investigation generally is added to the diet, as is shown in Table V. However, it would also be possible to give the test substance as discrete administrations at some designated time prior to the carcinogen administration. Within a period of 6–9 months after the initial dose of DMH, neoplasms of the large intestine are present in a large proportion of the animals subjected to this regime. In the mouse the vast majority of the tumors occur in the rectum and adjacent portion of the distal colon. A number of variations of this experimental procedure are possible. In place of DMH, two of its oxidative metabolites which are carcinogenic have been employed. These are azoxymethane and methylazoxymethanol (MAM) administered as the acetate (Zedeck *et al.*, 1972; Nigro *et al.*, 1973). A further variation is to use a direct-acting carcinogen, i.e., one not requiring metabolic activation, and to give this by the intrarectal route (Reddy *et al.*, 1974; Narisawa *et al.*, 1976).

An additional experimental model that can be employed for the study of inhibitors is carcinogen-induced epidermal neoplasia in the mouse. Both the carcinogen and the inhibitor can be administered topically. This experimental system has several advantages. The materials under investigation can be applied directly to the target tissue, and the neoplastic response can be followed readily by visualization. However, there are some disadvantages. One of these is that the carcinogen reaches the target tissue abruptly at a high concentration and generally dissolved in a solvent which itself might have some effect on the response of the system. Factors such as hair cycle and licking of the skin can alter the results obtained, although these factors can be controlled if care is taken. An additional problem is that some detoxification systems have weak activity in the epidermis, so that only low doses of carcinogen can be employed if their capacities are not to be exceeded. In addition to the test systems presented, many other possibilities exist. Their selection would be dependent on factors such as a particular interest in a specific target tissue and/or carcinogen. Some of the considerations discussed in the models described above may serve as guides for constructing effective new test procedures.

III. Inhibition of Chemical Carcinogenesis by Antioxidants and Some Related Compounds

A. Butylated Hydroxyanisole, Butylated Hydroxytoluene, and Ethoxyquin

The use of antioxidants as possible inhibitors of the chemical carcinogens has been based in general on the concept that the antioxidants may exert a scavenging effect on the reactive species of carcinogens thus protecting cellular constituents from attack. In early studies, wheat germ oil and α-tocopherol were employed. Experiments showing positive and negative results have been published. Confirmatory reports on the positive experiments have not appeared so that the implications of this work are not clear. These investigations as well as our own experience with α-tocopherol which has not shown it to be inhibitory, have been summarized previously (Wattenberg, 1972a). However, it is possible that under some appropriate conditions an inhibitory effect does occur.

During the past several years, studies have been carried out with other antioxidants. Several of these have been found to inhibit the effects of a substantial variety of chemical carcinogens (Fig. 1). The most extensive work of this type has been done with phenolic antioxidants; in particular, butylated hydroxyanisole (BHA) and butylated hydroxytoluene (BHT) (Table I). Inhibition occurs under a number of experimental conditions (Wattenberg, 1972a). It has been found in situations where the route of carcinogen administration results in direct contact of carcinogen with the target tissue. A number of experiments have been carried out in which the BHA or BHT were added to diets and polycyclic aromatic hydrocarbon carcinogens, such as BP and DMBA, were given either in the diet or by oral intubation. In these studies the target tissue in which neoplasia occurred was the forestomach. Those animals that received BHA or BHT in the diet

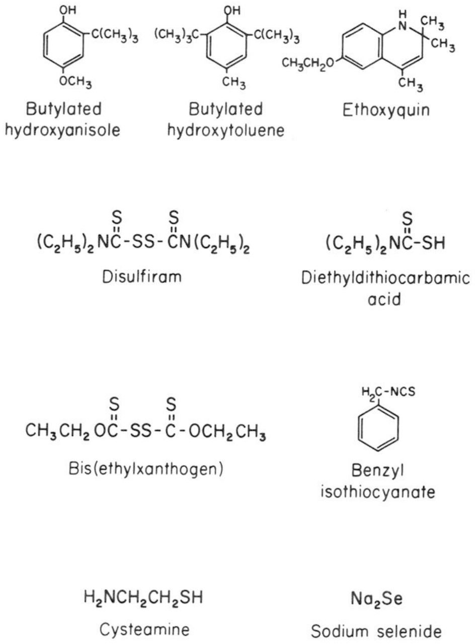

FIG. 1. Some compounds inhibiting chemical carcinogenesis.

TABLE I

INHIBITION OF CARCINOGEN-INDUCED NEOPLASIA BY BUTYLATED HYDROXYANISOLE (BHA), BUTYLATED HYDROXYTOLUENE (BHT), AND ETHOXYQUIN

Carcinogen	Antioxidant	Species	Site of neoplasm inhibited	References
Benzo [a] pyrene	BHA, ethoxyquin[a]	Mouse	Lung	Wattenberg (1973)
Benzo [a] pyrene	BHA, BHT	Mouse	Forestomach	Wattenberg (1972a)
7,12-Dimethylbenz [a] anthracene	BHA, ethoxyquin	Mouse	Forestomach	Wattenberg (1972a)
7,12-Dimethylbenz [a] anthracene	BHA, BHT	Mouse	Skin	Slaga and Bracken (1977)
7,12-Dimethylbenz [a] anthracene	BHA, BHT, ethoxyquin	Rat	Breast	Wattenberg (1972a)
7,12-Dimethylbenz [a] anthracene	BHA	Mouse	Lung	Wattenberg (1973)
7-Hydroxymethyl-12-methylbenz [a]-anthracene	BHA	Mouse	Lung	Wattenberg (1973)
Dibenz [a,h] anthracene	BHA	Mouse	Lung	Wattenberg (1973)
Diethylnitrosamine	BHA, ethoxyquin	Mouse	Lung	Wattenberg (1972b)
4-Nitroquinoline-N-oxide	BHA, ethoxyquin	Mouse	Lung	Wattenberg (1972b)
Uracil mustard	BHA	Mouse	Lung	Wattenberg (1973)
Urethane	BHA	Mouse	Lung	Wattenberg (1973)
N-2-Fluorenylacetamide	BHT	Rat	Liver	Ulland et al. (1973)
N-Hydroxy-N-2-fluorenylacetamide	BHT	Rat	Liver, breast	Ulland et al. (1973)
4-Dimethylaminoazobenzene	BHT	Rat	Liver	Frankfurt et al. (1967)
Azoxymethane	BHT	Rat	Large intestine	Weisburger et al. (1977)

[a] Unpublished.

TABLE II

EFFECTS OF BUTYLATED HYDROXYANISOLE (BHA) ON 7,12-DIMETHYLBENZ[a]-
ANTHRACENE (DMBA)-INDUCED NEOPLASIA OF THE FORESTOMACH OF
Ha/ICR MICE[a]

Experimental diet[b]		Number of mice at risk	Percentage of mice with tumors	Number of tumors per mouse
Carcinogen (per gram diet)	Antioxidant (per gram diet)			
DMBA, 0.05 mg	None	20	55	2.6
DMBA, 0.05 mg	BHA, 10 mg	18	0	0
DMBA, 0.05 mg	BHA, 2 mg	18	22	0.22

[a] Female Ha/ICR mice were fed experimental diets for 4 weeks, and the mice were sacrificed 14 weeks after the completion of this feeding period.

[b] Additions to a purified diet; casein, 27%; starch, 59%; vegetable oil, 10%; salts, 4% plus vitamins—"Normal Protein Diet," ICN Co., Cleveland, Ohio.

showed pronounced suppression of neoplasia at this site (Table II). Comparable levels of inhibition under the same conditions have also been obtained with ethoxyquin, an antioxidant widely used in commercial animal diets but only rarely for human food (Fig. 1). Suppression of neoplasia is also obtained in experiments in which the carcinogen is acting at a site remote from that of administration, i.e., inhibition of pulmonary neoplasia in experiments in which the carcinogen is given by oral intubation (Wattenberg, 1973). An illustrative experiment of this type is presented in Table III.

TABLE III

EFFECTS OF BUTYLATED HYDROXYANISOLE (BHA) ON BENZO[a]PYRENE
(BP)-INDUCED PULMONARY ADENOMA FORMATION[a]

Initial administration	Carcinogen administration	Number of mice at risk	Number of pulmonary adenomas per mouse
None	BP, 3 mg	13	15.8
Solvent (cottonseed oil)	BP, 3 mg	9	17.7
BHA, 7.5 mg	BP, 3 mg	11	5.4

[a] Eleven-week-old female A/HeJ mice were given an initial administration of 0.2 ml of solvent or test substance by oral intubation 4 hours prior to administration of the carcinogen, also by oral intubation. At 2-week intervals, a second and then a third such sequence of administrations was carried out. The experiment was terminated when the mice were 35 weeks of age.

BHA and BHT are of interest because of their extensive use as additives in food for human consumption. Of the two compounds, BHA is preferable because it is considerably less toxic than BHT. Studies in mice have been carried out in which BHA or BHT were added to the diet along with BP, a carcinogen widely encountered in the environment. At a concentration of either antioxidant of 5 mg per gram of diet, inhibition of the carcinogenic effect on the forestomach of the mouse occurs at a concentration of BP of 1 mg per gram of diet (Wattenberg, 1972a). In the United States, the human consumption of phenolic antioxidants is of the order of magnitude of several milligrams a day. Assuming that the results of the animal experiments hold for man, this amount of the antioxidants could be of importance in inhibiting the effects of chronic exposure to low doses of carcinogens, the type of exposure that is most likely to occur in human populations.

An early investigation aimed at determining the mechanism of inhibition of carcinogenesis of N-2-fluorenylacetamide (FAA) and N-hydroxy-N-2-fluorenylacetamide (N-OH-FAA) by BHT was carried out by Grantham et al. (1972). These investigators found that administration of BHT in the diet led to excretion in the urine of a larger percentage of each carcinogen. This higher level of excretion was accounted for chiefly by glucuronic acid conjugates. Animals receiving BHT showed lower levels of radioactivity in blood, liver, and liver DNA 48 hours after injection with labeled carcinogen. It was concluded that BHT increases detoxification of FAA and N-OH-FAA, thus lowering the amount available for activation reactions.

In later studies, work was initiated to determine the mechanism of inhibition of BP-induced carcinogenesis by BHA. Several possibilities were considered that can be divided into two major categories. The first involves direct chemical interaction between antioxidant and reactive species of carcinogen. The second possibility is that the antioxidant is acting in an indirect manner. Of primary interest in the latter regard is alteration of enzyme activity. Both types of mechanism have been under investigation. Data obtained thus far have shown that BHA administration produces enzyme alterations that appear to be consistent with its inhibitory effects.

BP is metabolized by the microsomal mixed-function oxidase system, which acts upon a wide variety of xenobiotic compounds including polycyclic aromatic hydrocarbons. Reactive metabolites as well as detoxification products are produced. The effects of dietary administration of BHA on microsomal metabolism of BP have been studied employing experimental conditions similar to those in which BHA inhibits neoplasia due to this carcinogen. Incubation of BP and DNA with liver microsomes from the BHA-fed mice results in approximately one-half the binding of BP metabolites to DNA as compared to that found employing microsomes from control mice (Speier and Wattenberg, 1975). Studies of a comparable nature have been carried out by Slaga and Bracken (1977) employing mouse skin. In this work, BHA or BHT was applied topically. Three or twelve hours later, the animals were sacrificed and the binding of [³H]BP or [³H]DMBA to DNA determined in epidermal homogenates. Both carcinogens showed approximately one half as much binding to DNA in homogenates from mice which had received BHA or BHT 3 hours before death than in homogenates from control mice. The inhibition of binding was still apparent at 12 hours but was a lesser order of magnitude.

Investigations have been undertaken to determine if differences in metabolites of BP are formed when this carcinogen is incubated with liver microsomes prepared from BHA-fed and control female A/HeJ mice. The metabolites were extracted from the incubation mixture and analyzed by high-pressure liquid chromatography. Of major interest were the effects of BHA feeding on epoxide formation. BP-4,5-oxide was isolated and identified. It was present in both the BHA-fed and control microsomal incubations but was substantially reduced in the former. BP-9,10-oxide and BP-7,8-oxide were not directly demonstrated. Data based on summation of diols and phenols resulting, respectively, from the enzymic and spontaneous conversions of these oxides indicate that they are present in reduced amounts in the microsomal incubations from BHA-fed mice. 3-Hydroxybenzo[a]pyrene (3-HOBP) was the major metabolite in microsomal incubations from BHA-fed and control mice. This metabolite constituted a significantly higher percentage of the total metabolites formed on incubating BP with microsomes from BHA-fed as compared to control mice. Thus BHA administration causes two metabolic alterations which could result in its exerting an inhibitory effect on BP-induced carcinogenesis. The first is a decrease in epoxidation, which is an activation process and the second is an increase in 3-HOBP, a metabolite of detoxification (Lam and Wattenberg, 1977).

B. DISULFIRAM AND RELATED COMPOUNDS

Experimental studies of the capacity of disulfiram (Antabuse, tetraethylthiuram disulfide) and some related compounds to inhibit chemical carcinogenesis have been carried out using the same experimental models employed for the phenolic antioxidants (Wattenberg, 1974). Like the phenolic antioxidants and ethoxyquin, disulfiram in the diet will inhibit neoplasia under conditions where the route of administration of the carcinogen results in direct contact with the target tissue. It is a potent inhibitor of BP-induced neoplasia of the forestomach (Table IV). This experimental model is being used in studies of mechanism of inhibition. Work carried out thus far has shown that administration of disulfiram in the diet results in an inhibition of binding of [^{3}H]BP and [^{14}C]BP to DNA, RNA, and protein of the forestomach (Borchert and Wattenberg, 1976). Inhibition of carcinogenesis occurring at a site remote from that of administration of the carcinogen is brought about by disulfiram. Thus this compound will inhibit mammary tumor formation in the rat resulting from oral administration of DMBA (Table IV). However, unlike BHA, BP-induced pulmonary neoplasia in the mouse is not inhibited by disulfiram.

Disulfiram and its reduction product diethyldithiocarbamate are exceedingly interesting in their effects on carcinogen-induced neoplasia of the large intestine (Wattenberg, 1975, 1976). In experiments of this nature, both disulfiram and diethyldithiocarbamate profoundly inhibit large-bowel neoplasia resulting from subcutaneous administration of DMH, as is illustrated in Table V. Work has been carried out with azoxymethane, an oxidative metabolite of DMH. This compound also produces neoplasia of the large intestine. Under comparable experimental conditions to those used for DMH, addition of disulfiram to the diet inhibits azoxymethane-induced neoplasia of the large intestine, but to a considerably lesser extent than it inhibits DMH (Wattenberg et al., 1977).

Studies bearing on the mechanism of inhibition of DMH-induced neoplasia of the large bowel have shown that both disulfiram and diethyldithiocarbamate inhibit the oxidation of this carcinogen in vivo (Fiala and Weisburger, 1976). The partial inhibition of azoxymethane-induced neoplasia by disulfiram introduces additional considerations. The fact that this antioxidant partially suppresses the neoplastic effects of azoxymethane, while under comparable conditions completely inhibiting DMH-induced neoplasia of the large bowel, suggests that it inhibits more than one oxidative step. If only DMH oxidation were being inhibited then no suppression of azoxymethane carcinogenesis should occur. If inhibition of azoxymethane were the sole effect, then comparable levels of inhibition of DMH and azoxymethane would be anticipated.

Work has been carried out bearing on the question whether the intact molecule of disulfiram is the inhibitor or if a metabolite of this compound has the inhibitory function (Fiala and Weisburger, 1976;

TABLE IV

INHIBITION OF CARCINOGEN-INDUCED NEOPLASIA BY SULFUR-CONTAINING COMPOUNDS

Carcinogen	Inhibitor	Species	Site of neoplasm inhibited	References
Benzo[a]pyrene	Disulfiram, bis(ethylxanthogen), 2-chloroallyl diethyldithiocarbamate, S-propyl dipropylthiocarbamate	Mouse	Forestomach	Wattenberg (1974); Borchert and Wattenberg (1976); Wattenberg et al. (1977)
Benzo[a]pyrene	Benzyl isothiocyanate, phenethyl isothiocyanate	Mouse	Forestomach	Wattenberg (1977)
7,12-Dimethylbenz[a]anthracene	Disulfiram, benzyl isothiocyanate, phenethyl isothiocyanate, phenyl isothiocyanate, benzyl thiocyanate, cysteamine	Rat	Breast	Wattenberg (1974, 1977); Marquardt et al. (1974)
1,2-Dimethylhydrazine	Disulfiram, diethyldithiocarbamate, bis(ethylxanthogen)	Mouse	Large intestine	Wattenberg (1975, 1976); Wattenberg et al. (1977)
Azoxymethane	Disulfiram	Mouse	Large intestine	Wattenberg et al. (1977)
N-2-Fluorenylacetamide	1-Naphthyl isothiocyanate	Rat	Liver, ear duct	Sidransky et al. (1966)
Ethionine	1-Naphthyl isothiocyanate	Rat	Liver	Sidransky et al. (1966)
3'-Methyl-4-dimethylaminoazobenzene	1-Naphthyl isothiocyanate	Rat	Liver	Sasaki (1963)
4-Dimethylaminoazobenzene	2-Naphthyl isothiocyanate	Rat	Liver	Lacassagne et al. (1970)

TABLE V

EFFECTS OF DISULFIRAM AND DIETHYLDITHIOCARBAMATE ON TUMOR
FORMATION IN THE LARGE INTESTINE OF FEMALE CF₁ MICE GIVEN 16
DOSES OF 1,2-DIMETHYLHYDRAZINE (DMH) SUBCUTANEOUSLY[a]

| Additions to the diet[b] | Number of mice at risk | Mice with tumors of the large intestine | | Number of tumors/mouse |
		Number	Percent	
None	20	18	90	4
Disulfiram, 5 mg/g	20	0	0	0
Sodium diethyldithiocarbamate, 7.5 mg/g	18	0	0	0

[a] Nine-week-old female CF₁ mice were given subcutaneous injections of 0.4 mg of DMH in the cervical area once a week for 16 weeks and sacrificed 14 weeks after the last administration (Wattenberg, 1975).

[b] Experimental diets consisting of powdered Purina Rat Chow with the indicated additions or without additions were started 11 days before the initial administration of DMH and continued until 4 days after the last administration.

Fiala *et al.*, 1977). These investigations have demonstrated that carbon disulfide (CS₂), a metabolite of disulfiram, inhibits the oxidation of DMH. The data obtained suggest that this may be the chemical species responsible for the inhibitory action of disulfiram and diethyldithiocarbamate on DMH-induced large-bowel neoplasia. In work carried out by others, it has been reported that incubation of microsomes with CS₂ in the presence of NADPH results in covalent binding of the sulfur to the microsomes. There is an accompanying decrease in cytochrome P-450 as measured spectroscopically (DeMatteis, 1974; Hunter and Neal, 1975). Several thiono-sulfur-containing compounds including disulfiram and diethyldithiocarbamate produce a similar decrease in cytochrome P-450 when incubated with microsomes under comparable conditions (Hunter and Neal, 1975). This raises the possibility that thiono-sulfur-containing compounds as a group may have the capacity to modify cytochrome P-450 so as to alter the microsomal metabolism of DMH and possibly other carcinogens in a manner which decreases their carcinogenicity.

The carcinogen-inhibiting effects brought about by disulfiram and diethyldithiocarbamate have drawn attention to the possibility that a number of widely used pesticides having dithiocarbamate or thiocarbamate groups might have similar properties. Several have been tested for their capacity to inhibit chemical carcinogenesis. Two of these when added to the diet were found to inhibit BP-induced neoplasia of the forestomach of the mouse. These are S-propyl dipropylthiocarbamate (Vernolate) and 2-chloroallyl diethyldithiocarbamate (CDEC). An additional pesticide, bis(ethylxanthogen) (Bexide) was also found to exert an inhibitory effect in this test system. Bis(ethylxanthogen) is the only one of these pesticides studied thus far for its effects on DMH-induced neoplasia of the large bowel. When added to the diet at a level of 5 mg/g, it completely inhibited DMH-induced large bowel neoplasia, and at a level of 1 mg/g reduced the number of animals bearing large bowel tumors to approximately one-half that occurring in the control group. Its inhibitory potency is of a similar order of magnitude to that of disulfiram (Wattenberg et al., 1977).

Bis(ethylxanthogen) has a feature that makes it of particular interest: the molecule does not contain nitrogen (Fig. 1). This is of importance since structurally similar dithiocarbamate pesticides have been shown to form nitrosamines, representing a hazard not occurring with bis(ethylxanthogen). A second relationship between disulfiram and nitrosamines has been reported recently (Schmähl et al., 1976). These investigators have found that disulfiram influences the organotropy of diethylnitrosamine (DENA) and dimethylnitrosamine (DMNA). In the case of DENA, disulfiram added to the diet inhibits liver tumor formation but enhances neoplasia of the esophagus. With DMNA, suppression of neoplasia of the liver is again found, but there is an increase in tumors of the paranasal sinuses.

C. Benzyl Isothiocyanate and Related Compounds

Along with studies of the inhibitory capacities of sulfur-containing antioxidants, experiments with benzyl isothiocyanate, phenethyl isothiocyanate, and benzyl thiocyanate have been carried out (Wattenberg, 1974, 1977). These three compounds are naturally occurring constituents of edible cruciferous plants (Virtanen, 1962; Lichtenstein et al., 1962). A fourth compound, phenyl isothiocyanate included in some of the experimental work, is synthetic. As with the phenolic antioxidants and disulfiram, benzyl isothiocyanate inhibits carcinogenesis when the carcinogen is administered so as to come into direct contact with the target tissue and also when it is acting at a remote site (Table IV). Addition of benzyl isothiocyanate to a diet containing BP results in inhibition of carcinogenesis of the forestomach in the mouse. Comparable inhibition is obtained if the BP is administered by oral intubation rather than in the diet. The inhibitory effects of benzyl isothiocyanate, phenethyl isothiocyanate, and benzyl thiocyanate on neoplasia of the forestomach resulting from administration of DMBA in the diet also has been investigated. Benzyl isothiocyanate and phenethyl isothiocyanate suppress gastric neoplasia whereas benzyl thiocyanate does not.

In studies of mammary tumor formation resulting from oral administration of DMBA to Sprague-Dawley rats, it was found that benzyl isothiocyanate, phenethyl isothiocyanate, phenyl isothiocyanate, and benzyl thiocyanate inhibit the occurrence of this neoplasm (Wattenberg, 1977). Inhibition is found if the compound is administered by oral intubation either 2 or 4 hours prior to the carcinogen, but not if it is given 24 hours before or 4 hours after the carcinogen (Table VI).

1-Naphthyl isothiocyanate has been shown to inhibit liver tumor formation resulting from administration of ethionine or FAA (Sid-

TABLE VI

EFFECTS OF BENZYL ISOTHIOCYANATE ON MAMMARY TUMOR FORMATION IN
SPRAGUE-DAWLEY RATS GIVEN DMBA BY ORAL INTUBATION

Expt. No.	Material administered by oral intubation[a]	Time of administration[b] (hours)	Number of rats at risk	Mammary tumors[c]	
				Percent of rats with tumors	Number of tumors per rat[d]
1	Benzyl isothiocyanate, 50 mg	−4	13	23[e]	0.23 ± 0.12[f]
	Vehicle	−4	13	85	2.2 ± 0.44
	Benzyl isothiocyanate, 50 mg	+4	13	62	1.3 ± 0.44
	Vehicle	+4	14	71	2.0 ± 0.50
	Nothing	—	13	77	1.8 ± 0.47
2	Benzyl isothiocyanate, 50 mg	−4	14	14[f]	0.14 ± 0.10[f]
	Vehicle	−4	12	100	2.6 ± 0.48
	Benzyl isothiocyanate, 50 mg	−24	11	71	1.1 ± 0.27
	Vehicle	−24	13	93	1.9 ± 0.29

[a] Benzyl isothiocyanate, 50 mg in 1 ml of olive oil or 1 ml of vehicle (olive oil) was administered by oral intubation.

[b] (−) Designates administration given prior to DMBA; (+) means that administration was after DMBA.

[c] Mammary tumor counts at completion of experiment, i.e., when rats were 25 weeks of age. This was 18 weeks after DMBA (12 mg in 1 ml of olive oil) was given by oral intubation.

[d] Mean ± SE.

[e] $P < 0.01$.

[f] $P < 0.001$.

ransky *et al.*, 1966). The carcinogens were added to the diet, which was fed for several months. Two conditions of inhibitor administration were effective. In one, the isothiocyanate and the carcinogen were fed simultaneously. In the second the isothiocyanate was fed for 4 or 8 weeks and then terminated immediately prior to the start of carcinogen administration. This latter regime is quite different from any employed with benzyl isothiocyanate so that there is a question whether similar mechanisms of inhibition are involved. A further difference is that the duration of 1-naphthyl isothiocyanate feeding was such as to produce hepatic pathology including moderate to marked degrees of bile duct proliferation and bile stasis. 1-Naphthyl isothiocyanate has also been reported to inhibit hepatocarcinogenicity resulting from feeding 3'-methyl-4-dimethylaminoazobenzene (Sasaki, 1963). 2-Naphthyl isothiocyanate suppresses the neoplastic effects of 4-dimethylaminoazobenzene on liver (Lacassagne *et al.*, 1970). At the present time, very little is known about the mechanism whereby any of the isothiocyanates described in this section inhibit chemical carcinogenesis. Of possible relevance are studies showing that 1-naphthyl isothiocyanate alters cytochrome P-450 in a manner comparable to that of thiono-sulfur-containing compounds (DeMatteis, 1974).

D. SELENIUM SALTS

Inhibition of chemical carcinogenesis by selenium salts has been reported. In an initial paper, the experimental system employed consisted of initiation of epidermal neoplasia with DMBA followed by promotion with croton oil. Sodium selenide added to the croton oil suppressed the development of skin tumors (Shamberger, 1966). In a subsequent paper repeated applications of 3-methylcholanthrene (MC) to the skin were carried out. Again, addition of sodium selenide inhibited epidermal neoplasia. In a further experiment, mice were placed on a selenium-deficient diet (*Torula* yeast) without supplements or with added sodium selenide or sodium selenite. BP was applied to the skin daily to produce epidermal neoplasia. Under these conditions a slight inhibition was found with both of the selenium salts (Shamberger, 1970). Evidence has been presented showing that there was an inverse relationship between selenium occurrence in soil and forage crops and human cancer death rates in the United States and Canada in 1965. Likewise an inverse relationship between human blood levels of selenium and human cancer death rates in several cities was found (Shamberger and Willis, 1971).

E. Cysteamine-HCl

Cysteamine-HCl has been shown to inhibit DMBA-induced mammary tumor formation in experiments in which the carcinogen was administered intravenously and the antioxidant i.p. In addition, the effects of this compound were studied on mouse fibroblasts (M2 line) in culture. Addition of cysteamine-HCl prior to or after addition of DMBA did not affect toxicity; however, this compound did reduce the number of transformed foci (Marquardt et al., 1974).

IV. Inhibition of Chemical Carcinogenesis by Inducers of Increased Microsomal Mixed-Function Oxidase Activity

A number of studies have demonstrated that it is possible to protect against chemical carcinogens by administration of inducers of increased microsomal mixed-function oxidase activity (Table VII). The inducers employed have varied from compounds such as polycyclic hydrocarbons, which themselves are noxious agents, to chemicals such as flavones, which have low toxicity (Wattenberg et al., 1976). In early studies it was shown that administration of polycyclic hydrocarbon inducers inhibited the occurrence of hepatic cancer resulting from feeding 3'-methyl-4-dimethylaminoazobenzene (Richardson et al., 1952; Miller et al., 1958). Likewise, it was demonstrated that polycyclic hydrocarbon inducers can markedly reduce the incidence of tumors of the liver, mammary gland, ear duct, and small intestine in rats fed FAA or 7-FL-FAA (Miller et al., 1958).

More recently, studies have been carried out in which protection against the carcinogenic effects of a number of other carcinogens has been observed (Table VII). Considerable work has been done with two polycyclic hydrocarbon carcinogens, DMBA and BP. Employing the pulmonary adenoma test system in the mouse, it has been shown that flavone inducers will inhibit the formation of these neoplasms resulting from oral administration of these two carcinogens (Wattenberg and Leong, 1968; Wattenberg and Leong, 1970). An experimental model that has been widely used in studies of the effects of inducers of increased mixed-function oxidase activity is mammary tumor formation in rats given DMBA. Several different types of inducers administered prior to DMBA will inhibit tumor formation. The inducers employed include the following: polycyclic hydrocarbons (Huggins et al., 1964; Wheatley, 1968), phenothiazines (Wattenberg and Leong, 1967), and flavones (Wattenberg and Leong, 1968).

In two experiments, inhibition of neoplasia of the small intestine

TABLE VII

INHIBITION OF CARCINOGENESIS BY INDUCERS OF INCREASED MICROSOMAL ENZYME ACTIVITY

Carcinogen	Inducer	Species	Organ	References
3'-Methyl-4-dimethylaminoazobenzene	Polycyclic hydrocarbons, α-benzene hexachloride, polychlorinated biphenyls	Rat	Liver	Richardson et al. (1952); Miller et al. (1958); Makiura et al. (1974); Thamavit et al. (1974).
N-2-Fluorenylacetamide	Polycyclic hydrocarbons, polychlorinated biphenyls	Rat	Liver, breast, small intestine	Miller et al. (1958); Makiura et al. (1974).
4-Dimethylaminostilbene	Polycyclic hydrocarbons	Rat	Ear duct	Tawfic (1965)
Urethane	Phenobarbital	Mouse	Lung	Adenis et al. (1970); Silva (1967)
Urethane	β-Naphthoflavone, chlordane, phenobarbital	Mouse	Lung	Wattenberg and Leong (1968); Yamamoto et al. (1971)
Benzo[a]pyrene	β-Naphthoflavone, quercetin pentamethylether	Mouse	Lung	Wattenberg and Leong (1970)
Benzo[a]pyrene	β-Naphthoflavone	Mouse	Skin	Wattenberg and Leong (1970)
7,12-Dimethylbenz[a]anthracene	β-Naphthoflavone	Mouse	Lung	Wattenberg and Leong (1968)
7,12-Dimethylbenz[a]anthracene	β-Naphthoflavone, phenothiazines, and polycyclic hydrocarbons	Rat	Breast	Huggins et al. (1964); Wattenberg and Leong (1967, 1968; Wheatley (1968)
Aflatoxin	Phenobarbital	Rat	Liver	McLean and Marshall (1971)
Bracken fern carcinogen	Phenothiazine	Rat	Small intestine, bladder	Pamukcu et al. (1971)

has been obtained by inducers of increased mixed-function oxidase activity (Table VII). One of these has been a study in which the carcinogen was FAA, and the inducers employed were polycyclic hydrocarbons. A second experiment involved the use of bracken fern as the carcinogen. This plant material when fed to rats causes cancer of the small intestine and urinary bladder. The addition to the diet of phenothiazine, a potent inducer of increased mixed-function oxidase activity, results in inhibition of neoplasia of both of these target sites (Pamukcu *et al.*, 1971).

A large number of synthetic compounds exist which induce increased mixed-function oxidase activity (Conney and Burns, 1972). In addition, there are natural materials that also have this capacity. One group of these are cruciferous vegetables. From this source several indoles with inducing activity have been identified (Loub *et al.*, 1975). The effects on chemical carcinogenesis of most of the known inducers has not been reported and might provide data of considerable interest.

Having presented the experiments listed in Table VII, which show a protective effect from administration of inducers of increased mixed-function oxidase activity, it is important to discuss an apparently conflicting set of data. It has been demonstrated for many chemical carcinogens that the microsomal mixed-function oxidase system converts these compounds to a proximate carcinogenic form (Miller and Miller, 1974). An initial thought might be that if a compound is activated by an enzyme system to a noxious form, then enhancement of the activity of this system would result in greater damage to the organism. This is true in situations involving a reversible effect in which there is a substantial threshold. Rapid activation could be important in achieving such a threshold. However, in the case of chemical carcinogenesis different conditions exist. In this instance, there appears to be either no threshold or a very low threshold (DiPaolo *et al.*, 1971). Thus, one might anticipate that slow activation would result in as great or even a greater carcinogenic effect than rapid activation, since there would be less likelihood of wastage of activated species from cells owing to production of an excess amount over that most effective for the number of critical binding sites available at a particular time. In addition, active carcinogenic species would be present over a longer period and therefore more likely to exist at a critical time or times in the cell cycle.

Another factor that may be of importance in explaining carcinogen inhibition by induction of increased mixed-function oxidase activity is that in many instances chemical carcinogens are subjected to detoxification reactions by this system as well as activation. The classic example of this is the aromatic amines. With these compounds, ring hydroxylation results in detoxification whereas hydroxylation of the nitrogen is an activation reaction (Miller and Miller, 1969). Thus, administration of inducers of mixed-function oxidase activity in these instances may result in a relatively greater proportion of the carcinogen being detoxified rather than activated to a carcinogenic metabolite. Changes in proportion of detoxified metabolites to carcinogenic metabolites could simply be the result of relative responses of the two pathways to the inducer. An alternative possibility suggested by the studies with BHA is that a basic alteration in metabolism may occur resulting in a changed metabolite pattern. In this instance, alteration of metabolite pattern could be independent of magnitude of induction and, in fact, as in the case of BHA, might occur without any overall increase in mixed-function oxidase activity. Further work is required to ascertain the mechanism of action of compounds discussed in this section which have already been shown to have the combined properties of increasing mixed-function oxidase activity and inhibiting chemical carcinogenesis.

V. Suppression of Chemical Carcinogenesis by Inhibition of Microsomal Mixed-Function Oxidase Activity

If the activity of the microsomal mixed-function oxidase system were totally absent, carcinogens requiring activation by this system would be inactive. Efforts have been made to achieve inhibition of chemical carcinogenesis by this mechanism. Studies of suppression of polycyclic hydrocarbon-induced epidermal neoplasia have been carried out employing 7,8-benzoflavone (α-naphthoflavone), a potent inhibitor of microsomal mixed-function oxidase activity. In experiments in which DMBA was the carcinogen, inhibition of epidermal neoplasia has been obtained (Gelboin *et al.*, 1970; Slaga and Bracken, 1977). A number of flavones are potent inducers of increased mixed-function oxidase activity as has been described in Section IV above. In contrast, 7,8-benzoflavone will cause inhibition of microsomal aryl hydrocarbon hydroxylase activity during a period shortly after its administration. A problem with exploitation of inhibition of mixed-function oxidase activity as a means of suppressing chemical carcinogenesis might occur if the enzyme inhibition were only partial. Under these conditions almost any result would be possible if the assumption is correct that slow activation of carcinogens can be effective in carcinogen activation. These considerations have been discussed in Section IV. An additional negative aspect of inhibiting the microsomal mixed-function oxidase system is that it would render the organism more susceptible to the noxious effects of xenobiotic compounds detoxified by this system.

Hoch-Ligeti *et al.* (1968) reported that administration of MC inhibits liver tumor formation in rats given dimethylnitrosamine simultaneously. Subsequently, Kunz *et al.* (1969) found that administration of phenobarbital inhibits the hepatocarcinogenicity of diethylnitrosamine and Hadjiolov (1971) and Hadjiolov and Mundt (1974) reported that administration of aminoacetonitrile inhibits the carcinogenicity of dimethylnitrosamine. The three compounds exerting inhibitory effects on nitrosamine-induced neoplasia of the liver all have been found to decrease dimethylnitrosamine demethylase activity in this organ. The suppression of demethylase activity has been regarded as the mechanism of inhibition. In further work it was found that the simultaneous administration of MC and dimethylnitrosamine resulted in a strong synergistic effect on lung tumor formation in both rats and mice. At the levels used in this study, neither the nitrosamine nor the hydrocarbon alone was carcinogenic for the lung. However, combined administration of the two agents brought about a significant incidence of pulmonary neoplasia. The mechanism of this synergism has not as yet been elucidated (Argus and Arcos, 1976).

VI. Miscellaneous Inhibitors of Chemical Carcinogenesis

There are a number of inhibitors of chemical carcinogenesis that have not been previously mentioned in this review. Many of these are somewhat difficult to classify and are presented in this section. 4-Nitroquinoline-N-oxide in low doses is a potent inhibitor of BP-induced epidermal neoplasia (Searle, 1965). Studies of Van Duuren *et al.* (1971) have shown that phenol, rutin, and morin will inhibit epidermal neoplasia from BP when applied simultaneously with this carcinogen. It has also been demonstrated that creosote oil fractions will suppress the formation of tumors of the mouse skin (Cabot *et al.*, 1940). Rogers (1957) has reported that pulmonary adenoma formation in the mouse resulting from urethane administration is inhibited by thymine, asparagine, orotic acid, dihydroorotic acid, ureidosuccinic acid, and cytidylic acid. The inhibition of this experimental system by thymine has been confirmed by Kaye and Trainin (1966). In other work, hydantoin has been shown to inhibit urethane-induced pulmonary adenoma formation (Levo, 1974). In investigation of hepatocarcinogens, Sidransky *et al.* (1963) reported that p-hydroxypropiophenone inhibits ethionine-induced liver tumors in rats, and Lacassagne and Hurst (1963) found that o,p'-dichlorodiphenyldichloroethane inhibits neoplasia of this organ resulting from 4-dimethylaminoazobenzene. Subcutaneous sarcoma formation resulting from administration of BP to mice has been reported to be inhibited by glyceraldehyde (Riley and Pettigew, 1944) and also by putrescine and *cis*-aconitic acid (Kallistratos and Fasske, 1975).

Carcinogenesis and inhibition of carcinogenesis can be brought about by inorganic compounds. Thus cadmium chloride when injected subcutaneously into rats will cause interstitial cell tumors of the testis. This neoplastic process is prevented by administration of zinc acetate (Gunn *et al.*, 1954).

VII. Discussion

A considerable number of compounds have been shown to inhibit chemical carcinogenesis. In most cases, the mechanism by which inhibition is brought about has not been established. In Table VIII major mechanisms thought to be of importance are listed. Thus far a substantial number of instances have been found in which the inhibitor alters the metabolism of the carcinogen. Clear evidence of inhibition by scavenging of active metabolites of a carcinogen *in vivo* has not yet been obtained, although this remains an attractive potential mechanism for inhibition. Several studies have been carried out in an effort to inhibit chemical carcinogenesis by prior administration of a competitive inhibitor. One of the uncertainties in this work is whether the inhibitors that are structurally related to carcinogens are actually acting by a competitive mechanism. Recent work of Poland *et al.* (1976) is of some interest with regard to competitive phenomena involving polycyclic aromatic hydrocarbons. Their studies have shown the presence of a binding protein in cytoplasm that is of importance for the induction of increased microsomal enzyme activity. Competition

TABLE VIII

MAJOR MECHANISMS FOR INHIBITING CHEMICAL CARCINOGENS

1. Alteration of metabolism of the carcinogen:
   (a) decreased activation
   (b) increased detoxification
   (c) combination of (a) and (b)
2. Scavenging of active molecular species of carcinogens so as to prevent their reaching critical target sites in the cell
3. Competitive inhibition

exists among various polycyclic aromatic hydrocarbons as well as other compounds for this binding site. Thus at least one *in vivo* situation exists in which an important group of carcinogens, i.e., the polycyclic aromatic hydrocarbons, are involved in competition for a defined binding site.

A perusal of Fig. 1 and Tables I, IV, and VII shows that compounds with a broad range of chemical structures inhibit chemical carcinogenesis. The diversity indicates that the capacity to inhibit this type of neoplastic process is not a restricted chemical characteristic, and that a considerable number of other inhibitors not yet identified probably exist. The quest to find these inhibitors is certainly worthwhile. Each time a new inhibitor is found, the potential increases for obtaining a broad range of further information. In terms of human exposure, there is a focus on determining whether the compound or related ones are present in the environment, and if so, in what form and amounts they occur, and how human intake is likely to take place. Basic investigations on mechanism of inhibition are obviously indicated. An example of a train of events occurring on identification of inhibitors is provided by the phenolic antioxidants. Two of these compounds, BHA and BHT, inhibit a large range of chemical carcinogens in animal models. Investigations of their occurrence in the environment revealed that they are widely used as antioxidants in food for human consumption. Thus an epidemiological base has been established for investigation of a potential role of the compounds in protecting against chemical carcinogenesis in human populations. Studies of the mechanism of inhibition of chemical carcinogens by these compounds has shown some interesting results. When these data on mechanism have been further substantiated, they could provide a basis for design of additional inhibitors and also for possibly predicting inhibitory capacities of both natural and synthetic compounds already present in the environment.

With the knowledge that inhibitors of chemical carcinogenesis exist, two questions arise. The first relates to the current role that these compounds are playing in reducing the impact of environmental carcinogens on man. The second is the optimal role that they might have. In order to assess their current role, additional information is required as to the actual range of compounds in the environment that have the capacity to inhibit carcinogens. Ancillary information including potency of inhibitors, range of carcinogens inhibited and magnitude of intake by individuals would also be necessary. For identifying inhibitors, information on mechanism(s) of inactivation is important to provide a basis for anticipating the effectiveness of chemical compounds. When adequate data are available on inhibitors, the definite evaluation of their role in man would be largely dependent upon epidemiological investigations.

Consideration of the optimal role that inhibitors of carcinogenesis might play entails evaluations of their deliberate use. At present, it would clearly be premature to undertake such measures because we simply do not have an adequate base of information. However, in the future, when more data are available on their mechanisms of inhibition, diversity, and toxicity, this course of action might be entertained. Accordingly, there would be some value in considering possible criteria to be met prior to deliberate usage of inhibitors of chemical carcinogenesis.

In Table IX, criteria are presented which I believe are prerequisites for seriously considering deliberate exposure of human populations to a particular inhibitor. For any normal group of individuals, a critical restraint is the possibility of toxicity. An inhibitor would have to be taken by individuals for many years in order to be effective so that even a low toxicity could outweigh any benefits. However, there are two situations which might result in this formidable obstacle being overcome. The first is the identification of inhibitors with trivial or no toxicity. One type of compound which might satisfy this rigid requirement for lack of toxicity is that which inhibits carcinogens occurring in the gastrointestinal contents without itself being absorbed. An inhibitor which is not absorbed could possibly be free of toxic properties. Other devices for avoiding toxicity might be equally effective.

A second basis for introduction of an inhibitor into the environment would be the aquisition of favorable data from epidemiological inves-

TABLE IX

CRITERIA PREREQUISITE TO CONSIDERATIONS OF EXPOSURE OF HUMAN
POPULATIONS TO INHIBITORS OF CHEMICAL CARCINOGENESIS[a]

Populations with "normal" risk of exposure to chemical carcinogens
1. The inhibitor has no toxicity or trivial toxicity—and/or
2. Human population groups have been exposed inadvertently to the inhibitor (a "natural" experiment in man) and it has been shown to be effective in reducing the incidence of carcinogen-induced neoplasia in appropriate epidemiological studies. In addition, there must be evidence of lack of toxic properties.
Populations with high risk of exposure to chemical carcinogens
1. Use of an inhibitor for which there is evidence that the benefits outweigh risks.

[a] It is important that any employment of inhibitors not be used as a device for either introduction of carcinogens into the environment or relaxing tolerance levels on the assumption that such exposures can be counteracted subsequently.

tigations. Such data would include firm evidence that a population group with a significant intake of a particular inhibitor has a diminished incidence of one or more neoplasms. It would be helpful to have mechanistic data relating the intake of the inhibitor to carcinogen inhibition. For example, if a population with a high consumption of a phenolic antioxidant such as BHA had a low cancer incidence, it would be of importance to be able to demonstrate that tissues from these individuals metabolize carcinogens to which they were likely to have been exposed in a manner so as to reduce their neoplastic potential. In addition, there should be clear evidence of lack of toxicity from the inhibitor. Under these conditions consideration of the use of the material bringing about the inhibition would be warranted. This, in essence, is a natural or unplanned type of experiment and depending on the magnitude of the inhibition and reliability of estimates of lack of adverse side effects could provide convincing data for deliberate use of the substance.

There do exist population groups with elevated exposures to chemical carcinogens. For individuals of this type less rigid requirements for lack of toxicity of inhibitors might be justified. With regard to this possibility, an exceedingly important prohibition is that inhibitors should not be used as a mechanism for allowing increased exposures to carcinogens or increasing tolerance levels to cancer producing substances.

VIII. Summary

Posed against the impact of environmental exposures to chemical carcinogens is the presence of compounds that inhibit these noxious agents. Many such inhibitors have now been demonstrated. The diversity of their chemical structures suggest that many more exist. The mechanisms by which these inhibitors operate is incompletely understood. In those instances in which information is available, the inhibitors act by virtue of altering the metabolism of the carcinogen. An evaluation of the current and potential role that these inhibitors may play is dependent on acquisition of further data on the range of compounds having the capacity to inhibit chemical carcinogenesis and mechanism(s) of inhibition.

REFERENCES

Adenis, L., Vlaeminck, M. N., and Driessens, J. (1970). *C. R. Seances Soc. Biol. Ses Fil.* **164,** 560–562.

Argus, M. F., and Arcos, J. C. (1976). *J. Theor. Biol.* **56,** 491–498.

Berenblum, I. (1929). *J. Pathol. Bacteriol.* **32**, 425–434.

Berenblum, I., and Haran, N. (1955). *Cancer Res.* **15**, 504–509.

Borchert, P., and Wattenberg, L. (1976). *J. Natl. Cancer Inst.* **57**, 173–179.

Cabot, S., Shear, N., and Shear, M. J. (1940). *Am. J. Pathol.* **16**, 301–312.

Conney, A. H., and Burns, J. J. (1972). *Science* **178**, 576–586.

Crabtree, H. B. (1941). *Cancer Res.* **1**, 39–43.

Crabtree, H. G. (1944). *Cancer Res.* **4**, 688–693.

Crabtree, H. G. (1945). *Cancer Res.* **5**, 346–351.

Crabtree, H. G. (1946). *Cancer Res.* **6**, 553–559.

DeMatteis, F. (1974). *Mol. Pharmacol.* **10**, 849–854.

DiPaolo, J. A., Donovan, P. J., and Nelson, R. L. (1971). *Nature (London), New Biol.* **230**, 240–242.

Falk, H. L., Kotin, P., and Thompson, S. (1964). *Arch Environ. Health* **9**, 169–179.

Fiala, E. S., and Weisburger, J. H. (1976). *Proc. Am. Assoc. Cancer Res.* **17**, 58.

Fiala, E. S., Bobotas, G., Kulakis, C., Wattenberg, L. W., and Weisburger, J. H. (1977). *Biochem. Pharmacol.* (in press).

Frankfurt, O., Lipchina, L., and Bunto, T. (1967). *Bull. Exp. Biol. Med. (Engl. Transl.)* **8**, 86–88.

Gelboin, H. V., Wiebel, F., and Diamond, L. (1970). *Science* **170**, 169–171.

Grantham, P. H., Weisburger, J. H., and Weisburger, E. K. (1972). *Food Cosmet. Toxicol.* **11**, 209–217.

Gunn, S. A., Gould, T. C., and Anderson, W. A. D. (1954). *Proc. Soc. Exp. Biol. Med.* **115**, 653–657.

Hadjiolov, D. (1971). *Z. Krebsforsch.* **76**, 91–92.

Hadjiolov, D., and Mundt, D. (1974). *J. Natl. Cancer Inst.* **52**, 753–756.

Hoch-Ligeti, C., Argus, M. F., and Arcos, J. E. (1968). *J. Natl. Cancer Inst.* **40**, 535–549.

Hozumi, M., Ogawa, M., Sugimura, T., Takeuchi, T., and Umezawa, H. (1972). *Cancer Res.* **32**, 1725–1728.

Huggins, C., Grand, L. C., and Brillantes, F. P. (1961). *Nature (London)* **189**, 204–207.

Huggins, C., Grand, L. C., and Fukunishi, R. (1964). *Proc. Natl. Acad. Sci. U.S.A.* **51**, 737–741.

Hunter, A. L., and Neal, R. A. (1975). *Biochem. Pharm.* **24**, 2199–2205.

Kallistratos, G., and Fasske, E. (1975). *Folia Biochim. Biol. Graeca* **13**, 94–107.

Kaye, A. M., and Trainin, N. (1966). *Cancer Res.* **26**, 2206–2212.

Klein, M. (1965). *J. Natl. Cancer Inst.* **34**, 175–183.

Kunz, W., Schaude, G., and Thomas, C. (1969). *Z. Krebsforsch.* **72**, 291–304.

Lacassagne, A., and Hurst, L. (1963). *C. R. Helid. Seance, Acad. Sci.* **256**, 5474–5476.

Lacassagne, A., Hurst, L., and Xuong, M. D. (1970). *C. R. Seance, Soc. Biol. Ses Fil.* **164**, 230–233.

Lam, L. K. T., and Wattenberg, L. (1977). *J. Natl. Cancer Inst.* (in press).

Levo, Y. (1974). *Naunyn-Schmiedeberg's Arch. Pharmacol.* **285**, 29–30.

Lichtenstein, E. P., Strong, F. M., and Borgan, D. G. (1962). *J. Agric. Food Chem.* **10**, 30–33.

Loub, W. D., Wattenberg, L. W., and Davis, D. W. (1975). *J. Natl. Cancer Inst.* **54**, 985–988.

MeLean, A. E., and Marshall, A. (1971). *Br. J. Exp. Pathol.* **52**, 322–329.

Maikiura, S. H., Aoe, S., Sugihara, S., Hirao, K., Masayuki, A., and Ito, N. (1974). *J. Natl. Cancer Inst.* **53**, 1253–1257.

Marquardt, H., Sapozink, M., and Zedeck, M. (1974). *Cancer Res.* **34**, 3387–3390.

Miller, E. C., and Miller, J. A. (1973). *In* "The Molecular Biology of Cancer" (H. Busch, ed.), pp. 377–402. Academic Press, New York.

Miller, E. C., Miller, J. A., Brown, R. R., and MacDonald, J. (1958). *Cancer Res.* **18**, 469–477.

Miller, J. A., and Miller, E. C. (1969). *Prog. Exp. Tumor Res.* **11**, 273–301.

Mirvish, S. S. (1975). *Ann. N.Y. Acad. Sci.* **258**, 175–179

Mirvish, S. S., Cardesa, A., Wallcave, L., and Shubik, P. (1975). *J. Natl. Cancer Inst.* **55**, 633–636.

Narisawa, T., Wong, C. Q., Maronpot, R. R., and Weisburger, J. H. (1976). *Cancer Res.* **36**, 505–510.

Neal, J., and Rigdon, R. H. (1967). *Tex. Rep. Biol. Med.* **25**, 553–557.

Nigro, N. D., Bhadrachari, N., and Ghomchai, C. (1973). *Dis. Colon Rectum* **16**, 438–443.

Pamukcu, A. M., Wattenberg, L. W., Price, J. M., and Bryan, G. T. (1971). *J. Natl. Cancer Inst.* **47**, 155–159.

Poland, A., Glover, E., and Kinde, A. S. (1976). *J. Biol. Chem.* **251**, 4936–4946.

Reddy, B. S., Weisburger, J. H., Narisawa, T., and Wynder, E. L. (1974). *Cancer Res.* **34**, 2368–2372.

Richardson, H. L., Stein, A. R., and Borson-Nacht-Nebel, E. (1952). *Cancer Res.* **12**, 356–361.

Riley, J. F., and Pettigrew, F. (1944). *Cancer Res.* **4**, 502–504.

Rogers, S. (1957). *J. Exp. Med.* **106**, 279–306.

Sasaki, S. (1963). *J. Nara Med. Assoc.* **14**, 101–115.

Schmähl, D., Krüger, F. W., Habs, M., and Diehl, B. (1976). *Z. Krebsforsch.* **85**, 271–276.

Searle, C. E. (1965). *Cancer Res.* **25**, 933–937.

Shamberger, R. J. (1966). *Experientia* **22**, 116.

Shamberger, R. J. (1970). *J. Natl. Cancer Inst.* **44**, 931–936.

Shamberger, R., and Willis, C. (1971). *Clin. Lab Sci.* **2**, 211–221.

Shamberger, R. M., Baughman, F. F., Kalchert, S. L., Willis, C. E., and Hoffman, G. C. (1973). *Proc. Natl. Acad. Sci. U.S.A.* **70**, 1461–1463.

Shimkin, M. B. (1955). *Adv. Cancer Res.* **3**, 223–267.

Sidransky, H., Clark, S., and Baba, T. (1963). *J. Natl. Cancer Inst.* **30**, 999–1008.

Sidransky, H., Ito, N., and Verney, E. (1966). *J. Natl. Cancer Inst.* **37**, 677–683.

Silva, E. A. (1967). *Hospital (Rio de Janeiro)* **71**, 1483–1493.

Slaga, T. J., and Bracken, W. M. (1977). *Cancer Res.* **37**, 1631–1635.

Speier, J., and Wattenberg, L. (1975). *J. Natl. Cancer Inst.* **55**, 469–472.

Sporn, M. B., Dunlop, N. M., Newton, D. L., and Smith, J. M. (1976). *Fed. Proc., Fed. Am. Soc. Exp. Biol.* **35**, 1332–1338.

Tawfic, H. N. (1965). *Acta Pathol. Jpn.* **15**, 255–260.

Thamavit, W., Hiasa, Y., Ito, N., and Phamarapravati, N. (1974). *Cancer Res.* **34**, 337–340.

Thurnherr, N., Deschner, E. E., Stonehill, E. H., and Lipkin, M. (1973). *Cancer Res.* **33**, 940–945.

Troll, W., Kassen, A., and Januff, A. (1971). *Science* **169**, 1211–1213.

Ulland, B., Weisburger, J., Yammamoto, R., and Weisburger, E. (1973). *Food Cosmet. Toxicol.* **11**, 199–207.

Van Duuren, B. L., Blazej, T., Goldschmidt, B. M., Katz, C., Melchionne, S., and Sivak, A. (1971). *J. Natl. Cancer Inst.* **46**, 1039–1043.

Virtanen, A. I. (1962). *Angew. Chem., Int. Ed. Engl.* **1**, 299–306.

Wattenberg, L. W. (1966). *Cancer Res.* **25**, 1520–1526.

Wattenberg, L. W. (1972a). *J. Natl. Cancer Inst.* **48**, 1425–1430.

Wattenberg, L. W. (1972b). *Fed. Proc., Fed. Am. Soc. Exp. Biol.* **31**, 633.

Wattenberg, L. W. (1973). *J. Natl. Cancer Inst.* **50**, 1541–1544.

Wattenberg, L. W. (1974). *J. Natl. Cancer Inst.* **52,** 1583–1587.

Wattenberg, L. W. (1975). *J. Natl. Cancer Inst.* **54,** 1005–1006.

Wattenberg, L. W. (1976). *In* "Fundamentals in Cancer Prevention" (P. N. Magee, ed.), Univ. Park Press, Baltimore, Maryland (in press).

Wattenberg, L. W. (1977). *J. Natl. Cancer Inst.* **58,** 395–398.

Wattenberg, L. W., and Leong, J. L. (1967). *Fed. Proc., Fed. Am. Soc. Exp. Biol.* **26,** 692.

Wattenberg, L. W., and Leong, J. L. (1968). *Proc. Soc. Exp. Biol. Med.* **128,** 940–943.

Wattenberg, L. W., and Leong, J. L. (1970). *Cancer Res.* **30,** 1922–1925.

Wattenberg, L. W., Loub, W. D., Lam, L. K. T., and Speier, J. L. (1976). *Fed. Proc., Fed. Am. Soc. Exp. Biol.* **35,** 1327–1331.

Wattenberg, L. W., Lam, L. K. T., Fladmoe, A., and Borchert, P. (1977). *Cancer* (in press).

Weisburger, E. K., Evarts, R. P., and Wenk, M. L. (1977). *Food Cosmet. Toxicol.* (in press).

Wheatley, D. N. (1968). *Br. J. Cancer* **22,** 787–792.

Yamamoto, R. S., Weisburger, J. H., and Weisburger, E. K. (1971). *Cancer Res.* **31,** 483–486.

Zedeck, M. S., Sternberg, S. S., McGowan, J., and Poynter, R. W. (1972). *Fed. Proc., Fed. Am. Soc. Exp. Biol.* **31,** 1485–1492.

LATENT CHARACTERISTICS OF SELECTED HERPESVIRUSES

Jack G. Stevens

Reed Neurological Research Center and Department of Microbiology and Immunology,
School of Medicine, University of California, Los Angeles, California

I. Introduction and Scope of the Review

The Herpesvirus group consists of many agents, individuals of which infect most members of the animal kingdom (cf. Kaplan, 1973). Although classification of an agent as a herpesvirus is now based almost entirely upon distinctive morphology of the virion, additional properties are also shared by most members of this group. Thus, herpesviruses undergo a replicative cycle that involves DNA expression and nucleocapsid assembly within the nucleus, the nascent nucleocapsid then acquiring an envelope when it "buds" through an inner nuclear membrane altered to contain viral specific proteins (reviewed by Ben-Porat and Kaplan, 1973). In addition to these morphological and replicative similarities, many herpesviruses have established a unique relationship with their host in which initial infection is followed by persistence of the agent, commonly for the life of

227

TABLE I

Common Herpes Viruses Grouped by Tissue in Which Latent Infection Exists[a]

Organ or tissue harboring latent virus	Virus	Status of evidence for the association	Reference[b]
Nervous system	Herpes simplex viruses types I and II	Strong	Stevens (1975a)
	Varicella-Zoster virus	Suggestive	Hope-Simpson (1965)
	Infectious bovine rhinotracheitis virus	Suggestive	Davies and Carmichael (1973)
	Herpesvirus simiae and other neurotropic simian herpesviruses	Strong	Hull (1973)
			McCarthy and Tosolini (1975)
	Pseudorabies virus	Suggestive	McKercher (1973)
	Equine Herpesvirus type I	Suggestive	McKercher (1973)
	Canine Herpesvirus	Suggestive	McKercher (1973)
Lymphoid tissue	Epstein–Barr Virus	Strong	Klein (1973)
			Roizman and Kieff (1975)
	Cytomegalovirus	Suggestive	Lang et al. (1976)
	Marek's disease virus	Strong	Biggs (1973)
			Kato and Akiyama (1975)
	Herpesvirus ateles, Herpesvirus saimiri	Strong	Deinhardt et al. (1973)
	Herpesvirus sylvilagus	Strong	Hinze and Wegner (1973)
Epithelial tissues	Lucké agent	Strong	Granoff (1973)
			Wolf et al. (1973)
	Epstein–Barr virus	Strong	Klein et al. (1974b)

[a] Insufficient evidence is available concerning some herpesviruses (infectious laryngotracheitis of chickens, feline rhinotracheitis virus, for example) to even tentatively classify them within this scheme.

[b] Where possible, recent comprehensive reviews summarizing the available evidence are presented. Therefore, no attempt has been made to establish precedence.

the host. This phenomenon is termed latency, and the herpesviruses, particularly as they are exemplified by the Herpes simplex agents, are usually presented as *the* classic example of latent viruses.[1]

If the tissues harboring latent viruses are considered, the herpesviruses may be further divided into three subgroups—those associated principally or exclusively with either nervous tissues, lymphoid tissues, or epithelial tissues. Table I represents a tentative grouping of the various agents according to this scheme; as can be seen, many agents infecting many animal species are represented. This review will present the herpesviruses within this context, but it will not be an exhaustive documentation of relevant studies concerning all agents. Rather, the focus will be on Herpes simplex virus (HSV), Epstein–Barr Virus (EBV), and the Lucké agent, which are presented as comparatively well-studied representatives from each subgroup. In the discussion, basic aspects of the latent state, particularly as they are known to exist in the intact host, will be of particular interest.

II. Herpes Simplex Virus

A. HISTORICAL

That Herpes simplex virus establishes latent infections from which it periodically reactivates to produce clinical disease has been inferred for many years, and a role for the nervous system in the phenomenon was suggested at the outset. However, only recently has direct evidence been gathered that supports the property of latency in general and a role for the nervous system in particular. The train of events which has led to our present knowledge concerning this phenomenon began early in this century when Howard (1903, 1905) documented three fatal cases of pneumonia and two of bacterial meningitis in which there were concurrent cutaneous herpetic lesions and inflammatory changes in the corresponding sensory ganglia. These observa-

---

[1] These working definitions of terms related to latent infections should be introduced here. In our laboratories, persistent infections are defined as infections in which virus (or at least the viral genome) is conserved in the host for long periods of time. A persistent infection in which the virus cannot be demonstrated by "conventional" virologic means (i.e., standard methods of viral cultivation) between episodes of acute disease in the host is termed a latent infection. This implies that the virus is maintained in some nonreplicating form. In contradistinction to a latent infection, a chronic infection is defined as one in which virus can be recovered by conventional methods from appropriate tissues at any time.

tions were followed closely by those of Cushing (1905), who, when treating 20 cases of trigeminal neuralgia by removing the corresponding ganglion, noted that two individuals subsequently developed lesions in areas supplied by contralateral nerves but none on the ipsilateral side. These findings suggested to both investigators that herpetic vesicles were somehow related to lesions in corresponding sensory ganglia. It is important to note, however, that even though herpetic lesions had previously been reported to be infectious (Vidal, 1873), neither Howard nor Cushing discussed their findings in this context. Thus, cutaneous herpetic disease was considered to be due to lesions in the corresponding sensory ganglion, but the fundamental basis for ganglionic and surface lesions was not considered.

Some 15 years later the infectious nature of the disease was firmly established with it was transmitted to the cornea of a rabbit (Grüter, 1920; Löwenstein, 1919). Immediately thereafter, initial studies concerning the agent and pathogenesis of disease following external inocualtion were begun. Initially, assays in rabbits showed that the infectious agent would pass a bacteria-tight filter, and it was therefore classified as a "filterable virus" (Levaditi and Harvier, 1920; Luger and Lauda, 1921). In addition to this finding, establishment of the rabbit model led almost immediately to the discovery by Doerr (1920; Doerr and Vöchting, 1920) that herpetic keratitis was often followed by signs referable to the nervous system (thus linking the infectious agent, lesions on the body surface, and neurologic disease). The nature of this relationship was investigated in great detail over the next 10-year period by several individuals, most notably Goodpasture and Teague. Of greatest significance here were the extensive and careful experiments which showed that the virus could be transported from peripheral sites to the central nervous system through nerve trunks (Goodpasture and Teague, 1923; Goodpasture, 1925). By the late 1920s then, there was evidence that the disease was caused by a "filterable virus" and that, after external inoculation, the agent traveled in nerves to the central nervous system where clinically apparent disease was produced. Thus, the general features concerning pathogenesis of acute herpetic disease in skin and nervous system were established.

Although recurrent disease remained unstudied, the foregoing investigations obviously led to hypotheses, and in 1929 Goodpasture correctly predicted experimental results that were obtained 40 years later. In a lecture delivered at Johns Hopkins University (Goodpasture, 1929), he noted that herpetic eruptions frequently occurred during the course of certain infectious diseases and other "intoxications" of various kinds, that they recurred in an equivalent site, and that the agent could not be recovered from skin when lesions were not present. This suggested to him that the processes were initiated by a latent virus, and that the latent agent did not reside in skin. Thus, the experiments involving nerve travel in animals indicated that the trigeminal (or other sensory ganglia) might well be the site at which virus was maintained. He further suggested that the virus remained latent in ganglionic neurons, and that the other diseases or "intoxications" sufficiently damaged the neuron to allow reactivation to occur.

It is of interest to note that in these discussions and most others of that time it was generally assumed that the virus was, in fact, latent and that recurrent lesions did not result from exogenous reinfection. Thus, the argument raised over the next 10-year period was not whether the virus was latent or not but, rather, whether the initial infection came from within the body [i.e., some sort of endogenous production of virus under the influence of certain physiological stimuli (Doerr, 1938)] or, alternatively, whether the virus was a typical infectious agent contracted in a usual manner. The latter alternative was proved correct when it was shown (Dodd *et al.*, 1938; Burnett and Williams, 1939) that an aphthous stomatitis due to the virus was often induced in those individuals who were without antibody and that this malady was then accompanied by the appearance of specific neutralizing antibody. The additional findings by Brain (1932), Andrewes and Carmichael (1930), and themselves (Burnett and Williams, 1939) showing that persons liable to suffer from recurrent disease always possessed serum antibody and sometimes had no history of a stomatitis suggested to Burnett and Williams that many primary infections were so mild as to go unnoticed. Finally, although they clearly favored a mechanism for recurrent disease based upon reactivation of the virus by various internal and external stimuli, Burnett and Carmichael did not suggest a site at which the latent infection might persist.

In subsequent years these early observations, when considered with the virologic consequences of surgical manipulation of the trigeminal tract in man (Carton and Kilbourne, 1952; Carton, 1953), have led to the following hypothesis to explain the natural history of recurrent herpetic disease in man. In general terms, infection has been postulated to follow a circuit from skin, mucous membrane, or eye (the primary infection) to the corresponding sensory ganglia via associated nerves. The virus would then become latent in the ganglia and later, as a result of one of the many provocations known to be associated with recurrences, virus would be reactivated, travel via the nerve to the surface and again produce lesions. As might be expected, this is not the only hypothesis that has been advanced; alternative hypotheses and their relative merits have been discussed elsewhere (Stevens, 1975a). Acceptance of the hypothesis involving sensory ganglia rests upon proof that the following phenomena obtain: (1) virus must be shown to establish latent infections in sensory ganglia; (2) virus must travel in some form and by some mechanism between the ganglion and the body surface in associated nerves; and (3) a diverse collection of "insults" must result in reactivation of virus from the ganglion and subsequent reappearance of specific lesions at the body surface. As I have detailed elsewhere (Stevens, 1975a,b), all phenomena, with the exception of reappearance of lesions following reactivation, have been shown to occur in experimental systems, and where they have been investigated, similar phenomena have been documented in man.

It is now well appreciated that persistent infections (which will now be termed latent since subsequent discussions will strongly support this designation) do occur in both the peripheral and central nervous systems (Stevens, 1975a,b; Cook and Stevens, 1976). Such infections were first demonstrated several years ago in our laboratories (Stevens and Cook, 1971). There, viral inoculation into the rear footpads of mice was shown to be followed by centripetal movement of the infection through the peripheral and central nervous systems to the brain. Animals that survived this infection harbored the virus in a "reactivable" form in the ipsilateral lumbosacral spinal ganglia. Although the virus could not be recovered from ganglia by direct assay, it could be "reactivated" and subsequently detected in a few days when the ganglia were explanted and maintained *in vitro*. Additionally, it was shown that the infection in these ganglia probably persisted for the life of the mouse, and appeared to be selectively associated with ganglia since similar techniques failed to reveal virus in the foot, sciatic nerve, and central nervous system of animals harboring virus in ganglia. Experiments of this general design have been successfully repeated by several laboratories for lumbosacral and other sensory ganglia in many species. Thus, latent infections have been established in trigeminal ganglia of rabbits (Stevens *et al.*, 1972) and mice (Knotts *et al.*, 1974; Walz *et al.*, 1974) following corneal inoculation; in trigeminal, cervical, and lumbosacral spinal ganglia of mice after inoculation of lip, ear, and vagina, respectively; and in lumbosacral spinal ganglia of guinea pigs following rear footpad inoculation (Scriba, 1975). Most important, virus was recovered from a significant number of human sensory ganglia when the techniques were applied to these tissues (Bastian *et al.*, 1972; Baringer and Swoveland, 1973; Rodda *et al.*, 1973; Baringer, 1974).

B. Tissues That Support the Latent Infection

In understanding the latent infection it is important first to determine the range of tissues that can support such an infection. One comprehensive study with this objective has been published (Cook and Stevens, 1976). There, mice were given a generalized infection by

TABLE II

In Vitro Reactivation of Latent Herpes Simplex Virus from Various Murine Tissues following Intravenous Inoculation of Virus

Animal no.	Tissues processed for detection of latent infections, and results[a]					
	Anterior brain	Posterior[b] brain	Spinal cord	Adrenal gland	Cervical and thoracic spinal ganglia	Lumbar and sacral spinal ganglia
1						
2					+	
3					+	
4			+			
5						+
6					+	
7			+		+	
8					+	
9					+	+
10		+			+	
11		+			+	+
12				+	+	
13	+	+			+	
14					+	
15						
16					+	
17				+	+	
18						+
19			+	+	+	
20					+	
21					+	
22						
23					+	

[a] No virus could be detected in trigeminal ganglia, bone marrow, lymph nodes, spleen, kidney, lung, or liver processed by the same methods. Blank spaces in the table also represent tissues from which virus could not be recovered. (From Cook and Stevens, 1976).

[b] "Posterior brain" was cerebellum and brainstem. The remainder constituted "anterior brain."

intravenous injection of sufficient virus to induce neurologic disease in 50–75% of inoculated mice, and then kill 10–70% of these animals with acute encephalitis. Nineteen to 109 days after infection, the mice were sacrificed and tissues of interest were explanted and maintained with monolayers of virus-susceptible cells. As can be seen in Table II, the persistent infection appeared to be restricted to nervous tissues, including adrenal medula. These results do not permit an unequivocal conclusion, however, since it can be argued that the methods of assay are not adequate to detect the latent infection in all tissues examined, or that the generalized infection, although severe, may not have been sufficient to adequately infect all tissues. However, similar infections established by "lymphotropic" herpesviruses in white blood cells can be detected by these methods (cf. Symposium on Herpesvirus and Cervical Cancer, 1973), and in the experiments presented here, diverse areas of the nervous system were involved—suggesting efficient spread of the virus. Therefore, it is reasonable to at least tentatively conclude that with Herpes simplex virus, latent infections are limited to nervous tissues.

C. CELL-TYPE HARBORING VIRUS, PHYSICAL STATE OF THE LATENT VIRUS

During the acute infection, it has been shown by several laboratories that Schwann, satellite, and other supporting cells in experimental animals undergo an abortive infection and that morphologically complete virions are replicated in neurons (reviewed by Stevens, 1975a). From these observations, it might be suggested that supporting cells would be the most likely cell type to harbor the virus. However, this appears not to be the case; the bulk of evidence, although indirect, indicates that latent virus is associated with neurons. Of several kinds of experiment that have been presented (cf. Stevens, 1975a), the most convincing are reports from two laboratories that, in sensory ganglia analyzed directly after removal from mice or rabbits, viral DNA can be detected only in neurons (Stevens and Cook, 1974; Stevens, 1975a,b; H. Schulte-Holthausen, 1975, cited by zur Hausen and Schulte-Holthausen, 1975).[2] In addition, reactivating ganglia demonstrate even more neurons in which viral DNA can be detected, and this DNA

---

[2] Passage of viral DNA from a nonproductive supporting cell to the neuron, coupled with subsequent replication in the neuron cannot be ruled out at this time. However, this is a burdensome and complicated hypothesis, and the sole basis for support at this time rests in the observation that supporting cells commonly undergo abortive (but, it must also be added, cytocidal) infections.

can be "chased" to supporting cells. The converse is not true (Cook *et al.*, 1974). The technique used for these analyses was *in situ* hybridization with subsequent autoradiography performed on sections of ganglia employing a probe of radioactive complementary RNA made from HSV DNA.

The state of the virus associated with these neurons has not been defined, but it appears most likely that some form of nonreplicating virus is conserved, thus indicating that the infection is, in fact, a latent one. The best evidence supporting this statement comes from two sources. First, as will be discussed in greater detail later, temperature-sensitive mutants of the virus whose restrictive temperature is mouse body temperature can establish long-term persistent infections in the mouse, and infectious virus cannot be demonstrated in involved tissues. Second, the only viral product that can be detected in persistently infected ganglia at the time of explant is the viral DNA alluded to above; extensive searches for infectious virus, and other viral specific products (detectable by immunofluorescent or ultrastructural methods), have with one exception consistently yielded negative results (reviewed by Stevens, 1975a). The one positive result obtained by these techniques was obtained by Baringer and Swoveland (1974), who, when searching serial sections of latently infected rabbit trigeminal ganglia by ultrastructural methods, found a rare neuron in which morphologically complete herpesviruses could be detected. Although this could be considered to be strong evidence that the infection is maintained by continuous replication of infectious virus, the following considerations make it seem at least equally likely that this finding represents spontaneous reactivation of a latent infection. In studies where the effects of antiviral IgG on latent infections in mouse lumbosacral ganglia were evaluated, latently infected ganglia were transplanted in Millipore chambers to the peritoneal cavities of passively immunized and unimmunized mice (Stevens and Cook, 1974). These ganglia were later removed and subjected to *in situ* nucleic acid hybridization techniques to search for viral DNA. Although the results with antisera will be discussed later, the relevant finding here is that in normal mice there was about a 100-fold increase (from ≤ 0.05 neuron per ganglionic section to 5–10 neurons per section) in the number of neurons in which viral DNA could be detected after ganglia had been maintained in the chambers for 3 days (conditions under which replication of infectious virus is "induced" and the virus is easily detected). These neurons were well separated, and the number binding viral specific cRNA did not increase significantly when the period of maintenance was increased to 6 days. These results suggest that, at the time of explant viral DNA was present in some "reactiva-ble" form in all neurons in which DNA was subsequently detected. Thus, for every neuron in which viral DNA could be detected at the time of explant, there were some 100 more in which the DNA was at a concentration too low to be detectable with the cRNA probe. In addi-tion, the number of silver grains referable to cRNA over the few neurons detected at the time of explant was roughly equivalent to the number over neurons which had been "induced" to replicate viral DNA by the transplantation procedure. From all of this, then, it seems likely that the specific grains detected at the time of explant were over neurons in which virus was spontaneously reactivating, that this is a murine counterpart of Baringer and Swoveland's ultrastructural fin-ding in rabbit trigeminal ganglia, and that the virus is, in fact, main-tained in some nonreplicating and therefore latent state in neurons of sensory ganglia.

The form in which the virus is maintained could range from per-sistence of the entire virion to conservation of the viral DNA only. Whatever the form, however, there is no *a priori* need to postulate integration of viral genetic material into cellular DNA as a means of perpetuation, since neurons do not divide.

D. ESTABLISHMENT, MAINTENANCE, AND REACTIVATION OF THE LATENT INFECTION

From the evidence presented earlier (principally morphologic), it seems likely that the virus is maintained in neurons, and in a nonrep-licating state. To study the interaction that takes place between neuron and virus in establishment, maintenance, and reactivation of the latent virus, an *in vitro* system more amenable to quantitative biochemical study than are ganglia is needed. Unfortunately, none has yet been developed, and this task may be difficult since, as noted above, la-tently infected neurons in ganglia are normally "induced" to produce virions when they are subjected to *in vitro* cultivation. However, since it may be possible to overcome this difficulty, we are intensively studying various clones of the mouse C-1300 neuroblastoma line maintained *in vitro* and manipulated by various techniques after in-fecting them with either wild-type or selected temperature-sensitive mutants of the virus which can establish latent infections *in vivo* (Lof-gren *et al.*, 1977).

A somewhat different approach also underway is the use of temperature-sensitive mutants with defined polypeptide phenotypes in *in vivo* systems. As we have discussed elsewhere (Lofgren *et al.*, 1977), given some basic assumptions, it may be predicted that mutants which cannot establish latent infections possess lesions in genes whose products are critical for establishment of the latent infection. Mutants restricted at 38°C (normal mouse temperature) in cell culture systems are available (Subak-Sharpe *et al.*, 1974), and some have been screened for their capacity to establish latent infections in the central and peripheral nervous systems of mice. This work is still in progress, and the results of preliminary investigations concerning five mutants (Lofgren *et al.*, 1977, and unpublished results) can be summarized as follows: (1) The mutants can be divided into two groups that differ in the capacity to establish latent infections. (2) Both DNA+ and DNA− mutants can establish latent infections, suggesting (but by no means proving) that DNA replication is irrelevant to establishment of latent infections. (3) Mutants that produce the fewest identifiable viral structural components during acute infection at the restrictive temperature in "differentiated" neuroblastoma cells maintained *in vitro* are the most likely to establish latent infections *in vivo*. However, this correlation does not extend to individual virus proteins since viruses with the most altered patterns of polypeptide synthesis are not necessarily the most likely to establish latent infections. The latter results are encouraging findings which imply specificity of involved functions. It is hoped that an analysis and comparison of remaining mutants will allow us to identify polypeptides related to establishment of latent infections, and studies concerning a definition of functions for these peptides can then be initiated.

Investigations of the mechanism(s) involved in maintaining the latent infection are just beginning, but there is a suggestion that antiviral IgG may play an important role. The evidence supporting this statement and its extensions is presented elsewhere (Stevens and Cook, 1974). In brief, it is based upon showing that viral DNA synthesis is inhibited in latently infected neurons populating ganglia which are transplanted in Millipore chambers to uninfected mice passively immunized with specific immune IgG, but not in mice given nonimmune IgG. How antiviral antibody might function in this inhibition is not known, but a model consistent with data derived for this and possibly related systems (Aoki *et al.*, 1972; Joseph and Oldstone, 1975) would involve specific interaction between the IgG and virus specific antigens on the surface of neurons. Through some as yet undefined intracellular effector molecule, this interaction could repress complete expression of the viral genome.

Reactivation of active infection following a defined manipulation has been accomplished in at least two model systems (Walz *et al.*, 1974; Stevens *et al.*, 1975) and occurs spontaneously in others (Nesburn *et al.*, 1967; Underwood and Weed, 1974; Sriba, 1975; Hill *et al.*, 1975). As might be expected, the biochemical basis for this phenomenon (overcoming the repressive effect of antibody) is completely unknown, and, as with other aspects, its ultimate resolution will depend upon development of a manipulable *in vitro* system.

Finally, several considerations that lead to an important and unresolved conceptual problem concerning the consequences of reactivation should be presented. First, it is well known that recurrent herpetic disease in man recurs at very close if not identical sites and that anesthesias of these sites are very uncommon. Second, in the experimental systems studied, reactivation is accompanied by productive infection of the neuron. Third, in all cell types studied to date, productive herpesvirus infection is accompanied by cell death and by morphologic criteria at least, neurons in the reactivating sensory ganglia of experimental animals are killed. If the results described in experimental animals mirror phenomena occurring in man, it is difficult to understand how the neuronal destruction associated with viral replication could be compatible with multiple recurrences at the same site and no accompanying anesthesias. Obviously, one explanation would involve proposing that, in this instance, the experimental models do not mirror the situation in man and that reactivation in man involves synthesis and passage to the body surface of an infectious subviral particle which does not kill the neuron.

E. SUMMARY AND CONCLUSIONS

After peripheral inoculation, Herpes simplex virus establishes persistent infections in both man and experimental animals. Experimentally, the infection is limited to nervous tissue and is particularly common in sensory ganglia where neurons appear to be the reservoir for a latent infection. The state in which the virus (or, more likely, some subviral form) exists is undefined, but specific immune IgG may play a role in maintenance. Reactivation in experimental systems results in productive infections of previously latently infected neurons. Whether this also is the case in man is not known. Finally, further significant definition of the latent state is likely to depend upon establishment of suitable cell culture systems which can be manipulated and analyzed by quantitative biochemical techniques.

III. Epstein–Barr Virus

A. HISTORICAL

As has been described, latent characteristics for Herpes simplex virus were suspected early on, principally because of the recurring nature of disease syndromes with which it was shown to be associated. The situation with Epstein–Barr virus was quite different. In this instance, the virus was conclusively shown to establish persistent infections at the time of its discovery. Indeed, this was the basis of its discovery—a persistently infected lymphoblastoid cell line was the initial source of virus.

Thus, the Burkitt lymphoma was thought almost from the time of its initial description to have an infectious etiology, and attempts were made to incriminate viruses. When tumor specimens taken from patients with Burkitt's lymphoma were examined by ultrastructural methods and no viruses were found, similar attempts were made using lymphoblastoid cell lines which had been established from the tumors. In 1964, in one of the first lines studied, a small number of cells were found by Epstein et al. (1964) to harbor virions with herpeslike morphology. Over the next couple of years, as a result of studies by several laboratories, particularly the Henles' (reviewed by Klein, 1973), this virus was shown to be unrelated to other herpesviruses and was also found in several other cell lines established from Burkitt tumors. In addition, antibodies to the agent were found both in individuals with Burkitt's lymphoma and in some "normal" people. From these results it was concluded that a previously undescribed lymphotropic Herpesvirus has been discovered and it was named the Epstein–Barr virus (EBV).

Since the time of initial description, a vast amount of effort, using a myriad of techniques and approaches, has been expended in many laboratories in attempts to determine whether this agent is etiologically involved in Burkett's lymphoma. Although a detailed discussion concerning the relationship of the virus to this and other diseases is outside the scope of this review, the present state of knowledge has been discussed in detail by Miller (1971), Klein (1973), and Roizman and Kieff (1975) and can be summarized as follows. A considerable amount of evidence (although circumstantial) indicates that EBV, either alone or, possibly in combination with another infectious agent, is responsible for Burkitt's lymphoma. Extensive serological studies have established that the virus is the causative agent of heterophile antibody-positive infectious mononucleosis, and evidence similar to that derived for Burkitt's lymphoma is mounting which indicates that EBV is responsible for nasopharyngeal carcinoma. Relationships with other conditions have been suggested, but supportive evidence is scanty.

To summarize from these considerations, it is clear that the evolution of knowledge concerning Epstein–Barr virus was quite different from that of Herpes simplex virus. First, Herpes simplex virus has been intimately associated with the overall historical development of concepts in viral disease; Epstein–Barr virus was discovered only recently. Second, diseases induced by Herpes simplex virus have been recognized and appreciated for years; those for which Epstein–Barr virus is responsible are still being defined. Third, much of the work with Herpes simplex virus has been involved with showing that it in fact does persist, whereas these properties were established with Epstein–Barr virus at the outset. Last, the viruses are latent in very dissimilar cell types; latent Herpes simplex virus is associated with a nondividing cell of ectodermal origin while Epstein–Barr virus persists in dividing cells of mesodermal origin. The functions of these cells, and the present state of knowledge concerning them, is quite different.

B. THE LATENT STATE

As was stressed earlier, persistent Epstein–Barr virus is associated with lymphocytes, and a few cells in lymphoblastoid cell lines established from Burkitt's lymphomas were shown to spontaneously replicate and release virus, being destroyed in the process. It is now well appreciated that similar cultures can be established from lymphocytes of seropositive individuals in the general population (Gerber and Monroe, 1968; Nilsson et al., 1971) and that lymphocytes can be established in continuous culture by addition of the virus to lymphocytes obtained either from fetuses or antibody-negative individuals (Gerber et al., 1969; Pope et al., 1969a,b; Henle and Henle, 1970). In addition, cloning experiments suggested early on that nonvirus-producing cells in virus carrying lines possessed the viral genome—descendants of these cells later also produced viral antigens and in a proportion similar to the parentlal line (Miller et al., 1970; Zajac and Kahn, 1970). Finally, it is now known that the virus-carrying lines have characteristics of B (bone marrow-derived) lymphocytes (Nilsson, 1971; E. Klein et al., 1972; Moore and Minowada, 1973); lymphoblastoid lines with T (thymus-derived) characteristics do not contain detectable EBV DNA (Kawai et al., 1973; Pagano, 1974) and do not possess viral receptors on the cell surface (Jondal and Klein, 1973). It should be noted, however, that not all lines with B-cell characteristics contain detectable amounts of the viral genome (Kawai et al., 1973; Klein et al., 1974a; Pagano, 1974). Thus, the presence of virus seems to be a sufficient but not universally necessary prerequisite for establishment of lymphoblastoid lines with B-cell characteristics.

Of particular importance to this discussion are the general findings that cell-free infectious virus cannot be recovered from either the Burkitt tumors or buffy coats from normal individuals at the time of explant. In addition, neither ultrastructural nor immunofluorescent evidence for the presence of virions or viral capsids can be found at this time; as with Herpes simplex virus, viral replication appears to take place following the "stress" of in vitro cultivation of cells carrying the viral genome (reviewed by Klein, 1972). Unlike the presently understood situation with Herpes simplex virus, however, virus-specific antigens[3] are detectable at two cellular sites in all biopsies of Burkitt's tumors. First, specific antigens detected by immunofluorescent methods exist on the surface of malignant lymphocytes (Klein et al., 1966, 1967, 1968). These are termed membrane antigens (MA). Second, an intranuclear antigen (Epstein–Barr nuclear antigen, or EBNA) detected initially by anticomplement staining methods (Reedman and Klein, 1973; Reedman et al., 1974), and more recently by radioimmunoassay techniques (Brown et al., 1975) is also present. Since the EBNA and MA antigens are present on essentially all lymphocytes in biopsies, and EBNA at least persists in all cells of lymphoblastoid lines irrespective of whether they are virus producers, the presence of these antigens is compatible with cell proliferation. It is perhaps noteworthy that viral specific antigens have not been detected in lymphoid cells observed directly after removal from normal seropositive individuals. However, antigens can be found in the lymphoblastoid lines derived from these cells. Whether the failures at the time of explantation are simply sampling errors or indicate a major difference in the relationship between virus and cell in individuals with tumors and normal individuals is not known. To summarize then, Epstein–Barr virus establishes a latent infection of malignant (and normal?) B lymphocytes, virus specific antigens are present in all of these cells, and in vitro cultivation is sufficient to induce virus replication from a portion of latently infected cells.

[3] Although the virus-specific antigens described here are generally considered to be products of the viral genome, the evidence supporting this conclusion is entirely circumstantial.

This simple and unifying view is satisfying, but there are complicating factors. Thus, it was appreciated early in the course of studies in which lymphoblastoid lines were established that not all produced viral particles or infectious virus and at the present time, cell lines which replicate significant amounts of infectious virus are the exception rather than the rule (reviewed by Roizman and Kieff, 1975). By appropriate immunologic techniques (principally the methods of immunofluorescence and complement fixation), it has been shown that cells in different lines characteristically are blocked at different stages of the viral infectious cycle, and the results of many analyses by many laboratories can be summarized as follows. Essentially all cells in all lines established possess the EBNA antigen (Reedman and Klein, 1973). There is also recent evidence suggesting that viral specific membrane antigens (a subset of MA?) recognizable only by specific immune T lymphocytes and termed lymphocyte-detected membrane antigen (LYDMA), is also present in each cell line (Svedmyr and Jondal, 1975). At any given time, a minority of cells (usually less than 5%) in certain lines may express additional virus-specific antigens, the antigen(s) expressed and the percentage of positive cells is characteristic of the line, and extends to clonal derivatives of the line (reviewed by Klein, 1972). In addition to EBNA and the membrane antigens detectable by lymphocytes, other antigens that may appear are: (1) early antigen (EA), a nuclear and cytoplasmic antigen detected by immunofluorescence, which has been further subdivided (W. Henle *et al.*, 1970; G. Henle *et al.*, 1971) into groups R (restricted, cytoplasmic clumps resistant to alcohol extraction) and D (diffuse, fairly dispersed in nucleus and cytoplasm, not alcohol extractable); (2) membrane antigen (MA), a multicomponent antigen (Svedmyr *et al.*, 1970) which has already been discussed; and (3) viral capsid antigen (VCA), also probably a multicomponent antigen detected by immunofluorescence techniques (Henle and Henle, 1966; Svedmyr and Demissie, 1971). The functions of EBNA and EA are not known; EBNA could be involved in induction and maintenance of the transformed state, while EA may be involved in regulatory processes during the lytic infection [EA containing cells cease to make host specified macromolecules and later die (Gergely *et al.*, 1971)]. VCA and most, if not all of MA are viral structural proteins (reviewed by Roizman and Kieff, 1975). Finally, a figure summarizing the sequence of appearance in productively infected cells of these antigens, and steps in synthesis where blocks are known to occur has been presented by Klein. This is reproduced (with the addition of LYDMA) as Fig. 1.

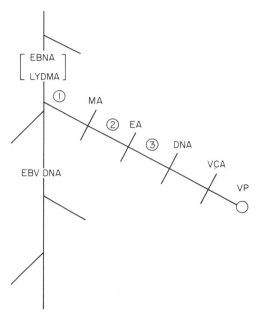

FIG. 1. Epstein–Barr virus-specific products, their relative time of appearance, and areas where blocks to further synthesis may occur in lymphoblastoid cell lines carrying the viral genome. All cell lines produce EBNA and harbor viral DNA. Depending upon the line studied, blocks to further syntheses may occur at the numbered points noted. The nature of these products is discussed in the text. From Klein (1975).

If it is assumed that all the EBV-associated antigens described above are indeed virus specified, then the extent to which the EBV genome is expressed varies significantly in different lymphoblastoid cell lines. The situation can vary from extremely limited expression (EBNA and possibly limited MA) to the replication of infectious virus. Why only a minority of cells in any culture produce more than EBNA at any time, and why the lines differ qualitatively in antigen expression is unknown but will be treated in greater detail below. Of course, it must be recognized that in some lines of limited inducibility only a portion of the viral genome may be present.

C. State of Viral DNA in Latently Infected Cells

Throughout the discussion so far, the assumption has been made that neoplastic Burkitt tumor cells, cell lines derived from the tumors and from seropositive individuals, and those established by addition of virus to lymphocytes taken from seronegative individuals do indeed carry viral genetic information. With rare exceptions, this is now known to be true. Initial evidence predicting this universal association came from studies performed by several laboratories on cells of the Raji line—a lymphoblastoid line derived from a Burkitt's tumor (Pulvertaft, 1965, Epstein *et al.*, 1966), which at the time of initial study was known to possess only a complement-fixing antigen (Pope *et al.*, 1969a,b; Gerber and Deal, 1970) specific for EBV. It should be noted in passing that this antigen is now recognized to likely be EBNA (Klein and Vonka, 1974).

As a result of studies involving nucleic acid hybridization techniques, it is now well established that each cell of the Raji line contains multiple copies of the viral genome. Initially, employing purified and radioactive EBV DNA as a probe, zur Hausen and Schulte-Holthausen (1970) showed that there was significant specific hybridization between viral DNA and DNA from the Raji line which had been immobilized on nitrocellulose filters. In addition, transcription of the EBV DNA in these cells was suggested since some Raji cell RNA bound to purified EBV DNA. More quantitative data were obtained by Nonoyama and Pagano (1971), who, using similar methods analyzed EBV specific radioactive complementary RNA (cRNA) transcribed *in vitro*. They, by employing appropriate reconstruction experiments, indicated that there were about 65 "genome equivalents" of EBV DNA per cell and that this was associated with cellular chromosomes. This number was corroborated when later investigations employing the generally more quantitative methods of DNA–DNA reassociation kinetics indicated that there were 50 genome equivalents per cell (Nonoyama and Pagano, 1973). When radioactive cRNA was employed in *in situ* hybridization studies in the Raji cells (zur Hausen, 1972; Nonoyama and Pagano, 1972; Pagano and Huang, 1974), it was shown that all nuclei contained viral DNA, and in about the same concentration. Whether the complete EBV genome is present in all these cells is not definitively known, but two types of experiments suggest that it is. First, when DNA from either Raji cells or purified EBV is used to drive a radioactive EBV DNA probe into hybrids in kinetic DNA–DNA reassociation experiments, the shape of the curves generated is identical (Nonoyama and Pagano, 1973; Pritchett *et al.*, 1976). Second, treatment of the Raji line with 5-bromodeoxyuridine results in the induction (in a very few cells) of virus particles which are morphologically intact (Hampar *et al.*, 1972) and infectious (Gerber, 1972).

It seems then, that all nuclei in a culture of virus negative Raji cells contain about 50 copies of most, if not all the EBV genome, and that these genomes are associated with cellular chromosomes. Subsequent studies have been concerned with a determination of the state in which these genomes exist. Initially, Nonoyama and Pagano (1972) isolated nuclei from [^{3}H] thymidine labeled Raji cells, lysed them on top of alkaline glycerol gradients, centrifuged the lysates under velocity conditions, and showed that 95% or more of the centrifuged viral DNA was in a position (≤ 70 S) significantly different from cellular DNA (130 S). Since this constituted evidence that the viral genome was not covalently linked to the host cell chromosome (at least in a conventional manner), they suggested that the DNA might well be existing as a plasmid. More recent evidence in which nonalkaline conditions were used in equilibrium centrifugation runs (Adams *et al.*, 1973) suggests that a significant proportion of EBV DNA molecules are, in fact, linearly integrated in the host cell chromosome in a form stable to Pronase and phenol, but not alkali. This finding is compatible with RNA linkage or hydrogen bonding. In extensions, Adams and Lindahl (1975), and Lindahl *et al.* (1976) looked at the nonintegrated EBV DNA sequences and found that they existed as circular molecules, of a length comparable to that of linear DNA derived from virus particles. Thus, it seems that in Raji cells, EBV sequences are present in two forms—one linearly associated with cellular DNA in an alkali-sensitive form, and the other a circular form free from cellular DNA. All viral genes may be present in the latter, since it has a contour length comparable with that of an entire viral genome. Nothing is known about the extent to which viral genes are present in the former. It should also be noted that these studies do not establish the physical status of the viral genome in each cultured cell.

Since cells in the Raji line in many ways resemble Burkitt cells *in vivo* (limited expression of the viral genome and no infectious virus produced), it might be predicted that the physical state of the viral genome in these cells should mirror that found *in vivo*. A report by Kaschka-Dierich *et al.* (1976) confirms this; as in the Raji line, both integrated and circular extrachromosomal viral DNA were found in relevant cells of Burkitt's tumors and nasopharyngeal carcinomas. The carcinoma cells were one-step removed from their natural habitat, however, since they had been passaged in nude mice to select against a significant population of contaminating lymphocytes. More recently, this same group has indicated that in two lymphoblastoid cell lines (Namalwa and AW-Ramos) harboring only a few viral genome equivalents per cell, all detectable viral DNA was integrated (Andersson and Lindahl, 1976; M. Andersson *et al.*, personal communication, 1976).

Thus, it may be that only integrated viral DNA is common to all cells latently infected with EBV. Finally, it should be noted that although these results of studies concerning viral DNA in the Raji line reflect the situation in the Burkitt tumor cells *in situ*, the state of DNA is latently infected cells present in normal individuals and those with infectious mononucleosis is unknown.

D. MAINTENANCE OF THE LATENT INFECTION

As with Herpes simplex virus, the regulatory mechanisms which maintain the latent infection have not been defined. From the previous discussions, it is clear that *in situ*, the viral genome is expressed minimally in Burkitt lymphoma cells—only EBNA and MA are known to be produced. When these cells are taken from the patient and placed *in vitro*, additional virus specific functions can be expressed in some cells—the extreme being production of infectious virus and destruction of the cell. Obviously, control mechanisms have been "upset" by *in vitro* cultivation, and there have been studies concerning the nature of these mechanisms. First, there is one report suggesting that, as was indicated for the HSV system, antiviral antibody plays a role in regulating viral expression in explanted lymphoblasts (Aoki *et al.*, 1972). In this system, addition of antibody depressed the synthesis of virus-specific antigens. Second, regulation of viral genetic expression has been studied by defining appropriate phenotypic characteristics of heterokaryons derived by fusion of various EBV genome carrying lines either to each other or to genome negative cells of various types. When the spontaneous appearance of viral products, or their appearance subsequent to 5-iododeoxyuridine induction or EBV superinfection was compared to the consequences of similar treatments of parental lines, several results were obtained. To summarize, the regulatory patterns were found to be exceedingly complex (Nyormoi *et al.*, 1973; Glaser and Nonoyama, 1974; Klein *et al.*, 1974b,c, 1976); there appeared to be multiple regulatory mechanisms instituted by both virus and cell and, in general, a straightforward definitive interpretation of the results is difficult to present. However, as Klein *et al.* (1976) point out, cell hybridization is one of but a few techniques currently available that can approach this important and complex problem in a meaningful way, and it seems likely that results establishing precise regulatory mechanisms will come from extensions of these experiments. Finally, it has been shown that in latently infected cells, the synthesis of viral DNA is coordinated with that of cellular DNA; it is replicated during early S phase of the cell cycle (Hampar *et al.*, 1974).

E. Permissive Infections in Man

Since EBV-associated diseases are readily transmitted in nature, there must be a naturally permissive cell comparable to the epithelial cell which replicates HSV. Such cells have not been identified, but they are likely to exist in the oropharynx, since infectious, cell-free throat washings can be obtained from individuals during the period of clinically apparent mononucleosis, and for prolonged periods after recovery (Gerber *et al.*, 1972; Miller *et al.*, 1973; Pagano, 1974). Similar excretion probably takes place after inapparent infection. These results make it reasonably certain that permissive cells do exist in the oropharynx, and, although the types have not been identified, there are two likely possibilities—epithelial cells and lymphocytes. In an analogy to the relationship between Marek's virus and the chicken (a system that has many other similarities to the EBV–human association), it could be predicted that the permissive cell is an epithelial cell since feather follicle epithelial cells are the permissive cells for Marek's virus (Calnek *et al.*, 1970, Nazerian and Witter, 1970). In this regard, it is now well established that the tumor cells in EBV-associated nasapharyngeal carcinomas carry EBV genetic information (Wolf *et al.*, 1973; Klein *et al.*, 1974a). However, there have been no reports that these tumor cells produce infectious virus, and it seems equally possible that, in analogy to some cell lines, viral genome-positive lymphoid cells populating the throat (tonsils?) would sometimes spontaneously become virus producers. Finally, it is important to note that, with the possible exception of tonsillitis (Veltri *et al.*, 1976), no disease syndrome has seriously been considered to be a consequence of reactivated EBV infections.

F. Summary and Conclusions

The Epstein–Barr virus genome is maintained in a latent state in neoplastic B lymphocytes of Burkitt's lymphomas and at least a portion is conserved in epithelial cells comprising nasopharyngeal carcinomas. These latent infections are accompanied by limited expression of the viral genome. The extent to which the viral genome is expressed in lymphocytes in normal individuals is unknown, but in either case, *in vitro* cultivation of genome carrying cells may be followed by replication of the virus. EBV derived from these cultures or from the throats of individuals with active infection, just as that derived from malignant lymphocytes can then latently infect and influence previously uninfected B lymphocytes to become capable of continuous cultivation. A minority of cells in EBV genome-carrying cultures may replicate infectious virus, but more commonly the cell lines are populated by cells that express various virus-specific antigens in varying numbers of cells. The pattern of antigen expression, however, is characteristic for a given cell line, and all established lines express a specific nuclear antigen and most possess multiple copies of the viral genome. Intensive studies concerning the state of the viral genome in one well-studied line (Raji) which contains about 50 genome equivalents of viral DNA indicates that a portion of the viral genomes are linearly associated by alkali-sensitive bonds with the host cell chromosomes, and the rest are present as circular molecules. Similar circular molecules have recently been found in nasopharyngeal carcinomas and Burkitt's tumors.

Although a considerable amount of information is now available concerning the status of the latent EBV genome and the extent to which it is expressed in latently infected cells, mechanisms by which the latent infections are established and reactivated are obscure. As with Herpes simplex virus, these problems can be approached most meaningfully when an *in vitro* system is found in which a large population of cells can be synchronously infected, influenced to undergo latent infection and then reactivated to active infection following a defined manipulation.

IV. Lucké Virus

A. HISTORICAL

Some 40 years ago, Balduin Lucké (1934) published pathologic descriptions of adenocarcinomas of the kidneys occurring in 158 leopard frogs *(Rana pipiens)*. Although these were for the most part nonmetastisizing, well-differentiated adenocarcinomas that only rarely underwent spontaneous regression, all gradations between adenomas and highly malignant adenocarcinomas were seen. In addition, in many tumors eosinophilic intranuclear inclusions could be found, and they appeared to be restricted to the neoplastic cells. Since these inclusions resembled those found in cells known to be infected by viruses, Lucké (1934) suggested that the tumors could well have been induced by a virus. Lucké's observations were accurate—he illustrated and described Cowdry's Type A inclusion bodies, now known to be pathognomonic for herpesvirus infections. In addition, it was also noted that tumors taken from frogs in June possessed fewer inclusion bodies than those observed during the period January to April. This observation, although unexplained at the time, was a very important one since, as will be noted below, virus replication (and the accompanying inclusion body formation) occurs only in frogs maintained at the lower temperatures.

In a later paper, Lucké (1938) provided additional evidence for the role of a virus when he described successful reproduction of the tumor by transmission of glycerinated and desiccated tumor material. A further suggestion of viral etiology came some 20 years later when Duryee (1956) indicated that tumor-inducing material could pass through bacteria-tight filters. At about the same time Fawcett (1956), in an important study, succeeded in demonstrating herpesvirus-like particles in thin sections of most tumors, but not in normal kidney cells examined by electron microscopic techniques. In addition, those tumors with inclusion bodies were found to contain the virus-like particles. Further evidence for the presence of a Herpes-like agent was presented in 1964 when Lunger succeeded in extracting a particle with this morphology from tumor material. These ultrastructural observations were later confirmed by others [Zambernard and Mizell (1965), Zambernard et al. (1966)], and there is now no doubt that a herpesvirus is associated with the Lucké tumor.

In subsequent years, vigorous attempts were made to determine whether the virus observed does, in fact, induce the tumor. During the course of these studies at least three other viruses, including an unrelated herpesvirus, have been isolated from tumors and then propagated in vitro; none of them induces tumors (reviewed by Granoff, 1973). Regrettably, with the exception of one preliminary report which has not been extended (Tweedell and Wong, 1974), there have been no demonstrations that the Lucké agent can be propagated in vitro. Therefore, it has not been possible to clone the virus in cell culture and Koch's postulates cannot yet be strictly tested. However, Naegele et al. (1974) have now successfully fulfilled all aspects except in vitro cultivation of the agent; virus recovered from tumor fragments maintained in vitro was oncogenic when injected into developing frog embryos. At present, this experiment probably constitutes the strongest evidence that the Lucké virus is in fact the etiologic agent responsible for the tumor, and it is supported by another earlier study (Mizell et al., 1969), in which virus purified by zonal ultracentrifugation was shown to induce the tumor.

B. Characteristics of the Latent Infection

As mentioned above, Lucké recognized early on that tumors derived from frogs studied during summer months demonstrated a paucity of inclusion bodies, and the opposite was true of tumors taken in the winter periods. This suggested a temperature dependence for inclusion body and, more important, virus formation, a phenomenon which has now been firmly established. Initially, Roberts (1963) found that neoplastic renal cells in frogs maintained at 20–25°C never developed intranuclear inclusions, while those from animals held at 5°C did, and Rafferty (1965) showed that inclusion-free tumors *in situ* developed into inclusion positive tumors after the frogs were maintained for 3–5 months at 4°C. These findings were later extended by Mizell *et al.* (1967) and Breidenbach *et al.* (1971), who found that maintenance of explants of virus-free tumor at 7.5°C for extended periods either in the anterior chamber of the frog's eye or *in vitro* resulted in production of virions. In addition, when portions of tumor were placed in the anterior eye chambers of frogs maintained at different temperatures, it was found that the "cutoff" temperature for virus production was 11.5°C (Skinner and Mizell, 1972). The opposite experiment has also been successfully executed; virus carrying tumors *in situ* or explanted to the anterior chamber of the eye "lose" the virus when held at 15–26°C (Zambernard and Mizell, 1965; Zambernard and Vatter, 1966; Skinner and Mizell, 1972). Whether these tumors again produce virus when placed at low temperatures has not been reported. Finally, there is also evidence that a portion of the viral genome is transcribed in the virus-free summer tumor. Collard *et al.* (1973) found that radioactively labeled RNA from virus-free tumors (but not normal kidneys) hybridized specifically with viral DNA. Recently this experiment has been extended; a virus specific antigen(s) has been found in the membrane of tumor cells maintained in warm temperatures—suggesting that at least a portion of the RNA is translated (Naegele and Granoff, 1977).

C. SUMMARY AND CONCLUSIONS

Taken together, these experiments indicate that in many ways, the Lucké agent behaves in a manner similar to those temperature-sensitive mutants of Herpes simplex virus that can successfully establish latent infections at restrictive temperatures. Thus, at restrictive temperatures latent infections are established, and virus replication is induced upon transfer of latently infected cells to permissive temperatures. However, since no latently infected nonneoplastic cells have yet been reported in the case of the Lucké agent, it is quite possible that latent infection is an accompaniment of neoplastic transformation. Finally, as with the two viruses previously described, a biochemical definition of the latent infection is of great importance. However, these

TABLE III

CHARACTERISTICS OF LATENT INFECTIONS ESTABLISHED BY HERPES SIMPLEX, EPSTEIN–BARR, AND LUCKÉ VIRUSES

Virus	Cell type harboring latent virus, or viral genetic information	Physical state of latent virus	Virus-specific antigens in latently infected cells	Permissive cells *in vivo*
Herpes simplex virus	Sensory and probably other neurons	Unknown, mature virus very unlikely	No antigens yet detected	Essentially all cell types, epithelium most important for transmission in nature
Epstein–Barr virus	Neoplastic B lymphocytes	1. Circular extrachromosomal DNA 2. DNA linearly integrated into cellular chromosome, association alkali labile	At least 2 antigens, Epstein–Barr nuclear antigen (EBNA), and membrane antigen (MA)	Probably lymphocytes and/or epithelial cells of nasopharynx
Lucké virus	Neoplastic kidney epithelial cells >12°C	Unknown, not mature virus	Membrane antigen	Neoplastic kidney epithelial cells <12°C

studies will be difficult to manage until the virus can be efficiently replicated *in vitro* and latently infected cell lines can be established.

V. Overall Summary and Extensions

As was suspected from the early observations and investigations with Herpes simplex virus, it is now clear that herpesviruses do establish latent infections from which they can be subsequently reactivated. A summary of this presentation concerning our present understanding of relevant aspects of the phenomena with HSV, EBV, and the Lucké virus is presented in Table III. Now that latent infections have been shown to take place and, as shown in Table III, the cellular reservoirs are known, future studies should be concerned with defining the biochemical phenomena associated with establishment, maintenance, and subsequent reactivation of latent infections. At the moment, these are most difficult tasks, since, to accomplish such studies, methods of obtaining large amounts of virus and then infecting pure cultures of relevant cells *in vitro* must be developed for each system. When this has been done, the infected cells can be manipulated by the various pharmacologic methods which have been suggested by *in vivo* investigations to play a role in viral latency and reactivation.

ACKNOWLEDGMENT

The work presented here which emanated from my laboratory was supported by the National Institutes of Health, United State Public Health Service (Grants Nos. AI-06246 and NS-08711).

REFERENCES

Adams, A., and Lindahl, T. (1975). *Proc. Natl. Acad. Sci. U.S.A.* **72**, 1477–1481.
Adams, A., Lindahl, T., and Klein, G. (1973). *Proc. Natl. Acad. Sci. U.S.A.* **70**, 2888–2892.
Andersson, M., and Lindahl, T. (1976). In preparation.
Andrewes, C. H., and Carmichael, E. A. (1930). *Lancet* **1**, 857–858.
Aoki, I., Geering, G., Beth, E., and Old, L. J. (1972). *In* "Recent Advances in Human Tumor Virology and Immunology" (W. Nakahara *et al.*, eds.), pp. 425–429. Univ. of Tokyo Press, Tokyo.
Baringer, J. R. (1974). *N. Engl. J. Med.* **291**, 828–830.
Baringer, J. R., and Swoveland, P. (1973). *N. Engl. J. Med.* **288**, 648–650.
Baringer, J. R., and Swoveland, P. (1974). *Lab. Invest.* **30**, 230–240.
Bastian, F. O., Rabson, A. S., Yee, C. L., and Tralka, T. S. (1972). *Science* **178**, 306–307.
Ben-Porat, T., and Kaplan, A. S. (1973). *In* "The Herpesviruses" (A. S. Kaplan, ed.), pp. 164–220. Academic Press, New York.
Brain, R. T. (1932). *Br. J. Exp. Pathol.* **13**, 166–171.
Breidenbach, G. P., Skinner, M. S., Wallace, J. H., and Mizell, M. (1971). *J. Virol.* **7**, 679–682.

Brown, T. D. K., Ernberg, I., and Klein, G. (1975). *Int. J. Cancer* 15, 606–616.
Burnett, F. M., and Williams, S. W. (1939). *Med. J. Aust.* 1, 637–642.
Calnek, B. W., Adldinger, H. K., and Kahn, D. E. (1970). *Avian Dis.* 14, 219–233.
Carton, C. A. (1953). *J. Neurosurg.* 10, 463–468.
Carton, C. A., and Kilbourne, E. D. (1952). *N. Engl. J. Med.* 246, 172–176.
Collard, W., Thornton, H., Mizell, M., and Green, M. (1973). *Science* 181, 448–449.
Cook, M. L., and Stevens, J. G. (1976). *J. Gen. Virol.* 31, 75–80.
Cook, M. L., Bastone, V. B., and Stevens, J. G. (1974). *Infect. Immun.* 9, 946–951.
Cushing, H. (1905). *J. Am. Med. Assoc.* 44, 773–779, 860–865, 920–929, 1002–1008, and 1088–1093.
Davies, D. H., and Carmichael, L. E. (1973). *Infect. Immun.* 8, 510–518.
Deinhardt, F., Falk, L. A., and Wolfe, L. G. (1973). *Cancer Res.* 33, 1424–1426.
Dodd, K., Johnston, L. M., and Buddingh, G. J. (1938). *J. Pediatr.* 12, 95–102.
Doerr, R. (1920). *Klin. Monatsbl. Augenheilkd.* 65, 104.
Doerr, R. (1938). *In* "Handbüch der Virusforschung" (R. Doerr and C. Hallauer, eds.), 1st ed., Vol. 1, pp. 41–45. Springer-Verlag, Vienna.
Doerr, R. and Vöchting, K. (1920). *Rev. Gen. Ophtalmol., Paris* 34, 409–421.
Duryee, W. R. (1956). *Ann. N.Y. Acad. Sci.* 63, 1280–1302.
Epstein, M. A., Achong, B. G., and Barr, Y. M. (1964). *Lancet* 2, 1702–1703.
Epstein, M. A., Achong, B. G., Barr, Y. M., Zajac, B., Henle, G., and Henle, W. (1966). *J. Natl. Cancer Inst.* 37, 547–559.
Fawcett, D. W. (1956). *J. Biophys. Biochem. Cytol.* 2, 725–742.
Gerber, P. (1972). *Proc. Natl. Acad. Sci. U.S.A.* 69, 83–85.
Gerber, P., and Deal, D. R. (1970). *Proc. Soc. Exp. Biol. Med.* 134, 748–751.
Gerber, P., and Monroe, J. H. (1968). *J. Natl. Cancer Inst.* 40, 855–866.
Gerber, P., Wang-Peng, J., and Monroe, J. H. (1969). *Proc. Natl. Acad. Sci. U.S.A.* 63, 740–747.
Gerber, P., Nonoyama, M., Lucas, S., Perlin, E., and Goldstein, L. I. (1972). *Lancet* 2, 988–989.
Gergely, J., Klein, G., and Ernberg, I. (1971). *Virology* 45, 22–29.
Glaser, R., and Nonoyama, M. (1974). *J. Virol.* 14, 174–176.
Goodpasture, E. W. (1925). *Am. J. Pathol.* 1, 11–28.
Goodpasture, E. W. (1929). *Medicine (Baltimore)* 7, 223–243.
Goodpasture, E. W., and Teague, O. (1923). *J. Med. Res.* 44, 139–184.
Granoff, A. (1973). *In* "The Herpesviruses" (A. S. Kaplan, ed.), pp. 627–640. Academic Press, New York.
Grüter, W. (1920). *Klin. Monatsbl. Augenheilkd.* 65, 398–399.
Hampar, B., Derge, J. G., Martos, L. M., and Walker, J. L. (1972). *Proc. Natl. Acad. Sci. U.S.A.* 69, 78–82.
Hampar, B., Tanaka, A., Nonoyama, M., and Derge, J. G. (1974). *Proc. Natl. Acad. Sci. U.S.A.* 71, 631–633.
Henle, G., and Henle, W. (1966). *J. Bacteriol.* 91, 1248–1256.
Henle, G., Henle, W., and Klein, G. (1971). *Int. J. Cancer* 8, 272–282.
Henle, W., and Henle, G. E. (1970). *Bibl. Haematol. (Basel)* 36, 706–713.
Henle, W., Henle, G., Pearson, C., Zajac, B., Waubke, R., and Scriba, M. (1970). *Science* 169, 188–190.
Hill, T. J., Field, H. J., and Blyth, W. A. (1975). *J. Gen. Virol.* 28, 341–353.
Hinze, H. C., and Wegner, K. L. (1973). *Cancer Res.* 33, 1434–1435.
Hope-Simpson, R. E. (1965). *Proc. R. Soc. Med.* 58, 9–25.
Howard, W. T. (1903). *Am. J. Med. Sci.* 125, 256–272.
Howard, W. T. (1905). *Am. J. Med. Sci.* 130, 1012–1019.

Hull, R. M. (1973). *In* "The Herpesviruses" (A. S. Kaplan, ed.), pp. 389–426. Academic Press, New York.

Jondal, M., and Klein, G. (1973). *J. Exp. Med.* **138**, 1365–1378.

Joseph, B. S., and Oldstone, M. B. A. (1975). *J. Exp. Med.* **142**, 864–876.

Kaplan, A. S., ed. (1973). "The Herpesviruses." Academic Press, New York.

Kaschka-Dierich, C., Adams, A., Lindahl, T., Bornkamm, G. W., Bjursell, G., Klein, G., Giovanella, B. C., and Singh, S. (1976). *Nature (London)* **260**, 302–306.

Kato, S., and Akiyama, Y. (1975). *IARC Publ.* **11**, Part 2, 101–108.

Kawai, Y., Nonoyama, M., and Pagano, J. (1973). *J. Virol.* **12**, 1006–1012.

Klein, E., VanFurth, R., Johannsen, B., Ernberg, I., and Clifford, T. (1972). *Oncogenesis Herpesviruses, Proc. Symp., 1971* Publ. No. 2, pp. 253–260.

Klein, G. (1972). *Proc. Natl. Acad. Sci. U.S.A.* **69**, 1956–1964.

Klein, G. (1973). *In* "The Herpesviruses" (A. S. Kaplan, ed.), pp. 521–555. Academic Press, New York.

Klein, G. (1975). *IARC Publ.* **11**, Part 2, 365–397.

Klein, G., and Vonka, V. (1974). *J. Natl. Cancer Inst.* **53**, 1645–1646.

Klein, G., Clifford, P., Klein, E., and Stjernsward, J. (1966). *Proc. Natl. Acad. Sci. U.S.A.* **55**, 1628–1635.

Klein, G., Clifford, P., Klein, E., Smith, R. T., Minowada, J., Kourilsky, F. M., and Gurchenal, J. G. (1967). *J. Natl. Cancer Inst.* **39**, 1027–1044.

Klein, G., Pearson, G., Nadkarni, J. S., Nadkarni, E., Klein, G., Henle, W., and Clifford, P. (1968). *J. Exp. Med.* **128**, 1011–1020.

Klein, G., Lindahl, T., Jondal, M., Leibold, W., Menezes, J., Nilsson, K., and Sundström, C. (1974a). *Proc. Natl. Acad. Sci. U.S.A.* **71**, 3283–3286.

Klein, G., Giovanella, B., Lindahl, T., Falkow, P., Singh, S., and Stehlin, J. (1974b). *Proc. Natl. Acad. Sci. U.S.A.* **71**, 4737–4741.

Klein, G., Wiener, F., Zech, L., zur Hausen, H., and Reedman, B. (1974c). *Int. J. Cancer* **14**, 54–64.

Klein, G., Clements, G., Zeuthen, J., and Westman, A. (1976). *Int. J. Cancer* **17**, 715–724.

Knotts, F. B., Cook, M. L., and Stevens, J. G. (1974). *J. Infect. Dis.* **130**, 16–27.

Lang, D. J., Cheung, K. S., Schwartz, J. M., Daniels, C. A., and Harwood, S. E. (1976) *Yale J. Biol. Med.* **49**, 45–58.

Levaditi, C., and Harvier, P. (1920). *Ann. Inst. Pasteur, Paris* **34**, 911–972.

Lindahl, T., Adams, A., Bjursell, G., Bornkamm, G. W., Kaschka-Dierich, C., and Jehn, U. (1976). *J. Mol. Biol.* **102**, 511–530.

Lofgren, K. W., Stevens, J. G., Marsden, H. S., and Subak-Sharpe, J. H. (1977). *Virology* **76**, 440–443.

Löwenstein, A. (1919). *Muench. Med. Wochenschr.* **66**, 769–770.

Lucké, B. (1934). *Am. J. Cancer* **20**, 352–379.

Lucké, B. (1938). *J. Exp. Med.* **68**, 457–468.

Luger, A., and Lauda, E. (1921). *Wien. Klin. Wochenschr.* **34**, 251.

Lunger, P. D. (1964). *Virology* **24**, 138–145.

McCarthy, K., and Tosolini, F. A. (1975). *Lancet* **1**, 649–650.

McKercher, D. G. (1973). *In* "The Herpesviruses" (A. S. Kaplan, ed.), pp. 427–493. Academic Press, New York.

Miller, G. (1971). *Yale J. Biol. Med.* **43**, 358–384.

Miller, G., Niederman, J. C., and Andrews, L. L. (1973). *N. Engl. J. Med.* **288**, 229–232.

Miller, M. H., Stitt, D., and Miller, G. (1970). *J. Virol.* **6**, 699–701.

Mizell, M., Stackpole, C. W., and Halpern, S. (1967). *Proc. Soc. Exp. Biol. Med.* **127**, 808–814.

Mizell, M., Toplin, I., and Isaacs, J. J. (1969). *Science* **165**, 1134–1137.

Moore, G. E., and Minowada, J. (1973). *N. Engl. J. Med.* **288**, 106.
Naegele, R. F., and Granoff, A. (1977). *Int. J. Cancer* (in press).
Naegle, R. F., Granoff, A., and Darlington, R. W. (1974). *Proc. Natl. Acad. Sci. U.S.A.* **71**, 830–834.
Nazerian, K., and Witter, R. L. (1970). *J. Virol.* **5**, 388–397.
Nesburn, A. B., Elliot, J. H., and Leibowitz, H. M. (1967). *Arch. Ophthalmol.* **78**, 523–529.
Nilsson, K. (1971). *Int. J. Cancer* **8**, 432–442.
Nilsson, K., Klein, G., Henle, W., and Henle, G. (1971). *Int. J. Cancer* **8**, 443–450.
Nonoyama, M., and Pagano, J. S. (1971). *Nature (London), New Biol.* **233**, 103–106.
Nonoyama, M., and Pagano J. S. (1972). *Nature (London), New Biol.* **238**, 169–171.
Nonoyama, M., and Pagano, J. S. (1973). *Nature (London)* **242**, 44–47.
Nyormoi, O., Klein, G., Adams, A., and Dombos, L. (1973). *Int. J. Cancer* **12**, 396–408.
Pagano, J. S. (1974). *In* "Viruses, Evolution and Cancer" (E. Kurstak and K. Maramorosch, eds.), pp. 8–116. Academic Press, New York.
Pagano, J. S., and Huang, E. S. (1974). *In* "Viral Immunodiagnosis" (E. Kurstak and R. Morisset, eds.), pp. 279–299. Academic Press, New York.
Pope, J. H., Horne, M. K., and Scott, W. (1969a). *Int. J. Cancer* **4**, 255–260.
Pope, J. H., Horne, M. K., and Wetter, E. J. (1969b). *Nature (London)* **222**, 186–187.
Pritchett, R., Pedersen, M., and Kieff, E. (1976). *Virology* **74**, 227–231.
Pulvertaft, R. J. V. (1965). *J. Clin. Pathol.* **18**, 261–273.
Rafferty, K. (1965). *Ann. N.Y. Acad. Sci.* **126**, 3–21.
Reedman, B. M., and Klein, G. (1973). *Int. J. Cancer* **11**, 499–520.
Reedman, B. M., Klein, G., Pope, J. H., Walter, M. K., Hilgers, J., Singh, S., and Johansson, B. (1974). *Int. J. Cancer* **13**, 755–763.
Roberts, M. E. (1963). *Cancer Res.* **23**, 1709–1714.
Rodda S., Jack, I., and White, D. O. (1973). *Lancet* **1**, 1394.
Roizman, B., and Kieff, E. D. (1975). *In* "Cancer, a Comprehensive Treatise" (F. F. Becker, ed.) Vol. 2, pp. 241–322. Plenum, New York.
Scriba, M. (1975). *Infect. Immun.* **12**, 162–165.
Skinner, M. S., and Mizell, M. (1972). *Lab. Invest.* **26**, 671–681.
Stevens, J. G. (1975a). *Curr. Top. Microbiol. Immunol.* **70**, 31–50.
Stevens, J. G. (1975b). *In* "Advances in Pathobiology 5, Cancer Biology III, Herpesvirus Epidemiology, Molecular Events, Oncogenicity and Therapy" (C. Borek and D. W. King, eds.), pp. 104–111. Stratton Intercontinental Medical Book, New York.
Stevens, J. G., and Cook, M. L. (1971). *Science* **173**, 843–845.
Stevens, J. G., and Cook, M. L. (1974). *J. Immunol.* **113**, 1685–1693.
Stevens, J. G., Nesburn, A. B., and Cook, M. L. (1972). *Nature (London), New Biol.* **235**, 216–217.
Stevens, J. G., Cook, M. L., and Jordan, M. C. (1975). *Infect. Immun.* **11**, 635–639.
Subak-Sharpe, J. H., Brown, S. M., Ritchie, D. A., Timbury, M. C., MacNab, J. C. M., Marsden, H. S., and Hay, J. (1974). *Cold Spring Harbor Symp. Quant. Biol.* **39**, 717–730.
Svedmyr, A., and Demissie, A. (1971). *Ann. N.Y. Acad. Sci.* **177**, 241–249.
Svedmyr, A., Demissie, A., Klein, G., and Clifford, P. (1970). *J. Natl. Cancer Inst.* **44**, 595–610.
Svedmyr, E., and Jondal, M. (1975). *Proc. Natl. Acad. Sci. U.S.A.* **72**, 1622–1626.
Symposium on Herpesvirus and Cervical Cancer. (1973). *Cancer Res.* **33**, 1351–1563.
Tweedell, K. S., and Wong, W. Y. (1974). *J. Nat. Cancer Inst.* **52**, 621–623.
Underwood, G. E., and Weed, S. D. (1974). *Infect. Immun.* **10**, 471–474.
Veltri, R. W., McClary, J. E., and Sprinkle, P. M. (1976). *J. Gen. Virol.* **32**, 455–460.

Vidal, E. (1873). *Ann. Dermatol. Sylphiligr.* **4**, 350–358.

Walz, M. A., Price, R. W., and Notkins, A. L. (1974). *Science* **184**, 1185–1187.

Wolf, H., zur Hausen, H., and Becker, V. (1973). *Nature (London), New Biol.* **244**, 245–247.

Zajac, A. B., and Kahn, G. (1970). *J. Natl. Cancer Inst.* **45**, 399–406.

Zambernard, J., and Mizell, M. (1965). *Ann. N.Y. Acad. Sci.* **126**, 127–145.

Zambernard, J., and Vatter, A. E. (1966). *Cancer Res.* **26**, 2148–2153.

Zambernard, J., Vatter, A. E., and McKinnell, R. G. (1966). *Cancer Res.* **26**, 1688–1700.

zur Hausen, H. (1972). *Int. Rev. Exp. Pathol.* **11**, 233–258.

zur Hausen. H., and Schulte-Holthausen, H. (1970). *Nature (London)* **227**, 245–247.

zur Hausen, H. and Schulte-Holthausen, H. (1975). *IARC Sci. Publ.* **11** (Part 1), 117–123.

ANTITUMOR ACTIVITY OF *Corynebacterium parvum*

Luka Milas and Martin T. Scott

Central Institute for Tumors and Allied Diseases, Zagreb, Croatia, Yugoslavia,
and Department of Experimental Immunobiology, Wellcome Research Laboratories, Beckenham, England

I. Introduction

Interest in the bacterium *Corynebacterium parvum* (CP) as an immunostimulant was first aroused after the demonstration by Halpern and colleagues (1964) that injection of killed organisms into mice caused intense stimulation of the lymphoreticuloendothelial system. This was at a time when other biological reticuloendothelial stimulants, e.g., zymosan (yeast cell walls) and Bacillus Calmette-Guérin (BCG) organisms were being found to be capable of inhibiting the growth of transplantable tumors in mice (Old *et al.*, 1960, 1961). CP was shown to be similarly effective in 1966 (Halpern *et al.*, 1966; Woodruff and Boak, 1966), and preliminary clinical trials were initiated in 1967 (Israel and Halpern, 1972).

The antitumor properties of CP in animals and preliminary clinical data were reviewed by Scott in 1974 (1974d), and the amount of data, concerning both its mode of action in animals and clinical experiences, that have accumulated during the past 2 years reflects the current level of interest in CP as a potential immunotherapeutic anticancer agent. This review considers first the immunological modifications resulting from CP administered in non-tumor-bearing animals. Animal tumor data and finally the clinical data are then considered. Throughout the reported studies the bacteria used have been in the form of either heat- or formalin-killed vaccines.

II. Terminology and Definitions

A number of anaerobic coryneforms known by the general designation *Corynebacterium parvum* possess lymphoreticular stimulating activity (Adlam and Scott, 1973; O'Neill *et al.*, 1973; McBride *et al.*, 1975a). However, until recently the taxonomic classification of these organisms has been confused and, in some instances, it has been difficult to establish the taxonomic identity or relationship between the different organisms used by various workers. Throughout this review the taxonomic descriptions of the original authors have been retained, this most often being CP. An alternative strain that has figured prominently in animal tumor studies is *Corynebacterium granulosum* (CG).

Johnson and Cummins (1972) and Cummins and Johnson (1974) have attempted to clarify the taxonomy of the anaerobic coryneforms using serology, cell wall composition, and DNA homology. Their conclusions were that they should be called Propionibacteria, since they produce propionic acid by fermentation, and should be divided into three groups—*P. acnes*, *P. granulosum*, and *P. avidum*. According to this scheme, the Burroughs Wellcome *C. parvum* vaccine strain 6134 is classified as *P. acnes* type I (C. Adlam, personal communication), and the Institut Merieux vaccine IM 1585 as *P. avidum* (Roumiantzeff *et al.*, 1975b). It is apparent that another group of anaerobic coryneforms, isolated mainly from dairy products and referred to as the "classical" Propionibacteria of van Niel (1928) are different from *P. acnes*, *P. granulosum*, and *P. avidum* (Johnson and Cummins, 1972). The "classical" Propionibacteria have thus far been uniformly negative in stimulatory activity (O'Neill *et al.*, 1973; McBride *et al.*, 1975a).

There have been studies to determine whether lymphoreticular stimulatory activity correlate with particular species. O'Neill *et al.* (1973) found activity among representative organisms from *P. acnes, P. granulosum,* and *P. avidum* with no single species showing outright superiority. McBride *et al.* (1975a) confirmed activity in organisms belonging to *P. acnes* and *P. avidum* and described a soluble cross-reacting antigen produced only by these strains.

III. Stimulation of the Lymphoreticuloendothelial System

A. CHANGES IN ORGAN WEIGHT AND HISTOLOGY

A single intravenous injection of CP into mice produces proliferation of lymphohistiocytic elements in the liver and spleen, resulting in a marked enlargement of these organs. The increase in organ weight is evident within a few days of CP injection, peaks in the second week, and then gradually returns to normal (Halpern *et al.,* 1964; Adlam and Scott, 1973). The degree of splenomegaly and hepatomegaly depends directly on the amount of CP injected, but the kinetics of the responses are relatively dose-independent (Adlam and Scott, 1973). Repeated injections provoke more intense, longer-lasting reactions (Halpern *et al.,* 1964).

In addition to the splenomegaly (Halpern *et al.,* 1964; Howard *et al.,* 1967; Adlam and Scott, 1973; O'Neill *et al.,* 1973; Woodruff and Dunbar, 1973; Bomford and Olivotto, 1974; Castro, 1974a; McBride *et al.,* 1974; Milas *et al.,* 1974a, 1975c) and hepatomegaly (Halpern *et al.,* 1964; Adlam and Scott, 1973; O'Neill *et al.,* 1973; Bomford and Olivotto, 1974; McBride *et al.,* 1974; Milas *et al.,* 1974a) that result from systemic injection of CP into mice, lung (Adlam and Scott, 1973) and lymph node (Castro, 1974a; McBride *et al,* 1974; Milas *et al.,* 1975c) weights are also increased. High doses of systemic CP may lead to thymic atrophy (Castro, 1974a; McBride *et al.,* 1974). The changes in spleen and liver weights following single subcutaneous injections of CP are minimal, but there is marked proliferation in, and enlargement of, the lymph node draining the injection site (Scott, 1974c; Tuttle and North, 1975).

Similar organ weight changes have been reported for other species: splenomegaly and hepatomegaly in the rat (Stiffel *et al.,* 1966; Brozovic *et al.,* 1975), rabbit (Pinckard *et al.,* 1968), and guinea pig (Stiffel *et al.,* 1966), and lung weight increase and splenomegaly in the rabbit (Collet, 1971) and an amphibian (Turner *et al.,* 1974), respectively.

Histologic changes in the spleen have commonly consisted of extensive proliferation of histiocytes, macrophages, lymphocytes, and hematopoietic cells: erythroid and myeloid cells and megakaryocytes (Halpern et al., 1964; Collet, 1971; Brozovic et al., 1975; Milas et al., 1975c). Proliferation occurred predominantly in the red pulp, whereas the white pulp of mice treated with CG has been reported to undergo lymphocyte depletion (Milas et al., 1975c).

Extensive proliferation of lymphocytes and histiocytes was found in the lymph nodes (Collet, 1971; O'Neill et al., 1973; Scott, 1974c; Tuttle and North, 1975) and in the lung (Collet, 1971; Pinckard et al., 1968).

Hepatomegaly is usually associated with mononuclear cell infiltrates (Halpern et al., 1964; Milas et al., 1974a; Brozovic et al., 1975). The cells are predominantly histiocytes, and they form granulomas or diffusely infiltrate liver parenchyma (Milas et al., 1974a). CP induces proliferation of liver macrophages and also increases the influx of extrahepatic macrophages (Warr and Šljivić, 1974c).

B. Hematopoietic Influence

CP increases hematopoietic activity in the spleen. In addition to the histological evidence already mentioned, an increased number of colony-forming units (CFU) has been demonstrated. A similar increase in CFU occurred in the bone marrow, although the total number of nucleated cells remained unchanged or was slightly reduced (Toujas et al., 1972, 1974, 1975). CP has also increased the number of CFU in the peripheral blood of mice (Bašić et al., 1975b).

Shortly after administration of CP, a transient leukopenia, affecting either lymphocytes alone (Milas et al., 1975c; Brozovic et al., 1975) or both lymphocytes and polymorphs (Woodruff and Dunbar, 1973), was found in the peripheral blood of mice. This may be related to the observation by Castro (1974a) that CP caused an absolute decrease in the number of Θ-positive lymphocytes in the thymus, and a reduced percentage in the spleen and lymph nodes. The reason for this reduction in T cells is not known; a direct effect of CP on lymphocytes, or an increased secretion of adrenal steroids due to stress have been suggested (Castro, 1974a).

Anemia may follow CP injection (Halpern and Fray, 1969; McCracken et al., 1971; Cox and Keast, 1974; McBride et al., 1974) and is accompanied by increased erythropoiesis in the spleen and a rise in reticulocyte count (Brozovic et al., 1975). The basis for this anemia is considered to be the enhanced phagocytosis and destruction of erythrocytes by the CP-stimulated reticuloendothelial system (Cox and Keast, 1974; McBride *et al.*, 1974). Soluble antigens from CP become attached to red cells *in vitro*, and any such attachment occuring *in vivo* would be expected to facilitate the phagocytic removal of the cells by virtue of their becoming opsonized by the anti-CP antibodies present in CP-treated mice (Cox and Keast, 1974; McBride *et al.*, 1974). An autoantibody directed against syngeneic red cell antigens has also been found after CP treatment (McCracken *et al.*, 1971).

C. Macrophage Activation

More macrophage colonies are formed from bone marrow cells from mice which received CP either subcutaneously (Wolmark and Fisher, 1974; Wolmark *et al.*, 1974) or systemically (Dimitrov *et al.*, 1975a; Baum and Breese, 1976). CP increases not only the number of macrophage precursors, but also their rate of proliferation (Baum and Breese 1976). The number of peritoneal (Bašić *et al.*, 1974; Yuhas and Ullrich, 1976) and alveolar (Collet, 1971) macrophages is also significantly increased after CP.

CP-activated macrophages show more rapid adherence to glass *in vitro* and increased spreading and vacuolation compared with normal macrophages (Olivotto and Bomford, 1974). Electron microscope studies have shown modifications in surface structure and distribution of lysosomes (Puvion *et al.*, 1976). Cytochemical analyses have detected increased (Wilkinson *et al.*, 1973a,b; McBride *et al.*, 1974) or modified (Puvion *et al.*, 1976) lysozomal enzyme activity and activation of phospholipase A (Munder and Modelell, 1974).

A further characteristic of the CP-activated macrophage is its acquired ability to kill, or inhibit the growth of, malignant cells *in vitro*, and this process will be described in detail in Section VII,G.

D. Phagocytic Activity

The increased phagocytic capabilities of CP-activated macrophages are reflected *in vivo* by increased clearance of particulate material from the blood: colloidal carbon (Halpern *et al.*, 1964; Prévot and Van Phi, 1964; Stiffel *et al.*, 1966; Raynaud *et al.*, 1972; Adlam and Scott, 1973; O'Neill *et al.*, 1973; McBride *et al.*, 1974; Warr and Šljivić, 1974b), bovine serum albumin (BSA) (McBride *et al.*, 1974), and ^{51}Cr-labeled sheep red blood cells (SRBC) (Warr and Šljivić, 1974b). Studies by Stiffel *et al.* (1970, 1971) have shown that the degree of phagocytic stimulation achieved with CP in mice depends on the strain of mice used.

The liver and spleen are the major organs responsible for the increased uptake of injected material (McBride *et al.*, 1974; Warr and Šljivić, 1974b), and the ability of different coryneforms to stimulate phagocytic clearance seems to correlate with their ability to cause splenomegaly and hepatomegaly (Adlam and Scott, 1973; O'Neill *et al.*, 1973). The *in vivo* antitumor activity of various strains has, however, correlated better with splenomegaly than with stimulation of phagocytic index (McBride *et al.*, 1975a).

IV. Immune Modulation

A. HUMORAL IMMUNITY

CP is a potent immunogen: specific anti-CP antibodies have been detected following injection of organisms into mice (Woodruff *et al.*, 1974; Scott and Warner, 1976), rabbits (Dawes and McBride, 1975), and man (James *et al.*, 1975; Minton *et al.*, 1976).

Systemic pretreatment of mice with CP amplifies the antibody response to various systemically injected, thymus-dependent antigens: SRBC (Biozzi *et al.*, 1968; Howard *et al.*, 1973a; James *et al.*, 1974; Warr and Šljivić, 1974a), rat erythrocytes (Howard *et al.*, 1973a), keyhole limpet hemocyanin (KLH) (Wiener and Bandieri, 1975), and BSA (James *et al.*, 1974). Both IgM and IgG responses are affected. The exclusively IgM responses of mice to thymus-independent antigens—dinitrophenol hapten coupled to a levan carrier (del Guercio, 1972) and pneumococcal polysaccharide SIII (Howard *et al.*, 1973b; James *et al.*, 1974; Warr and Šljivić, 1974a)—are also boosted.

Pinckard *et al.* (1967a,b, 1968) have studied the effects of a nonreticuloendothelial stimulating strain of CP on antibody production against BSA in rabbits. They found that systemic CP pretreatment increased the magnitude of primary and secondary responses and the relative binding affinities of the antibodies (Pinckard *et al.*, 1967a,b). Tolerance induction was also blocked (Pinckard *et al.*, 1968). The "inactive" strain of CP also increased homocytotropic antibody production whereas strains of CP with reticuloendothelial stimulating activity did not (Pinckard and Halonen, 1971). In mice, "active" strains of CP have increased the relative binding affinities of anti-BSA antibodies, but only when the mice had tumors (James *et al.*, 1974). The induction of tolerance by injection of large amounts of SIII polysaccharide was not affected by CP pretreatment (Howard *et al.*, 1973b).

Reports of adjuvant activity of CP in guinea pigs have concerned its injection mixed with antigen either in Freund's incomplete adjuvant (Neveu *et al.*, 1964) or as a water-in-oil emulsion (O'Neill *et al.*, 1973).

CP injected systemically a few days before systemic injection of optimally immunizing doses of antigen has usually resulted in increased antibody production; however, the modification of antibody responses by CP may depend on the dose of antigen, as well as the time of its administration in relation to CP. In mice immunized with a high dose of SRBC (10^8), CP given between 7 days and 1 day before antigen produced a marked increase in plaque-forming cells (PFC), days -7 and -4 having maximum effect. If the mice were immunized with 10^6 SRBC, CP given 7 days before only slightly increased PFC, and from 4 days before to 1 day after antigen, the PFC response was depressed. A similar dose-time dependence for CP adjuvant effects against SIII polysaccharide was also found (Warr and Šljivić, 1974a).

Published studies on the adjuvant activity of CP in mice have thus far been restricted to systemic injection of CP; however, subcutaneous injection of CP mixed with SRBC into the footpads of mice increased the number of IgM (direct) plaque-forming cells in the draining popliteal lymph node (R. Bomford, to be published). CP boosts antibody responses in guinea pigs when injected locally as a substitute for mycobacteria in Freund's incomplete adjuvant (Neveu *et al.*, 1964).

The stimulatory effects of CP on antibody production are most probably mediated via CP-activated macrophages. Wiener (1975) showed that macrophages from CP-treated mice were more effective than normal macrophages at promoting an *in vitro* primary response to SRBC by macrophage-depleted spleen cells. Watson and Šljivić (1976) confirmed these data and further demonstrated that antibody responses to a macrophage-independent antigen (DNP-POL) were not affected by CP. CP-activated macrophages retain large amounts of antigen on their surfaces, and this intensified presentation of antigen to lymphocytes may be a causal factor in the adjuvant activity of CP (Wiener and Bandieri, 1975). The interaction between antigen-laden macrophages and lymphocytes may be further intensified and prolonged in lymphoid organs as a result of the chronic trapping of lymphocytes that occurs in CP-treated mice (Frost and Lance, 1973).

The predominantly T-cell-dependent IgG response to SRBC in mice is amplified by CP in T-cell-deprived mice (Howard *et al.*, 1973a). This suggests that CP may be operating as a T-cell bypass mechanism, possibly through direct stimulation of B cells. Zola (1975) found that CP was mitogenic for B lymphocytes *in vitro;* however, another organism with no *in vivo* adjuvant properties was similarly active.

B. CELLULAR IMMUNITY

In addition to the anti-CP antibodies found after CP injection, mice also develop cell-mediated immunity to CP antigens. Delayed hypersensitivity (DTH) has resulted from subcutaneous injection of a wide range of CP doses (Scott, 1974c, 1976; Tuttle and North, 1975). No DTH was detected after intravenous injection of a single high dose of CP (Scott, 1974c), but multiple intravenous injections of low doses were effective (Scott and Warner, 1976).

CP treatment has been associated with depression of cell-mediated immune response to unrelated antigens. The DTH resulting from regional injections of picryl chloride or oxazolone (Asherson and Allwood, 1971; Allwood and Asherson, 1972) and SRBC (Scott, 1974a) was markedly depressed in mice pretreated systemically with CP. CP given after SRBC sensitization did not affect DTH reactivity (Scott, 1974a). Systemic CP pretreatment has also prolonged the survival of skin allografts. Skin grafts from A or C_3H mice survived several days longer when transplanted onto CBA mice which had received CP 1 day before or after grafting (Castro, 1974a). A similar prolongation of survival of BALB/c skin grafts was observed in C3Hf/Bu mice treated intravenously with CG, 2–28 days before, but not 2 or 7 days after, skin grafting. CG pretreatment did not affect the rejection time of second-set skin grafts (Milas *et al.*, 1975c). Skin grafting across the H-Y barrier (C57B1 ♂ → C57B1 ♀), Colapinto (1975) gave a more rapid rejection of skin grafts if CP was given before, or within a few days after, grafting, but prolongation occurred if CP was delayed until 10 days after grafting.

Scott (1974a) has attempted to analyze the mechanism(s) that may underlie the depressed DTH reactivity that results from a subcutaneous injection of SRBC in mice pretreated with intravenous CP. He found that anti-SRBC antibodies were not concomitantly increased, and that neither antigen sensitization at the draining lymph node level nor the subsequent loss of sensitized cells from the node was impaired by CP treatment. An increased uptake of sensitized cells by the CP-stimulated spleen was demonstrated, and DTH depression did not occur in splenectomized mice. These results were interpreted as showing that the peripheral expression of DTH was impaired in CP-stimulated mice owing to an effective depletion of sensitized cells that were trapped in the CP-stimulated spleen (Scott, 1974a).

Evidence for a further mechanism that may be involved in the CP-mediated depression of cell-mediated immunity has come from *in vitro* studies of cells from CP-stimulated mice. The performance of these cells in *in vitro* T-cell assays is impaired. Responsiveness to the T-cell mitogen phytohemagglutinin (PHA) of spleen and peripheral blood cells, but not lymph node cells, is depressed. The spleen cells are also less reactive in an *in vitro* mixed lymphocyte reaction (Scott, 1972a). The spleen cell response to the B-cell mitogen lipopolysaccharide is either unaffected by (Scott, 1972a) or less sensitive to (Kirchner *et al.*, 1975b) CP. Similar data are reported for spleen and peripheral blood cells from CG-stimulated mice by Milas *et al.* (1975c), who also showed that the PHA responsiveness of lymph node cells was augmented after very low doses of CG. The PHA reactivity of CP-stimulated spleen cells was completely restored after removal of macrophages by iron magnet techniques (Scott, 1972b; Kirchner *et al.*, 1975b), rayon adherence columns, and carageenin treatment, but not by treatment with anti-Θ serum and complement (Kirchner *et al.*, 1975b). These data suggest a nonspecific inhibition of T-lymphocyte function by CP-activated macrophages, the lack of correlation of macrophage numbers with degree of inhibition indicating a qualitative rather than quantitative change in the macrophage population (Scott, 1972b; Milas *et al.*, 1975c).

A further example of CP-mediated depressed T-cell activity has been the protection of F_1 recipient mice by intravenous CP against the lethal effects of graft versus host resulting from a subsequent injection of parental spleen cells (Biozzi *et al.*, 1965; Howard *et al.*, 1967). Karyotypic analysis revealed a strong inhibition of the proliferation of donor cells in the spleen of CP-treated recipients. The effect could not be attributed to any augmentation of an immune response against hypothetical parental antigens or to lack of space for donor cells in the host due to gross proliferation of lymphoreticular tissue (Howard *et al.*, 1967). The results do, however, seem compatible with a CP-activated macrophage-mediated inhibition of T-cell proliferation (Howard *et al.*, 1973a).

The depressive effects of CP on cell-mediated immunity have thus far been restricted to systemically injected CP. Scott (1974a) was unable to depress DTH to SRBC using subcutaneous CP, and the *in vitro* PHA response of cells from lymph nodes directly stimulated by regional injection of CP was not depressed (Scott, 1972a). Data are now accumulating that local interaction of CP with antigen may potentiate cell-mediated immunity. Subcutaneous injection of CP mixed with tumor antigens (irradiated tumor cells) results in strong specific cell-mediated antitumor immunity, whereas injection of CP or antigen alone are without effect (Bomford, 1975; Scott, 1975b). Subcutaneous injection of CP mixed with SRBC also potentiates DTH to SRBC (M. T. Scott, unpublished data). Subcutaneous injections of CP (Neveu *et al.*, 1964) or CG (Degrand and Raynaud, 1973), when mixed with antigen in Freund's incomplete adjuvant, have produced DTH in guinea pigs.

The fact that systemic CP pretreatment augments IgG antibody response to thymus-dependent antigens (see Section IV,A) implies that the normal cooperative activity of T cells is not impaired by CP.

V. Resistance to Infection

Pretreatment of mice with CP has protected them against subsequent infection with a variety of bacteria: *Staphylococcus aureus* and *Bordetella pertussis* (Adlam *et al.*, 1972), *Brucella abortus* (Adlam *et al.*, 1972; Halpern *et al.*, 1973), *Salmonella enteritidis* (Collins, 1974; Collins and Scott, 1974), *Listeria monocytogenes* (Fauve and Hevin, 1971; Swartzberg *et al.*, 1975; Ruitenberg and van Noorle Jansen, 1975). The effects have been evident both from prolonged survival or permanent protection against infection and from decreased bacterial counts in the liver and spleen. It is apparent that the CP-induced bacterial resistance is immunologically nonspecific and mediated by the enhanced bactericidal capabilities of the CP-activated spleen and liver macrophages (Fauve and Hevin, 1971, 1974; Collins and Scott, 1974; Fauve, 1975). Protection against *Salmonella enteritidis* did not correlate with any augmentation of specific anti-*Salmonella* immunity (Collins and Scott, 1974), and protection against *Listeria monocytogenes* still occurred in the athymic nude mouse (Ruitenberg and van Noorle Jansen, 1975). CP treatment after bacterial infection has not been protective (Philippon *et al.*, 1972; Collins and Scott, 1974).

CP also protects against protozoal infections. An increased resistance to malaria was caused by CP injected intravenously 6–19 days before intravenous injection of *Plasmodium berghei* sporozoites (Nussenzweig, 1967). The mice exhibited delay in the onset of detectable infection and prolonged survival, and some were completely protected. A similar protection against *P. vinckei* and *P. chabaudi*, but not *P. berghei*, has been reported by Clark *et al.* (1977). They also found that systemic CP pretreatment of mice afforded complete and chronic protection against infection with *Babesia microti* or *B. rodhaini*. Intraerythrocytic death of both *Plasmodium* and *Babesia* was evident in these studies (Clark *et al.*, 1977). Mice injected intravenously, but not intraperitoneally, with CP have shown increased resistance to the

Tulahuen strain of *Trypanosoma cruzi,* and significant protection still occurred if CP was delayed until 7 days after injection (Kierszenbaum, 1975). A macrophage-mediated mechanism was indicated by the interesting finding that CP protected against infection only with the reticulotropic Tulahuen strain, but not with the predominantly myotropic Y strain of *T. cruzi.* CP-pretreated mice are also resistant to *Toxoplasma gondii,* and peritoneal macrophages from these mice are capable *in vitro* of killing *Toxoplasma* (Swartzberg *et al.,* 1975).

In contrast to these protective findings, Bryceson *et al.* (1972) observed that subcutaneous pretreatment of guinea pigs with CP emulsified in Freund's incomplete adjuvant increased susceptibility to cutaneous infection with *Leishmania enriettii.* Treatment with CP did not influence delayed hypersensitivity to *Leishmania,* but caused production of anti-leishmanial antibodies. The authors explained their findings by "regional antigenic competition" between CP and leishmanial antigen, which may alter the distribution and processing of leishmanial antigen or the traffic of *Leishmania*-sensitive cells within draining lymph nodes. Intravenous inoculation of CP also depressed the resistance of rats to *Trichinella spiralis,* as expressed in a delay of expulsion of adult worms from rat intestinal tract. This may be related to a depression of the T-cell-mediated immunologic defense against *Trichinella spiralis* (Ruitenberg and Steerenberg, 1973). Depression of cell-mediated immunity by CP is discussed in Section IV,B.

The effects of CP against viral infections have also been studied. Intraperitoneal and intravenous inoculations of encephalomyocarditis virus caused the death of 95% of normal Swiss mice, but less than 50% of those treated intraperitoneally with 0.5 mg of CP 2 or 7 days earlier. Smaller and larger doses of CP were less effective (Cerutti, 1975). Peritoneal exudates of CP-treated mice contained a factor that inhibited multiplication of both encephalomyocarditis virus and vesicular stomatitis virus. The inhibitor was resistant to heating at 56°C for 30 minutes, but did not require the integrity of cell-protein synthesis, a characteristic of the biological activity of interferon. CP was also incapable of inducing interferon in an *in vivo* model (Cerutti, 1975). Other studies have shown that treatment of mice with *C. acnes,* an organism closely related to CP, suppresses the level of serum interferon induced by injection of Newcastle disease virus of Chikungunya virus (Farber and Glasgow, 1972; Fischbach and Glasgow, 1975).

VI. Other Effects

Systemically injected CP (Adlam *et al.,* 1972; Adlam, 1973; Adlam and Scott, 1973) is capable of sensitizing mice to histamine, a property previously considered to be unique for *Bordetella pertussis.* The ability of both CP and *B. pertussis* to sensitize depended on strain of mice used, strains sensitive to CP treatment being sensitive to *B. pertussis* and vice versa. Contrary to *B. pertussis,* CP-mediated histamine sensitivity was not associated with anaphylaxis. Anaphylaxis to horse serum, or ovalbumin, was not observed in mice receiving CP at various times before, after, or in combination with antigen (Adlam, 1973). The histamine-sensitizing activity of CP was not destroyed by heating or by treatment with formaldehyde. It was suggested that lysosome-rich CP-activated macrophages, because of their increased fragility, may release into the circulation large amounts of lysosomal enzymes, which then block the β-adrenergic receptors and (or) exert a direct effect on histamine levels (Adlam, 1973). A similar increase in sensitivity of CP-treated mice to endotoxin has been associated with a release of lysosomal enzymes (Howard, 1968).

Mice given high doses of intravenous CP have become lethally sensitive to normally safe doses of anesthetics, e.g., pentobarbitone and tribromoethanol, which are catabolized by the liver, but not ether (Mosedale and Smith, 1975). Using mice of a different strain, and lower doses of CP, Milas (1975) found no increased sensitivity to pentobarbitone. In rats, pretreatment with intravenous CP has increased the pentobarbitone-induced sleeping time by 100%, and this was associated with impairment of the hepatic microsomal enzyme system (Farquhar *et al.,* 1975). The anesthetic deaths reported may, therefore, be due to interference of detoxification processes in the liver by CP.

Certain strains of mice are capable of rejecting incompatible bone marrow grafts after lethal irradiation. If, however, these mice are given CP prior to irradiation, the bone marrow grafts are accepted (Cudkowicz and Bennett, 1971a,b; Lotzova and Cudkowicz, 1972; Rauchwerger *et al.,* 1976). The mode of action of CP under these circumstances is not understood.

VII. Effects on Experimental Neoplasia

A. CARCINOGENESIS

Baum and Baum (1974) reported that two subcutaneous injections of 0.7 mg of CP, a week apart, afforded mice protection against the carcinogenic effects of methylcholanthrene given at the time of the second CP injection. Sarcomas developed later, and their overall incidence was less than in untreated mice. Scott and Warner (1976) injected mice once a week for 14 weeks, either intravenously or sub-cutaneously, with 0.035 mg of CP. Eight days after the final injection they were challenged with either methylcholanthrene or ben-zopyrene. The pattern of development and final incidence of benzopyrene-induced tumors for both intravenous and subcutaneous CP-treated groups was similar to the control. Methylcholanthrene in-duced tumors in all intravenous CP-treated and control mice, but 25% of subcutaneous CP-treated mice remained tumor free at the end of the experiment. As detailed in later sections, CP-treated mice are capable of inhibiting the growth of cells transplanted from tumors that have been chemically induced in syngeneic mice. It is therefore unclear whether the reported protective effects of CP against chemical car-cinogens represent inhibition of the carcinogenic process, or merely inhibition of tumor growth once established.

There are reports that CP treatment reduces the incidence of tumors following the injection of oncogenic viruses; however, it is again un-clear to what extent these results may represent neutralization of the virus, interference with the oncogenic process or inhibition of estab-lished tumor growth. In an earlier section CP was described to protect against viral infection and a virus inhibitory factor was discussed (Cerutti, 1975). CG given systemically 4 days before systemic injec-tion of Friend leukemia virus markedly increased survival of mice (Kouznetzova *et al.*, 1974). CP also inhibits Moloney sarcoma virus (MSV) (N. H. Pazmino, M. Yuhas, and L. Milas, unpublished). Mice are sensitive to the oncogenic effects of MSV when newborn or aged. The final tumor incidence was not affected in newborn mice by CP either before or after virus inoculation, but the latent period before tumor appearance was significantly prolonged. In senescent mice, however, a 50% decrease in tumor incidence was induced by CP.

Aged DBA/2 mice have a high incidence (70%) of spontaneous mammary carcinomas. This incidence is decreased to 3–6% of the mice if, in adult life, they have rejected a subcutaneous transplant of syngeneic mammary carcinoma cells mixed with CP (Likhite, 1976). These mice are for a long time specifically resistant to tumor rechal-lenge and the ultimate decreased incidence of tumors may merely represent specific immunity to viral or tumor antigens.

B. IMMUNOPROPHYLAXIS

The first demonstration that CP pretreatment protected mice against challenge with syngeneic tumor cells was by Woodruff and Boak (1966). Intravenous CP 2 days before subcutaneous injections of either mammary carcinoma or methylcholanthrene-induced fibrosarcoma cells delayed the appearance of tumors and prolonged survival of the mice. Using allogeneic mouse tumor systems, Halpern et al. (1966) showed that intravenous CP retarded growth of subcutaneously injected Betz sarcoma cells, but only minimally affected the intraperitoneal growth of Ehrlich ascites carcinoma. The latter was, however, extremely sensitive to intraperitoneal CP pretreatment.

Numerous reports have since appeared describing the protective effects of anaerobic corynebacteria against many syngeneic mouse tumors: mammary carcinomas (Woodruff and Inchley, 1971; Milas et al., 1974c, 1975b), chemically induced fibrosarcomas (Fisher et al., 1970; Milas and Mujagić, 1972; Bomford and Olivotto, 1974; Castro, 1974b; Milas et al., 1974c; Bomford, 1975; McBride et al., 1975b), spontaneous fibrosarcomas (Smith and Scott, 1972; Bomford and Olivotto, 1974), osteosarcoma (van Putten et al., 1975), chemically induced ICIGCI$_1$ tumor (Mathé et al., 1973), mastocytoma (Scott, 1974b), plasmacytoma (Smith and Scott, 1972), line 1 lung carcinoma (Yuhas et al., 1975), Lewis lung carcinoma (Mathé et al., 1973), adenovirus 12-induced tumor (Rees and Potter, 1974), leukemias (Lamensans et al., 1968; Amiel et al., 1969; Smith and Scott, 1972; Mathé et al., 1973; Kouznetzova et al., 1974; Stiffel et al., 1974; Halpern et al., 1975; Roumiantzeff et al., 1975a), and lymphomas (Halpern et al., 1975; Roumiantzeff et al., 1975a).

Methylcholanthrene-induced fibrosarcomas have been extensively studied. Systemic CP (Bomford and Olivotto, 1974; Milas et al., 1974a) or CG (Milas et al., 1974a,c) prevented development of artificial metastases in the lung following intravenous injection of fibrosarcoma cells. Using ^{51}Cr-labeled tumor cells, Bomford and Olivotto (1974) have shown that the injected tumor cells that settled in the lungs of the CP-treated mice were killed more quickly. Subcutaneous pretreatment with CP also induced resistance to intravenous fibrosarcoma cell challenge (Milas and Mujagić, 1972). Both subcutaneous (Fisher et al., 1970) and systemic (Woodruff and Boak, 1966; Milas et al., 1974a,c) pretreatments have been shown to be effective against solid tumors arising from subcutaneous fibrosarcoma cell challenge. One particular fibrosarcoma was peculiarly sensitive to intraperitoneal CG pretreatment. The time of appearance of tumors was not affected, but, when they were 6–10 mm in diameter, more than 50% regressed (Milas et al., 1974c). Two comparative studies using mouse fibrosarcoma models have shown systemic pretreatment to be more effective than subcutaneous (Bomford and Olivotto, 1974; Milas et al., 1974a).

The protective effects of CP pretreatment against mouse leukemias depends on the relative routes of injection of CP and tumor cell challenge. Intraperitoneal CP pretreatment induced strong resistance against the intraperitoneal growth of AKR leukemia cells but was less effective against intravenous challenge (Lamensans *et al.*, 1968). Halpern *et al.* (1975) found that intraperitoneal CP was more effective against an intraperitoneal than an intravenous challenge with virus-induced YC8 leukemia cells. Intraperitoneal and intravenous injections are also more effective than subcutaneous or intradermal injections in protecting against intravenous L1210 leukemia (Mathé *et al.*, 1973).

Overall it is apparent that systemic injections have been superior to regional injections of CP in protecting against various tumor cell challenges, and this correlates well with the degree of lymphoreticular stimulation resulting from the two injection routes (Bomford and Olivotto, 1974; Milas *et al.*, 1974a). The role of the lymphoreticular system in CP-mediated antitumor effects is discussed in Section VII,G on modes of action. The stimulating effects of CP are relatively long lasting, and this is also true for some cases of CP-induced tumor protection. Although CP given 1–2 weeks before tumor cell challenge seems to be most effective, strong protection against AKR leukemia was still present after 35 days (Lamensans *et al.*, 1968). Good protection against fibrosarcoma cells was present at 25 days, but was lost by 50 days (Castro, 1974b) and, in another fibrosarcoma model, the effect of CG, although reduced, was still detected after 130 days (Milas *et al.*, 1975c). In contrast, the growth of poorly immunogenic line 1 lung carcinoma cells was inhibited only if injected within 10 days of CP (Yuhas and Ullrich, 1976). Smith and Scott (1972) suggested that the reduced susceptibility of different tumors to the protective effects of CP may be related to their immunogenicity. They screened several mouse tumors and found that better protection was achieved against the more immunogenic tumors.

The anatomical location of tumors may also influence their susceptibility. Yuhas and Ullrich (1976) showed that CP protected mice against subsequent intravenous or intraperitoneal injections of line 1 lung carcinoma, but not against subcutaneous or intramuscular tumor cells. Similar data have been reported for weekly immunogenic mammary carcinoma cells (Milas *et al.*, 1975b).

Although CP pretreatment usually protects better against low than high doses of tumor cells, in some instances it is relatively ineffective against very low numbers of tumor cells. Woodruff and Boak (1966) and Fisher *et al.* (1970) reported better protection against 10^4 than against 10^3 fibrosarcoma cells injected subcutaneously. Similarly 10^2

AKR leukemia cells grew better than 10^3 cells in mice pretreated with CP (Stiffel et al., 1971).

C. Immunotherapy

1. Systemic

In the same studies in which they first described the prophylactic effects of CP in syngeneic mice, Woodruff and Boak (1966) also first described its therapeutic action. A single dose of CP injected intravenously 8 or 12 days after subcutaneous injection of syngeneic mammary adenocarcinoma cells significantly delayed the appearance of the tumors. Once palpable, however, the subsequent growth of the tumors was unaffected. In later studies an actual inhibition of the growth rate of the same mammary adenocarcinoma, and two unrelated fibrosarcomas, was apparent when CP was injected intraperitoneally 3 days after tumor establishment (Woodruff et al., 1972). Intravenous CP treatment also caused a transitory, but significant, inhibition in the growth rate of a solid mastocytoma (Scott, 1974b). The growth of a solid mammary carcinoma has also been inhibited by biweekly intraperitoneal injections of CP starting either at the time of tumor injection (Likhite and Halpern, 1973) or 14 days later (Likhite and Halpern, 1974). Conflicting results have been reported for Lewis lung carcinoma. Intravenous CP given to mice within several days after subcutaneous transplantation of tumor cells either caused inhibition of tumor growth (Sadler and Castro, 1976) or had no effect (Morahan et al., 1976).

In none of the above studies were any tumor regressions observed, but, using a methylcholanthrene-induced fibrosarcoma in C3Hf/Bu mice, Milas et al. (1974d) obtained complete regressions of subcutaneously growing tumors when CG was injected intravenously 3 or 7 days after tumor cells. This tumor grows rapidly and by 7 days was about 6 mm in diameter. The responses of individual tumors were extremely variable. Some of them regressed completely and permanently, others regressed partially and regrew, and others grew slightly more slowly than in controls (Milas et al., 1974d). A characteristic of the regression of these tumors was that the tumor continued to grow at the same rate as in control mice for at least 10 days before the regression occurred. Systemic injections of CP also caused complete regressions of this tumor (Milas et al., 1974a; Suit et al., 1975, 1976b), its effect being equal to that of CG (Milas et al., 1974a).

In keeping with the pretreatment studies (Smith and Scott, 1972), it may also be that the immunogenicity of tumors affects their susceptibility to systemic CP therapy. Regressions have been achieved using intravenous CG against a poorly immunogenic mammary carcinoma, but, in contrast to a more immunogenic fibrosarcoma, they were extremely rare and only temporary (Milas *et al.*, 1975b). The efficiency of systemic CP may also depend on the site of tumor growth. Intravenous or intraperitoneal CP was more effective against a mouse fibrosarcoma growing intradermally or subcutaneously, than intramuscularly (Suit *et al.*, 1976b), and pulmonary deposits of this tumor were more susceptible than deposits that settled in the brain or heart (Milas *et al.*, 1974a).

The therapeutic effects of CP and CG against the artificial lung metastases that result from intravenous injection of fibrosarcoma cells have been extensively studied (Milas and Mujagić, 1972; Bomford and Olivotto, 1974; Milas *et al.*, 1974a; Milas and Withers, 1976). When the bacteria were injected systemically within a few days of tumor cell injection, they reduced the number of metastatic tumor nodules in the lung and completely cured many mice (Milas *et al.*, 1974a; Milas and Withers, 1976).

Variable results have been achieved with therapy of experimental leukemias using systemic CP. Intraperitoneal CP given as a single injection, or 5 times, at 4-day intervals, only minimally affected survival of mice which received subcutaneously L1210 leukemia cells 1 day prior to CP treatment (Mathé *et al.*, 1969). In another study using the same tumor, a significant effect was produced by multiple intravenous, or intraperitoneal, treatments of mice with CG; the treatment was started 3 or 4 days after tumor cell inoculation (Kouznetzova *et al.*, 1974). Systemic CP has retarded the growth of Moloney virus-induced YC 8 lymphoma (Halpern *et al.*, 1975; Roumiantzeff *et al.*, 1975a), but had no effect on Graffi leukemia (B. Halpern *et al.*, 1975).

All the above studies have used transplanted tumors. Thus far there is only one study concerning the therapeutic effects of CP on autochthonous tumors. Yuhas and Ullrich (1976) have described that three weekly intraperitoneal injections of CP caused temporary regressions of spontaneous mammary tumors growing in old, previously irradiated, mice.

Systemic CP treatment is most effective against small tumor masses, i.e., when injected soon after inoculation of tumor cells. The efficacy of both intravenous CG (Milas *et al.*, 1974d) and CP (Suit *et al.*, 1976b) treatment of C3H fibrosarcomas is substantially reduced for tumor sizes above 5–6 mm.

Doses of CP used for systemic injection have varied, but have been mostly in the range of 0.1–1 mg dry weight of organisms, the most frequent dose being around 0.5 mg. Milas *et al.* (1974d, 1975a) used single injections of 0.25 or 0.5 mg to cause complete tumor regressions in their mouse fibrosarcoma model. Suit *et al.* (1976b) studied the dose response of the single injection of intravenous CP given 4 days after the same tumor. There was a fall in efficacy as the dose was decreased from 0.35 to 0.1 mg. Doses of 0.7 and 1 mg were no better than 0.35 mg but were more toxic. Toxicity of high doses of systemic CP has been reported by others (Currie and Bagshawe, 1970; Fisher *et al.*, 1970; Milas *et al.*, 1974c; Scott, 1974b). Scott (1974b) observed that the highest single intravenous dose of CP that could be tolerated (0.7 mg) was most effective in inhibiting the growth of solid murine mastocytoma. Multiple high doses of CP have usually not resulted in better antitumor activity (Scott, 1974b; Milas *et al.*, 1975b; Suit *et al.*, 1976b) but may be more toxic (Fisher *et al.*, 1970). In a fibrosarcoma therapy model, Suit *et al.* (1976b) have shown that multiple doses of intravenous CP, individually ineffective, were effective. The same finding has been described for a pretreatment situation (Milas *et al.*, 1975c). Multiple low doses of systemic CP have been shown to cause lymphoreticular stimulation and immunologic modifications similar to those of a single high dose (Scott and Warner, 1976), and this mode of application of CP may provide a means of avoiding toxicity in clinical situations.

Oral administration of CP has been tested and found to be ineffective in the therapy of the subcutaneously growing Lewis lung carcinoma. This route of injection also failed to cause splenomegaly (Sadler and Castro, 1975).

2. *Local*

Direct injection of CP into growing solid tumors has been a particularly effective form of therapy, complete and permanent regressions being a common observation in many different tumor models. When a murine (Likhite and Halpern, 1974) or rat (Likhite, 1974) mammary carcinoma growing for 14 and 20 days, respectively, was injected with CP they all regressed permanently. Not only did the injected tumors regress, but their metastases as well. Strong inhibition of tumor growth, or some complete regressions, following intralesional CP or CG therapy have also been described for mouse fibrosarcomas (Milas *et al.*, 1975b; Tuttle and North, 1975; Woodruff and Dunbar, 1975; Morahan *et al.*, 1976; Suit *et al.*, 1976b), a mouse mastocytoma (Scott, 1974c, 1976), and a hamster melanoma (Paslin *et al.*, 1974). Subcutaneous injections of CP at sites distant from the growing tumor only minimally affect its growth, whereas injections into the region of the tumor cause marked inhibition of growth but are less effective than intralesional injections (Likhite and Halpern, 1974; Scott, 1974c; Woodruff and Dunbar, 1975).

Animals whose tumors have undergone complete regressions following intralesional CP therapy are specifically resistant to reinoculation of cells from the same tumor (Likhite, 1974; Scott, 1974c; Woodruff and Dunbar, 1975). Mice which have rejected tumors that develop from tumor cells admixed with CP are similarly, specifically immune (Likhite and Halpern, 1974; Likhite, 1976). The immunity is strong and long lasting (at least 20 months), and immune mice ultimately develop fewer spontaneous tumors (Likhite, 1976). The nature of this immunity is discussed in detail in Section VII,G.

Doses of intralesional CP that have been used, and found to be effective, have varied between 0.02 and 0.7 mg, however, different tumor models and sizes of tumor have been studied. Scott (1974c) investigated the optimal dose of intralesional CP for a mouse mastocytoma and found that, within the dose range 0.007–0.35 mg, 0.07 mg was optimal. The reduced effectiveness of higher doses of intralesional CP contrasted with the effects of intravenous CP against this tumor where the highest doses were found to be most effective (Scott, 1974b).

In keeping with systemic CP therapy, better results are achieved with intralesional therapy by shortening the time interval between tumor cell transplantation and CP. CP injected 6 days after tumor cell inoculation caused 4 out of 6 mouse mastocytomas to regress completely, and only 1 out of 6 after 10 days (Scott, 1974c). Similar data have been reported for a mouse fibrosarcoma (Woodruff and Dunbar, 1975).

Using the C3H fibrosarcoma model, which is extremely sensitive to systemic CP, i.e., complete regressions are achieved, Suit *et al.* (1976b) compared the efficacy of intravenous with intralesional CP therapy and found more regressions after intravenous treatment. With tumors less sensitive to systemic CP, intralesional CP has been found to be superior: mouse mammary carcinoma (Likhite and Halpern, 1974), rat mammary carcinoma (Likhite, 1974), mouse mastocytoma (Scott, 1974c), and mouse fibrosarcoma (Woodruff and Dunbar, 1975). Milas *et al.* (1976) reported the two routes to be equally effective against a mouse mammary carcinoma. Morahan *et al.* (1976) found that intravenous CP had no effect against Lewis lung carcinoma, and results with intralesional CP were variable, ranging from enhanced tumor growth to complete regressions.

The overall results with intralesional CP in animal tumor models are impressive, but it is again apparent that some tumors are more suscep-tible than others. This variability may again be related to the individ-ual immunogenicities of the tumors; a component of the local tumor destruction caused by CP is considered to be immunologically mediated (see Section VII,G). The degree of local tumor destruction would also be expected to be related to the distribution of CP within the tumor, and differences in the individual injection techniques may be another source of variation.

There have been few studies combining systemic and intratumor therapy with CP. Scott (1974c) reported that intravenous CP reduced the antitumor effects of a subsequent injection of CP against a weakly immunogenic murine mastocytoma. In contrast, Suit et al. (1976b) demonstrated that a relatively strong immunogenic mouse fibrosar-coma responded better to the combination of intravenous and intrale-sional CP, regardless of whether the intravenous inoculation preceded or followed intralesional CP, than to the individual treatments alone.

D. COMBINATION WITH SPECIFIC ACTIVE IMMUNOTHERAPY

The local interaction of CP with live or irradiated tumor cells results in strong, specific, long-lasting, cell-mediated tumor immunity (see Section VII,G). Specific active immunotherapy using mixtures of CP and irradiated tumor cells has been shown to inhibit or prevent the growth of mouse mastocytomas (Scott, 1975b) and mouse fibrosar-comas (Bomford, 1975), respectively. Subcutaneous injection of CP mixed with irradiated fibrosarcoma cells inhibited the growth of live tumor cells injected at a distant site 2 or 6 days previously. Therapy delayed until 10 days was ineffective. Successful therapy required a minimal number of irradiated tumor cells ($\geqslant 5 \times 10^4$), with no upper limit being detected, and only small doses of CP (0.0014–0.1 mg). There was an upper limit for the amount of CP in the mixtures which increased with the number of tumor cells. This suggests a necessity for a balance between the amount of CP and tumor antigen for optimal immunity. The small doses of CP that, in combination with irradiated tumor cells, completely inhibited tumor growth, contrasted with the larger amounts (0.35 mg) that were considerably less effective after intravenous injection (Bomford, 1975). Similar observations on the efficacy of very small doses (0.0035 mg) of CP injected in combination with irradiated mastocytoma cells are those of Scott (1975b).

Scott (1975b) was unable to potentiate tumor specific immunity using systemic injections of irradiated mastocytoma cells mixed with CP. The CP did, however, abolish the enhancing effect of the irradiated tumor cells alone. Likhite and Halpern (1973) using a mouse mammary carcinoma and rat Shay chloroma also found that biweekly therapeutic intraperitoneal injections of CP and killed tumor cells were no more inhibitory than intraperitoneal injections of tumor cells alone. That tumor immunity may be stimulated using systemic CP injections is, however, evident from other studies. Combination of CP and heavily irradiated tumor cells, both given intraperitoneally, protected mice against viable sarcoma cells inoculated intravenously more effectively than the individual treatments (Milas *et al.*, 1975d). Yuhas *et al.* (1975) also reported that combination of intraperitoneal injection of CP and intravenous immunization with viable tumor cells inhibited the subcutaneous growth of line 1 lung carcinoma more effectively than either treatment alone. Combination of systemic CP and localized tumor antigen may also result in augmented tumor immunity. Woodruff and Dunbar (1973) report strong inhibition of the growth of a mouse fibrosarcoma using simultaneous injections of intraperitoneal CP and subcutaneous mitomycin C-treated tumor cells, which had been further treated with neuraminidase to increase their immunogenicity.

Under some circumstances combination of CP with irradiated tumor cells may depress, rather than potentiate, tumor immunity. Smith and Scott (1972) have shown that CP given intravenously to mice 7 days before intraperitoneal immunization with irradiated leukemia cells depressed the protective effects of the immunization. This may be related to the depressive effects of systemic CP pretreatment on various T-cell-mediated immune phenomena that we have already discussed.

E. COMBINATION WITH CONVENTIONAL MODALITIES OF CANCER TREATMENT

The foregoing studies have shown that immunotherapy with CP, in keeping with immunotherapy in general, is effective only against relatively small tumor masses. Clinically, this is likely to represent a minimal disease situation, i.e., when the primary tumor burden has been reduced by more conventional forms of therapy—radiotherapy, chemotherapy, or surgery. This section describes the animal data concerning combination of CP with these treatments.

1. *Combination with Radiotherapy*

Tumor response to radiotherapy depends not only on radiobiological factors (Withers, 1974), but also on the immune competence of the tumor hosts (for more details, see Milas *et al.*, 1975a). Both CP and CG have been combined with local irradiation in the therapy of experimental tumors (Milas *et al.*, 1975a,e; Suit *et al.*, 1975, 1976a,b; Moroson and Schechter, 1976). Intravenous CP (0.1–0.5 mg) reduced the radiation dose necessary to achieve local control of a relatively strongly immunogenic 8-mm mouse fibrosarcoma in 50% of treated animals (TCD 50 values) (Milas *et al.*, 1975a; Suit *et al.*, 1976b). Tumors were irradiated with single doses of γ-irradiation ranging from 200 to 4400 rads. CP also significantly augmented radiocurability of fractionated irradiation: 500 rads given for 3, 6, or 10 consecutive days (Milas *et al.*, 1975e) or 10 equal doses ranging from 50 to 950 rads with 2 days between irradiations (Suit *et al.*, 1976b). Tumors that were not cured by these combinations grew more slowly, and metastasized less frequently than tumors treated with irradiation alone. An interesting observation was that CP greatly augmented radiocurability of doses between 200 and 2500 rads whereas little improvement occurred when tumors were being controlled with about 80% probability. The TCD_{50} value for this tumor in normal mice is approximately 3400 rads. Higher irradiation doses significantly injure stromal tissues including blood vessels, and this may result in inaccessibility of surviving tumor cells to the immune defense mechanisms. High irradiation doses may also inactivate local lymphocytes or macrophages.

Suit *et al.* (1976b) studied the effects of several routes of CP administration, dose levels of CP, and time relationships between treatments of CP and irradiation. Intravenous CP regularly potentiated radiocurability. Intralesional and subcutaneous CP were, however, more effective against tumors if applied alone. When CP was given intralesionally and intravenously when tumors were 5 and 8 mm, respectively, followed by 200 rads local irradiation, the effect was less than with CP alone. In the reverse situation, i.e., first CP intravenously and then intralesionally, augmentation of radiocurability was observed. Single intravenous doses of CP smaller than 0.1 mg were ineffective. The sequence of CP and irradiation was also important. CP given to mice 2–4 days before irradiation was more effective than when given 2 days after irradiation.

CP is not as effective in augmenting radiocurability of weakly immunogenic murine tumors. In studies by Suit *et al.* (1976a) the effects of the combined treatment were barely evident against a mammary carcinoma, but the TCD_{50} values for two squamous cell carcinomas were significantly reduced. Local irradiation of a highly metastasizing mammary carcinoma with 6000 rads, single dose, caused complete regression of irradiated tumors, but, surprisingly, greatly increased the number of metastases in the lung compared to that in mice whose tumors were surgically removed (Milas *et al.*, 1976). Treatment with CP before, but not after, irradiation not only prevented this effect, but reduced the number of metastases below that in amputated mice.

Under certain circumstances radiotherapy may be immunosuppressive and enhance tumor spread (Stjernswärd *et al.*, 1972). CP given before irradiation may prevent such deleterious effects. Milas *et al.* (1974b,c) found that enhancement of pulmonary metastases caused by whole-body irradiation of mice 1 day before intravenous injection of fibrosarcoma cells, can be prevented by CG treatment within 2 weeks prior to irradiation. CG was ineffective when given after radiation. Similar observations were reported for CP by Bomford and Olivotto (1974).

2. *Combination with Chemotherapy*

Despite the immunosuppressive nature of most cancer chemotherapy drugs, animal studies show that immunostimulation using CP can be successfully combined with drug therapy, often with additive, or even synergistic effects.

Most studies have used cyclophosphamide. Intradermal treatment of mice with CP 12 days after intraperitoneal injection of cyclophosphamide caused complete regression of a subcutaneously growing fibrosarcoma in about 70% of treated mice (Currie and Bagshawe, 1970). No complete regressions were achieved, although a significant retardation in the tumor growth was still present, when CP was injected 6 or 16 days after chemotherapy. When given before, or simultaneously with cyclophosphamide, CP was not effective but caused high toxicity. Using a similar tumor system Woodruff and Dunbar (1973) obtained results similar to those of Currie and Bagshawe (1970). In their experiments CP was given intraperitoneally and the best effect was achieved when injected 9 days after cyclophosphamide. Treatment of a murine leukemia with cyclophosphamide in combination with intraperitoneal CP was optimal when intraperitoneal CP was given 4 or 8 days after cyclophosphamide. This was when the leukemia was in remission. CP 12 days after cyclophosphamide, immediately prior to relapse, was ineffective (Pearson *et al.*, 1975). Intradermal injections of CG, either 3 or 6 days after cyclophosphamide treatment of a rat leukemia has been described to be no more effective than drug treatment alone (Pearson *et al.*, 1974a). The unpublished results of one of the authors (M. T. S.) are that the most effective treatment of a subcutaneously growing mouse fibrosarcoma occurs when a single dose of CP is given intravenously, or given subcutaneously mixed with irradiated tumor cells, 4 days after a single intraperitoneal injection of cyclophosphamide. Fisher *et al.* (1975a,b) have studied the effects of prolonged administration of CP alone, and in combination with cyclophosphamide, on the treatment of mouse mammary carcinomas. The best effects were obtained when systemic CP was administered asynchronously at weekly intervals in combination with cyclophosphamide. The optimal time interval between cyclophosphamide injections was 7 days, and so was the interval between CP injections. Best results were obtained when the CP was given 4 days after cyclophosphamide, i.e., cyclophosphamide on days 0, 7, 14 and CP on days 4, 11, 18, etc.

There are also data describing CP in combination with other drugs. A murine leukemia has also been successfully treated, with 76% complete remissions, using a combination of 1,3-bis(2-chloroethyl)-1-nitrosourea (BCNU) followed 3 days later by intradermal CG: injections of drug or CG alone were considerably less effective, as was CG 6 or 12 days after BCNU (Pearson *et al.*, 1972). A different mouse leukemia responded well to a single intradermal injection of CG 3 days after BCNU, but repeated injections of CG at 3, 7, 9, and 11 days after drug were less effective (Pearson *et al.*, 1974b). Intravenous injection of CP 1 day after procarbazine fully protected all mice against leukemia cells, whereas with procarbazine alone there were no survivors (Amiel and Berardet, 1970). There is also a preliminary report that adriamycin in combination with CP is more effective in increasing the life-span of mice with leukemia than either drug or CP alone (Houchens and Gaston, 1976).

It is apparent that the combination of CP with drugs may be a promising form of cancer therapy and data concerning the principles underlying this form of therapy are clearly required: e.g., what are the drug susceptibilites of the various CP antitumor effects? The protective effect of intravenous CP against the formation of lung metastases following intravenous injection of tumor cells is still detectable in cyclophosphamide-treated mice, and CP almost entirely abolishes the enhancement of metastases by cyclophosphamide (van Putten *et al.*, 1975). Scott (1975a) has shown that an injection of cortisone acetate in CP-stimulated mice transiently inhibited the *in vitro* nonspecific antitumor activity of their macrophages and was sufficient to abolish *in vivo* resistance to a live tumor cell challenge. Studies by Fisher *et al.* (1976a) have, however, combined prolonged administration of cortisone acetate with repeated cyclophosphamide and CP injections and shown no inhibition of antitumor effects.

CP has already been described to increase the number of colony-forming cells in the bone marrow, and a possible indirect antitumor effect in future clinical situations may be the toleration of more intensive chemotherapy due to a marrow protective effect. Further data in this area are also required, since a recent report describes that CP-stimulated mice are more susceptible to the toxic effects of high doses of 5 fluorouracil (Foster, 1976).

3. *Combination with Surgery*

No general principles underlying the combination of CP treatment with the surgical removal of solid tumors are yet apparent from the few animal data available.

Combined intradermal and intraperitoneal CP at 7 and 14 days after surgical removal of a subcutaneously growing rat hepatoma inhibited the formation of lung metastases. CP injected before amputation was ineffective. If large numbers of irradiated hepatoma cells were injected before surgery the number of lung metastases was increased, and this effect was abolished by simultaneous injection of CP (Proctor *et al.*, 1973). CP before amputation has been found to be effective in mouse models. Sadler and Castro (1976) reported that single intravenous or intraperitoneal, but not subcutaneous, injections of CP within 4 days before surgery reduced the incidence of lung metastases from a Lewis lung carcinoma. Similar data for systemic CP in a mouse mammary carcinoma model has been presented by Milas *et al.* (1976). CP or CG injected after removal of the mammary carcinoma were ineffective, and injections of CG 4 and 10 days after surgery slightly enhanced metastases.

F. ANTITUMOR ACTIVITY OF CP FRACTIONS

It will be apparent from the clinical data (see Section VIII,B) that some of the side effects commonly observed with whole bacterial vaccines are serious. It is hoped that studies attempting to characterize the active principle of CP will result in retention of antitumor activity with a reduction in toxicity.

A phospholipid extract of CP has been reported to be less toxic than whole organisms in mice. It failed to cause splenomegaly and hepatomegaly but did inhibit the multiplication of bacteria in the liver and spleen. Its antitumor properties were not examined (Fauve and Hevin, 1974). A lipid extracted from the surface of CP has also been shown to be a chemoattractant for mouse and guinea pig macrophages and for human monocytes (Russel *et al.*, 1976). An extract of CP produced by mild hydrolysis has retained some antitumor activity, although considerably less than whole organisms. A lipid component seemed to be responsible, and antitumor activity was increased if the extract was adsorbed onto latex to facilitate its phagocytosis (McBride *et al.*, 1976). Zola (1975) has shown that the *in vitro* B-cell mitogenic property of CP is lacking in a delipidated preparation of cell walls. If stimulatory activity is associated with a lipid component, then other components may be similarly active. Adlam *et al.* (1975) have shown that lipid-free cell walls of CP retained their lymphoreticular stimulating and antitumor activity against allogeneic sarcoma 180. Water-soluble extracts prepared from delipidated cell walls of CP have also been shown to stimulate carbon clearance, antibody formation and DTH, as well as protecting against encephalomyocarditis virus and MSV (Migliore-Samour *et al.*, 1974; Jollès *et al.*, 1975).

Various cell wall preparations of anaerobic corynebacteria were shown by Kouznetzova *et al.* (1974) to possess reticuloendothelial stimulating activity, adjuvant properties, and protective effects against experimental mouse leukemias. A chemical analysis of CP cell walls has been presented by Azuma *et al.* (1975), who also found that adjuvant activity for antibody formation and DTH was present in cell walls, but that cell-mediated antitumor immunity was not augmented. The adjuvant active unit of the cell wall structure is considered to be a peptidoglycan, and a similar dissociation between adjuvant and antitumor activity has been described for synthetic peptidoglycans (Azuma *et al.*, 1976; Yamamura *et al.*, 1976).

G. MODES OF ACTION

1. *Nonspecific Activity of CP-Activated Macrophages*

The *in vivo* antitumor effects of systemically injected CP in mice have been shown to be resistant to a variety of immunosuppressive procedures, suggesting an immunologically nonspecific mechanism (i.e., not amplifying a specific antitumor response) to be operating. They are resistant to subsequent whole-body irradiation (Bomford and Olivotto, 1974; Milas *et al.*, 1974b). They are also still apparent in mice deprived of T lymphocytes by thymectomy, irradiation, and bone marrow reconstitution (TIR) (Woodruff *et al.*, 1973; Scott, 1974b) and antilymphocyte serum treatment (Hattori and Mori, 1973; Castro, 1974b). The inhibitory effects of systemic CP on various T-cell-dependent immune phenomena (discussed in Section IV,B) are also in keeping with a noninvolvement of lymphocytes in the CP-mediated antitumor response. That antibody is unlikely to be involved is suggested by the demonstration that splenectomy, a procedure likely to impair antibody production, did not abrogate the *in vivo* antitumor effects of a subsequent injection of CP (Castro, 1974b; Mazurek *et al.*, 1976). CP effects were also apparent in mice genetically selected for low antibody responses (Biozzi *et al.*, 1972).

The resistance of systemic CP effects to immunosuppression is compatible with a macrophage-mediated response, and CP-activated macrophages exert antitumor effects *in vitro*. This is not a property unique to anaerobic corynebacteria, but is shared by many other microorganisms, such as BCG (Hibbs *et al.*, 1972; Hibbs, 1973; Cleveland *et al.*, 1974). *Toxoplasma gondii* (Hibbs *et al.*, 1972; Hibbs, 1973; Krahenbuhl and Remington, 1974), *Listeria monocytogenes* (Hibbs *et al.*, 1972; Hibbs, 1973; Krahenbuhl and Remington, 1974), and *Besnoitia jellisoni* (Krahenbuhl and Remington, 1974).

Peritoneal macrophages from mice treated with CP inhibit the *in vitro* growth and DNA synthesis of syngeneic mastocytoma cells (Scott, 1974b), radiation-induced leukemia cells (Olivotto and Bomford, 1974; Bomford and Christie, 1975; Christie and Bomford, 1975), fibrosarcoma cells (Olivotto and Bomford, 1974; Ghaffar *et al.*, 1974, 1975), and RBL-5 lymphoma cells (Kirchner *et al.*, 1975b). The ultimate fate of the target tumor cells in such cytostatic assays is not clear, but a direct cytotoxic effect of CP-activated macrophages on Lewis lung carcinoma has been described by Morahan and Kaplan (1976). Similarly, Bašić *et al.* (1974, 1975a) found that peritoneal macrophages from mice treated with CG destroy *in vitro* cultures of a syngeneic fibrosarcoma, tumorigenic mouse L-P 59 cells, transformed Chinese hamster ovary cells, and human melanoma cells.

The antitumor activity of peritoneal macrophages has been detected within 2 days following intravenous injection of CP, was maximal after 5 days, and thereafter declined but was still present at 20 days. In contrast, the antitumor activity of lung macrophages was maximal 14 days after CP (Olivotto and Bomford, 1974). The activity of splenic macrophages could be first detected 7 days after intraperitoneal CP; it peaked at 14 days and usually disappeared after 18–21 days (Kirchner *et al.*, 1975b).

It is apparent that these *in vitro* cytostatic or cytotoxic effects are exclusive to the macrophages. The effector cells used by Olivotto and Bomford (1974) were almost exclusively macrophages by both morphologic and functional criteria. Nonadherent peritoneal cells from CP-stimulated mice did not inhibit tumor cell growth *in vitro* (Ghaffar *et al.*, 1974), and procedures for removing lymphocytes from peritoneal cells, such as extensive washing, trypsinization, or irradiation, did not impair their antitumor activity (Ghaffar *et al.*, 1974; Scott, 1974b; Bašić *et al.*, 1975a). Similarly, the activity of spleen cells was found to be unaffected by treatment with anti-θ-serum and complement, whereas macrophage removal using rayon adherence columns, iron-magnetic techniques, or carageenin treatment, almost entirely abolished it (Kirchner *et al.*, 1975b).

The mechanisms by which CP-activated macrophages kill, or inhibit the growth of, tumor cells *in vitro* is not clear. Medium removed from cultures of activated macrophages (Olivotto and Bomford, 1974; Bašić *et al.*, 1975a) or from cultures containing both, CP-stimulated macrophages and tumor cells (Ghaffar *et al.*, 1974) did not inhibit the growth of tumor cells *in vitro*. This suggested that the antitumor activity of activated macrophages was not mediated through substances released into the growth medium, and that macrophage-tumor cell contact may be required. After several hours of culture, adherence of macrophages to tumor cells is already apparent (Olivotto and Bomford, 1974; Bašić *et al.*, 1975a), and electron microscopy studies have shown a close apposition between the two cell surfaces (Puvion *et al.*, 1975, 1976). Adherent tumor cells subsequently undergo lysis (Bašić *et al.*, 1975a). Hibbs (1974) reported that, upon contact with target cells, macrophages activated by BCG or *Toxoplasma* appear to secrete lysosomal enzymes directly into the cytoplasm of target cells, which then lyse. This was inhibited by trypan blue, an inhibitor of lysosomal enzyme function (Hibbs, 1974). The *in vivo* antitumor effects of systemic CP are similarly sensitive to trypan blue (Morahan and Kaplan, 1976). Cortisone acetate also inhibits the *in vitro* antitumor activity of CP-activated macrophages (Scott, 1975a), the presumed effect being the prevention of exocytosis of lysosomal enzymes through stabilization of the macrophage membrane (Weissmann and Dingle, 1961; de Duve *et al.*, 1962; Allison and Davies, 1972). The lysosomal enzymes that may be involved in the *in vitro* killing of tumor cells by activated macrophages are not known. However, Puvion *et al.* (1976) recently reported no correlation between the level of acid phosphatase in CP-activated macrophages and tumor cell-killing ability.

The mechanisms of macrophage activation by CP have been the subject of recent studies by Christie and Bomford (1975) and Bomford and Christie (1975). Normal mouse peritoneal macrophages could not be activated *in vitro*, as assayed by inhibition of tumor cell proliferation, by exposure to CP alone, but only by mixtures of CP and spleen cells from CP-immune mice. Treatment of the spleen cells with anti-θ serum and complement abolished this activation. Supernatants from cultures of the CP-immune spleen cells and CP were also capable of activating normal macrophages. This indicated an immunological pathway of macrophage activation mediated by a release of soluble factors from CP-sensitized T lymphocytes on contact with the antigen. Participation of such an immune mechanism in the *in vivo* CP activation of macrophages was evidenced by the acceleration of macrophage activation by CP in mice which had been immunized with CP 60 or 130 days earlier. Macrophages from normal mice became cytostatic 5 days after CP treatment, but those from previously sensitized mice were already cytostatic within 1 day (Bomford and Christie, 1975). It seems that CP can also activate macrophages *in vivo* by an alternative, immunologically independent pathway, since macrophage activation in both TIR mice (Bomford and Christie, 1975) and athymic nude mice (Ghaffar *et al.*, 1975) is equal to that in normal mice.

The fact that CP activates complement by the alternative pathway in both normal human and guinea pig serum (McBride *et al.*, 1975c) allows speculation as to a further pathway of macrophage activation mediated by cleavage products of complement component C3. Activation of complement by the alternative pathway generates the C3 cleavage product C3b, and Schorlemmer *et al.* (1976) report experiments in which attachment of C3b to mouse macrophages in culture results in macrophage activation as evidenced by release of lysosomal enzymes into the culture. Similarly, activated mouse macrophages have recently been shown to nonspecifically inhibit mouse tumor cell growth *in vitro* (A. C. Allison, personal communication).

The *in vitro* cytotoxicity mediated by macrophages stimulated with anaerobic corynebacteria seems to be limited to cells with malignant growth characteristics. CG-stimulated macrophages do not destroy syngeneic or allogeneic fibroblasts, or allogeneic kidney epithelial cells *in vitro* (Bašić *et al.*, 1975a). These observations accord with findings by Hibbs' group that *in vitro* cultures of normal allogeneic cells, but not cultures of cells with neoplastic properties, were resistant to destruction by murine macrophages activated with *Toxoplasma, Listeria monocytogenes,* or BCG (Hibbs *et al.*, 1972; Hibbs, 1973). The reasons for this discriminatory behavior of activated macrophages are not known but may be related to membrane properties of both activated macrophages and neoplastic cells facilitating, or initiating, close contact between them. Membranes of malignant and transformed cells differ from normal cells in electrical charge (Ambrose *et al.*, 1956), surface glucoprotein (Roberts *et al.*, 1973), glycolipid and glycosyltransferase activity (Hakomori and Murakami, 1968; Roth and White, 1972), and lectin agglutinability (Aub *et al.*, 1963; Burger, 1969). Activated macrophages exhibit increased stickiness (Bašić et al., 1975a), membrane motility (Nathan et al., 1971), and membrane glycosamine incorporation (Hammond and Dvorak, 1972).

What is the evidence that a nonspecific destruction of tumor cells by CP-activated macrophages operates in vivo? Most of the evidence to date is indirect. The resistance of the in vivo antitumor effects of systemic CP to various immunosuppressive procedures, including radiation, has already been commented upon. Mouse tumors regressing following intravenous CP or CG treatment are heavily infiltrated with macrophages (Milas et al., 1974a,d). It is, however possible that these cells may merely be removing the remnants of tumor cells killed by other host mechanisms. An involvement of macrophages is implied by the findings of McBride et al. (1975b). They showed that gold salts (sodium aurothiomalate), which inhibit macrophage lysosomal enzyme activity, suppressed the in vivo protective action of CP against both intravenously and subcutaneously injected mouse fibrosarcoma cells. Scott (1975a) has also reported similar suppressive effect using cortisone in a murine mastocytoma model. Current experiments in one of our laboratories (Peters et al., 1977) provide more direct evidence for in vivo involvement of activated macrophages. Addition of peritoneal macrophages from CP-stimulated mice to fibrosarcoma cells resulted in the suppression of tumor growth when this mixture was transferred intraperitoneally or subcutaneously into syngeneic recipients. Normal peritoneal cells or heat-killed activated cells had no effect.

It should be borne in mind that these nonspecifically activated macrophages which kill tumor cells in vitro, and are presumed to have a similar role in vivo, may be the same cells that have already been described to inhibit T lymphocyte responses in vitro (Scott, 1972a,b; Kirchner et al., 1975b). Kirchner et al. (1975a) have presented data that CP-activated macrophages may also be the cell type responsible for suppressing the specific secondary cytotoxic response of immune spleen cells against tumor cells in vitro. Systemic CP pretreatment has been described to depress the in vivo protective effects of specific immunization with irradiated tumor cells in an experimental leukemia model (Smith and Scott, 1972), and there thus may be a balance between the beneficial antitumor effects of CP and its immunosuppressive effects.

2. Potentiation of Tumor-Specific Immunity

Studies using local injections of CP have revealed a further mode of action which is immunologically specific, i.e., potentiates the host's immune response to tumor-specific antigens.

Subcutaneous injection of mixtures of CP with viable mouse mammary carcinoma or rat Shay chloroma cells into the corresponding syngeneic hosts resulted in the development of tumors that grew for about 2 weeks and then rapidly regressed. Animals whose tumors had undergone regression were found to be specifically resistant to tumor rechallenge (Likhite and Halpern, 1973). An analogous situation is the injection of CP directly into an established tumor, and animals whose tumors have undergone regression following intralesional CP therapy are similarly specifically immune to rechallenge (Likhite and Halpern, 1974; Scott, 1974c). The specific resistance resulting from local CP-tumor cell interaction is long lasting and has been detected up to 20 months after injection of CP mixed with viable mouse mammary carcinoma cells (Likhite, 1976).

The foregoing studies suggested that, under conditions of close contact between CP and tumor cells, CP may be augmenting a specific antitumor immune response. Fisher *et al.* (1974) observed that the *in vitro* cytotoxicity of tumor draining lymph node cells for mouse mammary carcinoma cells was increased after injection of CP directly into the tumor or between the tumor and the draining lymph node. Since treatment of normal mice with CP did not result in any cytotoxicity, the augmentation in tumor-bearing mice was ascribed to a CP-mediated potentiation of the specific tumor immune response. Potentiation of specific antitumor activity by CP is also evident from experiments in which subcutaneous injections of CP mixed with irradiated mastocytoma cells have specifically immunized mice against tumor rechallenge, while injections of CP or irradiated cells alone were without effect. The injection sites of CP and irradiated tumor cells did not need to be coincident but required common lymphoid drainage for immunity to occur (Scott, 1975b). Similar specific immunity arising from therapeutic injections of CP-irradiated mouse fibrosarcoma cell mixtures have been reported by Bomford (1975). It was reduced in T cell-deprived mice (Bomford, 1975; Scott, 1975b) and could be transferred by lymph node cells draining the site of mixture injection, but not by serum (Scott, 1975b). Tuttle and North (1976a,b) were also unable to transfer immunity with serum and further presented evidence that the lymphoid cell involved was a relatively short-lived T cell, which probably does not require macrophages or other lymphocytes to effect its antitumor activity. That such a cell-mediated immune mechanism may be operative in the local destruction of tumor cells following intralesional injection of CP is suggested by the complete T cell dependence of this form of CP therapy (Scott, 1974c; Woodruff and Dunbar, 1975). Tumors regressing following intralesional injection of

CP are heavily infiltrated with lymphocytes and macrophages (Likhite and Halpern, 1973, 1974).

In Section VII,G,1 it has been reasoned that the antitumor effects of systemically injected CP are predominantly nonspecific and macrophage-mediated. There are data, however, showing that potentiation of specific immunity is not exclusive to locally injected CP but may also be a component in systemic CP therapy. Halpern *et al.* (1973) reported that the *in vitro* specific cytotoxicity of lymph node cells of mice bearing leukemia was greatly augmented and prolonged by intraperitoneal treatment of mice with CP. Yuhas *et al.* (1975) observed that neither specific immunization of mice with tumor cells nor treatments with intravenous CP caused resistance to line 1 carcinoma cells, but that combination of the two was very efficient. Furthermore, CP has required the presence of T cells to induce optimal resistance to pulmonary deposits of a murine fibrosarcoma (Milas *et al.*, 1975d).

The role of antitumor antibodies in CP-induced resistance is less certain than that of immune cells. Transfer of serum from mice positively immunized by mixtures of CP and irradiated tumor cells was ineffective in conferring resistance upon normal mice (Scott, 1975b). Cytotoxic antibodies have been reported after regression of living tumor cells mixed with CP (Likhite, 1975), but these may be a result of the temporary growth of the tumor itself. In an allogeneic mouse tumor model, CP pretreatment did not modify the level of complement-dependent cytolytic antibody. It did, however, increase the antibody-dependent cellular cytotoxicity (ADCC) of spleen cells (Mantovani *et al.*, 1976). We are aware of no similar data concerning ADCC in a syngeneic tumor system. A noninvolvement of antibodies may be inferred from the undiminished protective effects of CP in splenectomized mice (Castro, 1974b; Mazurek *et al.*, 1976) and genetically low antibody producers (Biozzi *et al.*, 1972).

The mechanism(s) of the potentiating activity of CP on specific antitumor immunity is as yet unclear. The processing of tumor antigens within CP-stimulated lymphoid organs may be modified. Wiener and Bandieri (1975) have shown that macrophages from CP-treated mice retain more antigen on their surface than normal macrophages which may improve antigen presentation to lymphocytes. Another contributing factor could be the increased and prolonged lymphocyte trapping in lymph nodes of CP-stimulated mice (Frost and Lance, 1973).

3. *Immunity to CP*

In addition to its adjuvant properties, CP is itself a potent immunogen producing both agglutinating antibodies (Woodruff *et al.*, 1974;

Scott and Warner, 1976) and DTH (Scott, 1974a,c; Tuttle and North, 1975). There is evidence that the expression of an immunological response to CP antigens is important for local destruction of tumor cells following intralesional CP injection. Scott (1974c) described that the therapeutic effects of an intralesional injection of CP into an established mouse mastocytoma were reduced if the specific reactivity of the tumor-draining node to CP had been preempted by a large amount of the bacteria injected intravenously. Tuttle and North (1975) were unable to achieve regressions of a mouse fibrosarcoma following intralesional injection of CP unless the mice had been previously sensitized to show DTH to CP, and the intralesional injection was at the time of maximum CP sensitivity. The destruction of tumor cells at the site of a DTH reaction to CP was associated with the influx of phagocytic mononuclear cells. These may be activated macrophages since Christie and Bomford (1975) have shown that *in vitro* macrophages can be nonspecifically activated to kill tumor cells as a result of local interaction of CP with CP-sensitized T lymphocytes.

Immunity to CP would also be likely to influence its antitumor activity in any situation where tumor antigens might cross-react with CP antigens (James *et al.*, 1976). Another situation would be if CP antigens were to become absorbed onto the surface of tumor cells. They have been shown to be absorbed onto syngeneic red cells *in vitro* (Cox and Keast, 1974).

4. *Other Considerations*

Tumor-bearing mice contain in their circulation soluble tumor antigens and antibody–antigen complexes that may block the efficiency of immune effector cells. CP treatment may, through nonspecific stimulation of phagocytic activity, cause these factors to be removed. Examples of this may be the abolition of enhancing effects of active immunization with irradiated tumor cells reported for a rat hepatoma (Proctor *et al.*, 1973) and a murine mastocytoma (Scott, 1975b). A related observation may be the abrogation by CP of the enhanced spontaneous pulmonary metastases that resulted from local irradiation of a primary tumor (Milas *et al.*, 1976). CP treatment also alters distribution of tumor cells released into circulation (Bomford and Olivotto, 1974) and may affect the process of metastases in this manner.

Serum from mice treated with CP and several days later with endotoxin contains a substance which, upon injection into tumor-bearing mice, causes tumor necrosis (Carswell *et al.*, 1975; Green *et al.*, 1976). This tumor necrosis factor (TNF) is not produced by treatments with CP or endotoxin alone and is considered to be released by host CP-activated macrophages on contact with endotoxin (Carswell *et al.*, 1975). Whether TNF represents a component of the *in vivo* CP-activated macrophage antitumor process remains to be determined.

Processes facilitating the accumulation of host effector cells at a tumor site would be expected to contribute to the degree of damage inflicted by immunotherapy. In this respect, two such reports seem relevant to the effects of locally injected CP. Various strains of anaerobic coryneforms, including CP, have been found to produce chemotactic factors that attract macrophages specifically (Wilkinson *et al.*, 1973b). Moore and Hall (1973) have also observed that local injections of CP caused a local change in capillaries resulting in extravasation of lymphoblasts.

Most of the data presented in this section may be considered as evidence that the CP organism is not itself toxic for tumor cells, and our own unpublished results support this. CG added to mouse sarcoma cells *in vitro* did not alter their subsequent ability to form colonies *in vitro* (L. M.), and CP added to mouse mastocytoma cells *in vitro* did not inhibit their DNA synthesis (M. T. S.).

VIII. Clinical Experience

A. THERAPEUTIC EFFECTS

The first preliminary study of the clinical use of CP involved 141 patients with various metastatic carcinomas who received either chemotherapy (cytoxan, 5-fluorouracil, methotrexate, vinblastine, and rufocromomycin) or a combination of chemotherapy with CP twice a month (Halpern and Israel, 1971; Israel and Halpern, 1972). Two milligrams of CP were given subcutaneously in each arm every week. Therapy was continued throughout the lifetime of patients, except when discontinued during periods of low white blood cell and thrombocyte counts. The patients were monitored only for survival, and CP was found to have a significant effect. The mean survival time was 3.8 months for patients receiving chemotherapy alone, and 8.7 months for those who received CP and chemotherapy.

Further studies by the same group (Israel, 1973, 1975; Israel and Edelstein, 1975) showed that CP could be used effectively as an adjunct to chemotherapy of lung tumors, breast carcinomas, sarcomas, and melanomas. Mean survival of patients with disseminated carcinoma of epidermoid origin under chemotherapy alone was 5.6 months; it was 9.8 months if treatment with CP was included. Similarly, patients with oat-cell carcinoma survived 9.1 months if given CP and chemotherapy, but only 5.0 months if they were on chemotherapy alone. In advanced breast carcinoma, survival of patients treated with the combined modalities was 85% at 1 year and 41% at 2 years, compared with 41% and 16% of patients receiving chemotherapy alone. The 1-year survival of patients with advanced nonlymphomatous sarcomas and malignant melanomas was also significantly increased by addition of CP (Israel and Edelstein, 1975).

Immunocompetent patients, as judged by the positivity of purified protein derivative of tuberculin (PPD) skin testing, responded better to treatment with CP. An interesting observation was that CP was capable of converting negative skin tests (PPD, mumps, candidin, killed BCG, and DNCB) in about 50% of patients previously nonresponsive to these antigens.

A further observation in studies by the Israel group was that CP treatment greatly improved hematopoietic tolerance to chemotherapy. The number of chemotherapeutic interruptions due to low white blood cell and platelet counts was one-half as frequent as that in the group receiving chemotherapy alone (Israel and Edelstein, 1975), and patients treated with CP also tolerated larger doses of chemotherapy. Some recent studies have not confirmed these findings. Myelosuppression was no less severe, and the amount of chemotherapy tolerated was no greater in breast carcinoma patients who were given weekly subcutaneous injections of 4 mg of CP in addition to cyclophosphamide, adriamycin, methotrexate, and 5-fluorouracil (De Jager *et al.*, 1976). In this study CP also did not improve the effectiveness of chemotherapy. Intravenous CP (2.5 mg/m^2) also failed to reduce the myelosuppressive effects of chemotherapy in patients with breast carcinoma (Haskell *et al.*, 1976).

Subcutaneous injections of CP and CG have been used as an adjuvant to radiotherapy with ^{60}Co of patients with head and neck malignant tumors, and, in comparison with irradiation alone, slightly increased the survival rate (Mahé *et al.*, 1975). Treatment with 1mg of the bacteria commenced 6 weeks after completion of the radiation therapy. Bacteria were administered weekly for the first 6 weeks, and then once every 2 weeks for the duration of the trial.

Other preliminary reports have provided encouraging results concerning the use of subcutaneous CP in combination with surgical resection of malignant melanoma (Ishmael *et al.*, 1976) and in combination with chemotherapy of advanced ovarian cancer (Ochoa *et al.*, 1976).

Intramuscular injections of anaerobic corynebacteria have been used in immunotherapy of patients with acute lymphoid leukemia

(Schwarzenberg and Mathé, 1975). Immunotherapy was started after remission was achieved by previous chemoradiotherapy. One group of 13 patients received BCG and irradiated leukemic cells, and another 12 received this therapy plus CG once a week, given on the day of administration of BCG and tumor cells. Two-year survival was increased in the group receiving CG. Adults were given 1.5 mg of CG and children 0.75 mg of CG per injection.

Intravenous injections of CP have also been used clinically. Most studies have thus far dealt with the toxicologic and immunologic effects of CP (see below); however, several preliminary reports describing antitumor activity have already appeared. Band *et al.* (1975) treated 19 patients with various progressive metastatic solid tumors who had previously been treated with either chemotherapy, radiation therapy, or both. Doses of CP ranged from 0.5 to 6 mg/m^2 and were given by intravenous infusions daily for 10 days. Objective regressions were observed in 4 patients and include the following tumors: colon carcinomas, breast cancer, and pulmonary metastases of bone sarcoma. Israel *et al.* (1975) treated 20 terminally ill patients with various solid tumors in whom previous chemotherapy treatment had failed. Intravenous CP at a dose of 4 mg was given daily, 5 times a week, for 4–16 weeks. In 8 patients (40%) the tumors regressed to more than 50% of their original size. These were all metastases at various anatomical locations from lung adenocarcinoma, malignant melanomas, reticulum cell sarcoma, gastric cancer, testicular seminoma, and mediastinal teratoma. Partial regressions caused by CP were successfully maintained by subsequent chemotherapy and weekly subcutaneous injections of CP. Different immunological functions were evaluated during immunotherapy, and the most characteristic finding was a decrease in C3 complement which correlated directly with the clinical improvement of patients.

Impressive data on CP therapy of disseminated malignant melanoma were recently reported by Reed (1976). Single intravenous injections of CP at 5 mg/m^2 were given 19 days after chemotherapy with imidazole carboxamide (DTIC). In addition to CP, irradiated cultured melanoma cells (6×10^7 cells) were given subcutaneously. Seven of 11 patients (64%) treated in this way showed objective regression of liver metastases, compared with only 2 of 13 (15%) responses in patients treated with DTIC alone ($P < 0.05$). Patients who received the combined treatment lived longer than patients in the chemotherapy group: median survival 7.5 and 4 months, respectively. The effect on lung metastases was not as striking; 45% of patients responded to immunochemotherapy and 25% to chemotherapy.

Another study involving malignant melanoma showed that intravenous CP (2 injections of 5 mg/m² given a week apart) can increase the therapeutic effect of cyclophosphamide and DTIC (Presant *et al.*, 1976).

Single intravenous treatments with CP, 5 mg/m², decreased tumor growth and prolonged survival of patients with metastatic breast cancer (Minton *et al.*, 1976), and appreciably improved chemotherapy treatments of lung carcinoma (Takita and Moayeri, 1976; Valdivieso *et al.*, 1976).

Intratumor injection of CP, which is very efficient at producing complete regression of experimental animal tumors, has also been tried in patients (Cunningham-Rundles *et al.*, 1975; Hirshaut *et al.*, 1975; Israel, 1975). Israel (1975) reported that 11 out of 11 cutaneous melanomas and 1 out of 2 skin metastases of oat-cell carcinoma completely regressed when injected with 4–8 mg of CP for 5 consecutive days. Intratumor injections induced local inflammation within a few days, and this was sometimes followed by suppuration. Injections were also painful, causing discontinuation of prolonged treatment. In studies by Cunningham-Rundles *et al.* (1975), the mean maximum tolerated dose of intralesional CP was 18 mg. In their study 3 out of 14 injected tumors underwent complete regression and another 3 partially regressed. All six patients who responded to CP had tumors localized in the skin, whereas nonresponders had tumors which, in addition to the skin, involved subcutaneous tissues and visceral organs. The growth of uninjected tumors was not affected by this treatment.

B. Toxicity

Many Phase I clinical studies with CP have recently been conducted, and most of these have used the intravenous route of injection (Band *et al.*, 1975; Hirshaut *et al.*, 1975; Israel *et al.*, 1975; Ossorio *et al.*, 1975; Reed *et al.*, 1975b; Woodruff *et al.*, 1975; Cheng *et al.*, 1976; Fisher *et al.*, 1976b; Humphrey *et al.*, 1976; Minton *et al.*, 1976). Patients involved in these studies had various malignant tumors of very advanced clinical stages and were resistant to currently available therapies. The first study (Reed *et al.*, 1975b) employed the initial intravenous CP dose of 1 mg/m²; after this dose was shown to be safe, 2, 3, 5, and 7.5 mg/m² were investigated. The bacteria were given by infusions in 5% dextrose in water over a period ranging from 1 to 4 hours. The doses of CP employed by other investigators were usually 5 mg/m² or lower and have been administered by infusion in 250–500 ml of either saline or 5% dextrose in water over 1–4 hours. We shall summarize the side effects of intravenous CP reported in the various published studies. For the initial 2–3 hours after the start of the infusion patients have no symptoms. A chill reaction then develops in most patients, which, in an appreciable number, can be vigorous, lasting from 20 to 40 minutes. Occasionally, recurrent chills may appear after a few minutes or hours after cessation of the first chill. A high proportion of patients develop peripheral vasoconstriction manifested as a mild cyanosis or blanched appearance. Following the onset of the chill reaction, mild hypertension may occur and an increase in the pulse rate is regularly observed. Toward the end of the chill period most patients develop a fever up to 105°F, and at this time most patients have nausea, vomiting, and mild headache. Some patients may feel slightly apprehensive. The temperature usually subsides within a few hours, but may last up to 3 days. Some patients sweat profusely during the regressive phase of the fever and some of them become mildly hypotensive. Myalgias and muscle weakness are rarer symptoms that develop at higher doses of CP. The overall symptoms associated with intravenous CP are usually more intensive with increasing doses of CP. Patients receiving a second intravenous dose of CP develop the same, but less intensive, symptoms. After a few repeated infusions of CP, the symptoms are minimal or may not appear at all. Even progressively increasing daily doses soon result in decreased toxicity symptoms. Fisher et al. (1976b) observed that a single intravenous administration of 100 mg of hydrocortisone 0.5 hour prior to CP infusion markedly diminished CP toxicity.

In most studies renal and hepatic functions were not affected. However, with very high single doses of CP (more than 20 mg per patient), slight rises in serum alanine aminotransferase levels and jaundice have been detected (Woodruff et al., 1975).

A case of angina pectoris associated with a sudden rise of blood pressure (Band et al., 1975) and of a generalized Schwartzman reaction with acute azotemia and severe thrombocytopenia (Reed et al., 1975b) was also reported. Although cardiovascular changes have generally been minimal, they may be sufficient to contraindicate CP in patients with compromised cardiovascular status (Band et al., 1975).

Most of the symptoms that accompany intravenous CP injection are also associated with subcutaneous injections, but in a milder form. Fever, headache, and malaise are observed most often. At the injection sites, soreness, induration, and erythema develop and may last from several hours to a few days (Reed et al., 1975b). Local soreness has persisted occasionally for about a week. To counteract pain at the injection sites, CP has been mixed with 2% xylocaine or 1% lignocaine (Israel and Halpern, 1972; Israel and Edelstein, 1975). Similar symptoms are associated with the intralesional injections of CP (Cunningham and Rundles *et al.*, 1975).

C. Immunologic Parameters

Various immunologic parameters have been monitored in patients undergoing therapy with CP. Total white blood cell counts are rarely affected; however, alterations in the absolute number of lymphocytes and monocytes frequently occur. A decrease is already apparent within a day of CP infusion, but cell numbers return to normal within a week (Ossorio *et al.*, 1975; Reed *et al.*, 1975a; Woodruff *et al.*, 1975; Cheng *et al.*, 1976; Minton *et al.*, 1976; Ochoa *et al.*, 1976). Several investigators have reported great variability in individual total lymphocyte and T-cell counts (Israel *et al.*, 1975; Hirshaut *et al.*, 1975; Humphrey *et al.*, 1976); however, Ochoa *et al.* (1976) found decreased lymphocyte and T-cell counts in all patients. The number of circulating B cells may be increased moderately (Hirshaut *et al.*, 1975).

The PHA responsiveness of peripheral blood lymphocytes is depressed 1–5 days after intravenous CP but then recovers, occasionally rising above the base line (Reed *et al.*, 1975a; Minton *et al.*, 1976). After 1–2 months, patients receiving multiple CP injections have shown increased reactivity to T-cell mitogens, PHA, and concanavalin A (Con A), whereas responses to poke weed mitogen and streptolysin "O" have remained unchanged (Reed *et al.*, 1975b). A similar tendency toward increased PHA and Con A reactivity has also been described by Israel *et al.* (1975).

The effects of CP on skin testing with delayed-hypersensitivity antigens: dermatophytin, candida, streptokinase-streptodornase, mumps, DNCB, and others have been monitored. In studies by Reed *et al.* (1975b), 9 of 25 patients receiving intravenous CP showed an improvement in skin test responses. Cheng *et al.* (1976) reported that 10 positive reactions were converted to negative and 4 negative reactions to positive. Variable results on skin tests were also reported by Israel *et al.* (1975) and by Hirshaut *et al.* (1975). Of 6 patients initially unresponsive to DNCB, 4 became positive to the same antigen shortly after receiving their first CP dose (Hirshaut *et al.*, 1975).

James *et al.* (1975) found a constant increase in the circulating IgG levels of all patients with malignant melanoma, breast or gastric cancer who had received 20 mg of CP intravenously followed by weekly intramuscular injections of 2 mg for 10–11 weeks. All 4 subclasses of

IgG were increased, but particularly IgG$_2$. IgA, IgM, and IgE levels were inconsistently affected. The rise in immunoglobulin levels was attributed largely to the development of antibodies against CP. Preexisting antibodies were noted in all patients and titers rose within 2 weeks after the initial CP injection and remained elevated throughout the 100-day period of observation. Development of anti CP antibodies in CP-treated patients has also been observed by Minton *et al.* (1976), and they found no correlation with the antitumor activity of CP. Other studies dealing with the effects of CP on antibody production in patients with various malignant tumors have shown no significant changes in immunoglobulin levels (Dimitrov *et al.*, 1975b; Israel *et al.*, 1975; Hirshaut *et al.*, 1975). Only occasionally IgE (Woodruff *et al.*, 1975) and IgM (Hirshaut *et al.*, 1975) may be elevated.

Intravenous CP may be associated with complement activation in cancer patients. Serum levels of C3 (Dimitrov *et al.*, 1975b; Israel *et al.*, 1975) and C3 and C4 (Biran *et al.*, 1975) have been found to be decreased after intravenous CP. A similar depletion in C3 and C4 levels has occurred in normal human serum *in vitro* after addition of CP. Addition of CP to guinea pig serum, which, unlike the human serum did not contain antibodies against CP, only resulted in decreased C4 levels (McBride *et al.*, 1975c). The depletion of C3 and C4 levels in patients occurred more frequently if the patients were immunocompetent, and the suggestion is that CP activates complement in patients both directly via the alternative pathway (C3), and via the classical pathway (C1, 4, 2, . . .) when natural or induced anti-CP antibodies are present (Biran *et al.*, 1975; McBride *et al.*, 1975c). Israel *et al.* (1975) found that decrease in C3 levels in the serum of patients correlated directly with the effectiveness of CP therapy. We have already discussed a possible role for C3 cleavage products in the activation of mouse macrophages (Schorlemmer *et al.*, 1976).

IX. Perspectives and Prospects

The results achieved using CP in the treatment of experimental animal tumors have been impressive, and the overall clinical results to date are encouraging. Other than for the toxicity studies, however, the human data are as yet too preliminary to form the basis for discussing future perspectives. For this we have drawn on the large amount of animal data available, but, in doing so, are aware that there are, thus far, no human data indicating whether or not what we consider to be the modes of action of CP in animals, also operate in man. Results concerning the *in vitro* performance of macrophages and lymphocytes from CP-treated patients in both nonspecific and specific antitumor assays are eagerly awaited.

Tumor size is a critical consideration in CP immunotherapy. Throughout the animal studies, small tumor masses, even strongly antigenic ones, have responded best to treatment. Clinically these situations are likely to be seen in patients with newly diagnosed tumors at early stages, or those whose tumor burden has been reduced by prior irradiation, surgery, or chemotherapy.

The combination of CP with chemotherapy in the treatment of some animal tumors has been extremely successful, the individual antitumor effects being additive, or even synergistic. Clinical studies using CP as an adjunct to chemotherapy have been preliminary, but at least they indicate that immunostimulant therapy is not incompatible with immunosuppressive chemotherapy. The combination chemoimmunotherapy approach is likely to benefit from further animal studies using appropriate tumor models. Screening for potential synergistic or antagonistic CP-drug combinations could be rewarding. It may be that CP potentiates the antitumor activity of some drugs as it does the effects of local irradiation, or that CP-mediated antitumor effects, once established, are sensitive to subsequent drug treatment.

It is apparent that some of the therapeutic effects of CP may not be a direct result of its antitumor activity. Infection is the cause of death in some cancer patients immunosuppressed either directly as a result of the disease, or because of conventional therapies. Increased survival of any such patients receiving CP may be attributable, at least in part, to enhanced bacterial resistance resulting from reticuloendothelial stimulation. Another "indirect" antitumor effect might be that more intensive radio- or chemotherapy can be tolerated because of CP-mediated protection against their myelodepressive side effects.

Small disseminated microfoci of tumor cells persisting or appearing after successful treatment of the primary tumor mass are often the ultimate cause of death in cancer patients. It is for this reason that the establishment of systemic antitumor immunity should be the ultimate goal of any immunotherapeutic regimen. The designers of clinical trials involving CP should take into consideration the fact that different kinds of systemic antitumor immunity (specific or nonspecific) may be preferentially selected under different circumstances. The intensity and durability of the specific cell-mediated antitumor immunity that has resulted from local interaction of CP and tumor antigen in mice suggests this to be a desirable situation to achieve clinically. Optimal immunity may be restricted to situations where either direct intralesional injection or stimulation of the tumor-draining nodes is practical, or specific active immune therapy using CP mixed with attenuated tumor cells when these are obtainable. In some cases a surgically resectable tumor may be accessible to preoperative intralesional CP injection, e.g., gastric cancers via endoscopy, thereby establishing specific tumor immunity that may not result from surgical resection alone. A reasonably strong tumor-associated antigen and high degree of patient immunocompetence would both be expected to facilitate specific immunization. Animal studies indicate that optimal immunization requires a balance between the amount of CP and tumor antigen. However, given our poor understanding of the antigenicity of human tumors, clinical trials attempting specific immunization must be empirical.

The immunologically nonspecific, macrophage-mediated, systemic antitumor activity that seems to predominate after systemic injections of CP does not require close contact between CP and tumor and is likely to be independent of tumor antigenicity and patient immunocompetence. Theoretically, therefore, in the case of tumors at inaccessible sites, those of low antigenicity, and patients with poor immunocompetence, nonspecific therapy may be appropriate. Anergic patients may benefit particularly from the antibacterial effects that have been described for systemic CP. Although little nonspecific systemic stimulation has resulted from a single subcutaneous injection of CP in mice, the systemic effects of repeated subcutaneous injections have been shown to be additive. The final degree of stimulation achieved, however, was less than for the same amount of CP given as repeated systemic injections (Scott and Warner, 1976). In widely disseminated tumors, the wider distribution of CP following systemic injection would be expected to maximize the chance of CP reaching either tumor sites or draining nodes, thereby engaging specific immune mechanisms as well. Combination of systemic and regional CP injections designed to elicit both nonspecific and specific immunity may prove to be particularly effective. Suit et al. (1976b) found combination of intralesional and systemic CP to be more effective in mice than either individual treatment. Scott (1974c), however, has shown that systemic CP may diminish the effectiveness of subsequent intralesional therapy, although it did not diminish the ability of CP-irradiated tumor cell mixtures to immunize (Scott, 1975b).

The individual doses of CP that can be administered systemically in humans are considerably less than those required for effective tumor therapy in mice. However, unlike the mouse situation with rapidly growing experimental tumors, the human situation allows for repeated injections over an extended period. The effects of repeated low doses, both systemic and subcutaneous are additive in the mouse and interestingly the antitumor protection afforded by repeated low doses of CP may be greater than the total dose given as a single injection (Milas *et al.*, 1975c). In specific cell-mediated immunity resulting from CP-irradiated tumor cell mixtures in mice, the doses of CP have been in the human equivalent range (Bomford, 1975; Scott, 1975b).

Despite the fact that experimental conditions in CP animal tumor studies have been extremely uniform—i.e., the same tumor cells, in similar sites in genetically uniform, often specific pathogen-free animals—the responses of individual tumors to CP have varied. Some have regressed completely and some partially, whereas others have been unaffected (Milas *et al.*, 1974d). That CP responsiveness is affected also by genetic constitution is apparent from the differing degrees of lymphoreticular stimulation that occur in different strains of inbred mice (Stiffel *et al.*, 1970). This may be associated with differing degrees of natural immunity to CP. All these considerations would indicate that, in the considerably less uniform human situation, a wide range in the responses of "similar" tumors to CP therapy may be expected.

The identification of clinical situations in which CP may be effective is a major problem. It is apparent, however, that the basic mechanisms underlying the antitumor activity of CP, i.e., macrophage activation and potentiation of specific cell-mediated immunity, are similar to those described for BCG (see review by Bast *et al.*, 1974). The clinical assessment of BCG is more advanced than that of CP, and, given the basic similarities between the two organisms, the evaluation of CP in situations where results with BCG have been promising seems logical.

ACKNOWLEDGMENTS

We thank Professor N. Allegretti, Drs. C. Adlam, R. Bomford, and J. K. Whisnant for their criticisms and helpful suggestions during the preparation of this manuscript.

REFERENCES

Adlam, C. (1973). *J. Med. Microbiol.* **6**, 527.
Adlam, C., and Scott, M. T. (1973). *J. Med. Microbiol.* **6**, 261.
Adlam, C., Broughton, E. S., and Scott, M. T. (1972). *Nature (London), New Biol.* **235**, 219.
Adlam, C., Reid, D. E., and Torkington, P. (1975). *In* "*Corynebacterium parvum:* Applications in Experimental and Clinical Oncology" (B. Halpern, ed.), p. 35. Plenum, New York.
Allison, A. C., and Davies, P. (1971). *In* "Biological Council Symposium on Effects of

Drugs on Cellular Control Mechanisms" (B. R. Rabin and R. B. Friedman, eds.), p. 49. Macmillan, London.

Allwood, G. G., and Asherson, G. L. (1972). *Clin. Exp. Immunol.* **11**, 579.

Ambrose, E. J., James, A. M., and Lowick, J. H. (1956). *Nature (London)* **177**, 576.

Amiel, J. L., and Berardet, M. (1970). *Eur. J. Cancer* **6**, 557.

Amiel, J. L., Litwin, J., and Berardet, M. (1969). *Eur. J. Clin. Biol. Res.* **14**, 909.

Asherson, G. L., and Allwood, G. G. (1971). *Clin. Exp. Immunol.* **9**, 249.

Aub, J. C., Tieslan, C., and Lankaster, A. (1963). *Proc. Natl. Acad. Sci. U.S.A.* **50**, 613.

Azuma, I., Sugimura, K., Taniyama, T., Aladin, A., and Yamamura, Y. (1975). *Jpn. J. Microbiol.* **19**, 265.

Azuma, I., Sugimura, K., Taniyama, T., Yamawaki, M., Yamamura, Y., Kusomoto, S., Okada, S., and Shiba, T. (1976). *Infect. Immun.* **14**, 18.

Band, P. R., Jao-King, C., Urtasun, R. C., and Haraphongse, M. (1975). *Cancer Chemother. Rep.* **59**, 1139.

Bašić, I., Milas, L., Grdina, D. J., and Withers, H. R. (1974). *J. Natl. Cancer Inst.* **52**, 1839.

Bašić, I., Milas, L., Grdina, D. J., and Withers, H. R. (1975a). *J. Natl. Cancer Inst.* **55**, 589.

Bašić, I., Milas, L., and Withers, R. H. (1975b). *4th Annu. Conf. Int. Soc. Exp. Hematol.* p. 3.

Bast, R. C., Zbar, B., Borsos, T., and Rapp, H. J. (1974). *N. Engl. J. Med.* **290**, 1413 and 1496.

Baum, H., and Baum, M. (1974). *Lancet* **2**, 1397.

Baum, M., and Breese, M. (1976). *Br. J. Cancer* **33**, 468.

Biozzi, G., Howard, J. G., Mouton, D., and Stiffel, C. (1965). *Transplantation* **3**, 170.

Biozzi, G., Stiffel, C., Mouton, D., Bouthillier, Y., and Decreusefond, C. (1968). *Immunology* **14**, 7.

Biozzi, G., Stiffel, C., Mouton, D., Bouthillier, Y., and Decreusefond, C. (1972). *Ann. Inst. Pasteur, Paris* **122**, 685.

Biran, H., Moake, J. L., Reed, R., and Freireich, E. J. (1975). *Clin. Res.* **23**, 409A.

Bomford, R. (1975). *Br. J. Cancer* **32**, 551.

Bomford, R. (1977). To be published.

Bomford, R., and Christie, G. H. (1975). *Cell. Immunol.* **17**, 150.

Bomford, R., and Olivotto, M. (1974). *Int. J. Cancer* **14**, 226

Brozovic, B., Šljivić, V. S., and Warr, G. W. (1975). *Br. J. Exp. Pathol.* **56**, 183

Bryceson, A. D. M., Preston, P. M., Bray, R. S., and Dumonde, D. C. (1972). *Clin. Exp. Immunol.* **10**, 305.

Burger, M. M. (1969). *Proc. Natl. Acad. Sci. U.S.A.* **62**, 994.

Carswell, E. A., Old, L. J., Kassel, R. L., Green, S., Fiore, N., and Williamson, B. (1975). *Proc. Natl. Acad. Sci. U.S.A.* **72**, 3666.

Castro, J. E. (1974a). *Eur. J. Cancer* **10**, 115.

Castro, J. E. (1974b). *Eur. J. Cancer* **10**, 121.

Cerutti, I. (1975). *In* "*Corynebacterium parvum:* Applications in Experimental and Clinical Oncology" (B. Halpern, ed.), p. 84. Plenum, New York.

Cheng, V. S. T., Suit, H. D., Wang, C. C., and Cummings, C. (1976). *Cancer* **37**, 1687.

Christie, G. H., and Bomford, R. (1975). *Cell. Immunol.* **17**, 141.

Clark, I. A., Cox, F. E. G., and Allison, A. C. (1977). *Parasitology* **74**, 9.

Cleveland, R. P., Meltzer, M. S., and Zbar, B. (1974). *J. Natl. Cancer Inst.* **52**, 1887.

Colapinto, N. D. (1975). *Proc. R. Soc. London, Ser.* **189B**, 107.

Collet, A. J. (1971). *RES, J. Reticuloendothel. Soc.* **9**, 424.

Collins, F. M. (1974). *Bacteriol. Rev.* **38**, 371.

Collins, F. M., and Scott, M. T. (1974). *Infect. Immun.* **9**, 863.

Cox, K. O., and Keast, D. (1974). *Clin. Exp. Immunol.* **17**, 199.

Cudkowicz, G., and Bennett, M. (1971a). *J. Exp. Med.* **134**, 83.

Cudkowicz, G., and Bennett, M. (1971b). *J. Exp. Med.* **134**, 1513.

Cummins, C. S., and Johnson, J. L. (1974). *J. Gen. Microbiol.* **80**, 433.

Cunningham-Rundles, W. F., Hirshaut, Y., Pinsky, C. M., and Oettgen, H. F. (1975). *Clin. Res.* **23**, 337A.

Currie, G. A., and Bagshawe, K. D. (1970). *Br. Med. J.* **1**, 541.

Dawes, J., and McBride, W. H. (1975). *Immunochemistry* **12**, 855.

de Duve, C., Wattiaux, R., and Wibo, M. (1962). *Biochem. Pharmacol.* **9**, 97.

Degrand, F., and Raynaud, M. (1973). *Eur. J. Immunol.* **3**, 660.

De Jager, R., Pinsky, C., Kaufman, R., Ochoa, M., Oettgen, H., and Krakoff, I. (1976). *Proc. Am. Soc. Clin. Oncol.* **17**, 296.

del Guercio, P. (1972). *Nature (London), New Biol.* **238**, 213.

Dimitrov, N. V., Andre, S., Eliopoulos, G., and Halpern, B. (1975a). *Proc. Soc. Exp. Biol. Med.* **148**, 440.

Dimitrov, N. V., Israel, L., and Peltier, A. (1975b). *Proc. Am. Soc. Clin. Oncol.* **16**, 258.

Farber, P. A., and Glasgow, L. A. (1972). *Infect. Immun.* **6**, 272.

Farquhar, D., Loo, T. L., Reed, R., and Luna, M. (1975). *Lancet* **1**, 914.

Fauve, R. M. (1975). In *"Corynebacterium parvum:* Applications in Experimental and Clinical Oncology" (B. Halpern, ed.), p. 77. Plenum, New York.

Fauve, R. M., and Hevin, M. B. (1971). *Ann. Inst. Pasteur, Paris* **120**, 399.

Fauve, R. M., and Hevin, B. (1974). *Proc. Natl. Acad. Sci. U.S.A.* **71**, 573.

Fischbach, J., and Glasgow, L. A. (1975). *Infect. Immun.* **11**, 80.

Fisher, B., Wolmark, N., and Coyle, J. (1974). *J. Natl. Cancer Inst.* **53**, 1793.

Fisher, B., Wolmark, N., Rubin, H., and Saffer, E. (1975a). *J. Natl. Cancer Inst.* **55**, 1147.

Fisher, B., Wolmark, N., Saffer, E., and Fisher, E. R. (1975b). *Cancer* **35**, 134.

Fisher, B., Rubin, H., Saffer, E., and Wolmark, N. (1976a). *J. Natl. Cancer Inst.* **56**, 571.

Fisher, B., Rubin, H., Sartiano, G., Ennis, L., and Wolmark, N. (1976b). *Cancer* **38**, 119.

Fisher, J. C., Grace, W. R., and Mannick, J. A. (1970). *Cancer* **26**, 1379.

Foster, R. S., Jr. (1976). *Proc. Am. Assoc. Cancer Res.* **17**, 203.

Frost, P., and Lance, E. M. (1973). *Immunopotentiation, Ciba Found. Symp., 1973* No. 18, p. 29.

Ghaffar, A., Cullen, R. T., Dunbar, N., and Woodruff, M. F. A. (1974). *Br. J. Cancer* **29**, 199.

Ghaffar, A., Cullen, R. T., and Woodruff, M. F. A. (1975). *Br. J. Cancer* **31**, 15.

Green, S., Dobrjansky, A., Chiasson, M. A., Carswell, E. A., Helson, L., Schwartz, M. K., and Old, L. J. (1976). *Proc. Am. Assoc. Cancer Res.* **17**, 84.

Hakomori, S., and Murakami, W. T. (1968). *Proc. Natl. Acad. Sci. U.S.A.* **59**, 254.

Halpern, B., and Fray, A. (1969). *Ann. Inst. Pasteur, Paris* **117**, 778.

Halpern, B., Fray, A., Crépin, Y., Platica, O., Lorinet, A. M., Rabourdin, A., Sparros, L., and Isac, R. (1973). *Immunopotentiation, Ciba Found. Symp., 1973* No. 18, p. 217.

Halpern, B., Crépin, Y., and Rabourdin, A. (1975). In *"Corynebacterium parvum:* Applications in Experimental and Clinical Oncology" (B. Halpern, ed.), p. 191. Plenum, New York.

Halpern, B. N., and Israel, L. (1971). *C. R. Hebd. Seances Acad. Sci.* **273**, 2186.

Halpern, B. N., Prévot, A. R., Biozzi, G., Stiffel, C., Mouton, D., Morard, J. C., Bouthillier, Y., and Decreusefond, C. (1964). *RES, J. Reticuloendothel. Soc.* **1**, 77.

Halpern, B. N., Biozzi, G., Stiffel, C., and Mouton, D. (1966). *Nature (London)* **212**, 853.

Hammond, E. M., and Dvorak, H. F. (1972). *J. Exp. Med.* **136**, 1518.
Haskell, C. M., Ossorio, C., Sarna, G. P., and Fahey, J. L. (1976). *Proc. Am. Soc. Clin. Oncol.* **17**, 265.
Hattori, T., and Mori, A. (1973). *Gann* **64**, 15.
Hibbs, J. B., Jr. (1973). *Science* **180**, 868.
Hibbs, J. B., Jr. (1974). *Science* **184**, 468.
Hibbs, J. B. Jr., Lambert, L., Jr., and Remington, J. S. (1972). *Nature (London), New Biol.* **235**, 48.
Hirshaut, Y., Pinsky, C., Cunningham-Rundles, W., Rao, B., Fried, J., and Oettgen, H. (1975). *Proc. Am. Assoc. Cancer Res.* **16**, 181.
Houchens, D. P., and Gaston, M. R. (1976). *Proc. Am. Assoc. Cancer Res.* **17**, 53.
Howard, J. G. (1968). *In* "Structure et éffect biologique de produits bacteriens provenant de bacilles gram negatifs " (L. Chedid ed.) p. 331. CNRS, Paris.
Howard, J. G., Biozzi, G., Stiffel, C., Mouton, D., and Liacopoulos, P. (1967). *Transplantation* **5**, 1510.
Howard, J. G., Scott, M. T., and Christie, G. H. (1973a). *Immunopotentiation, Ciba Found. Symp., 1973* No. 18, p. 101.
Howard, J. G., Christie, G. H., and Scott, M. T. (1973b). *Cell. Immunol.* **7**, 290.
Humphrey, G., Nitschke, R., Oleinick, S., Wells, J., Cox, C., and Lankford, J. (1976). *Proc. Am. Assoc. Cancer Res.* **17**, 198.
Ishmael, D. R., Bottomley, R. H., Hoge, A. F., and Zieren, J. D. (1976). *Proc. Am. Assoc. Cancer Res.* **17**, 105.
Israel, L. (1973). *Cancer Chemother. Rep.* **4**, 283.
Israel, L. (1975). *In* "Corynebacterium parvum: Applications in Experimental and Clinical Oncology" (B. Halpern, ed.) p. 389. Plenum, New York.
Israel, L., and Edelstein, R. L. (1975). *Collect. Pap. Annu. Symp. Fundam. Cancer Res.* **26**, 485.
Israel, L., and Halpern, B. N. (1972). *Nouv. Presse Med.* **1**, 19.
Israel, L., Edelstein, R., Depierre, A., and Dimitrov, N. (1975). *J. Natl. Cancer Inst.* **55**, 29.
James, K., Ghaffar, A., and Milne, I. (1974). *Br. J. Cancer* **29**, 11.
James, K., Clunie, G. J. A., Woodruff, M. F. A., McBride, W. H., Stimson, W. H., Drew, R., and Catty, D. (1975). *Br. J. Cancer* **32**, 310.
James, K., Willmott, N., Milne, I., and McBride, W. H. (1976). *J. Natl. Cancer Inst.* **56**, 1035.
Johnson, J. L., and Cummins, C. S. (1972). *J. Bacteriol.* **109**, 1047.
Jollès, P., Megliore-Samour, D., Korontzis, M., Floc'h, F., Maral, R., and Werner, G. N. (1975). *In* "Corynebacterium parvum: Applications in Experimental and Clinical Oncology" (B. Halpern ed.), p. 40. Plenum, New York.
Kierszenbaum, F. (1975). *Infect. Immun.* **12**, 1227.
Kirchner, H., Glaser, M., and Herberman, R. B. (1975a). *Nature (London)* **257**, 396.
Kirchner, H., Holden, H. T., and Herberman, R. B. (1975b). *J. Immunol.* **115**, 1212.
Kouznetzova, B., Bizzini, B., Chermann, J. C., Degrand, F., Prévot, A. R., and Raynand, M. (1974). *Recent Results Cancer Res.* **47**, 275.
Krahenbuhl, J. L., and Remington, J. S. (1974). *J. Immunol.* **113**, 507.
Lamensans, A., Stiffel, C., Mollier, M. F., Mouton, D., and Biozzi, G. (1968). *Eur. J. Clin. Biol. Res.* **13**, 773.
Likhite, V. V. (1974). *Int. J. Cancer* **14**, 684.
Likhite, V. V. (1975). *J. Immunol.* **114**, 1736.
Likhite, V. V. (1976). *Nature (London)* **259**, 397.
Likhite, V. V., and Halpern, B. N. (1973). *Int. J. Cancer* **12**, 699.

Likhite, V. V., and Halpern, B. N. (1974). *Cancer Res.* **34**, 341.

Lotzova, E., and Cudkowicz, G. (1972). *Transplantation* **13** 256.

McBride, W. H., Jones, J. T., and Weir, D. M. (1974). *Br. J. Exp. Pathol.* **55**, 38.

McBride, W. H., Dawes, J., Dunbar, N., Ghaffar, A., and Woodruff, M. F. A. (1975a). *Immunology* **28**, 49.

McBride, W. H., Tuach, S., and Marmion, B. P. (1975b). *Br. J. Cancer* **32**, 558.

McBride, W. H., Weir, D. M., Kay, A. B., Pearce, D., and Caldwell, J. R. (1975c). *Clin. Exp. Immunol.* **19**, 143.

McBride, W. H., Daves, J., and Tuach, S. (1976). *J. Natl. Cancer Inst.* **56**, 437.

McCracken, A., McBride, W. H., and Weir, D. M. (1971). *Clin. Exp. Immunol.* **8**, 949.

Mahé, E., Bourdin, J. S., Gest, J., Saracino, R., Brunet, M., Halpern, G., Deband, B., and Roth, F. (1975). *In* "*Corynebacterium parvum:* Applications in Experimental and Clinical Oncology" (B. Halpern, ed.), p. 376. Plenum, New York.

Mantovani, A., Tagliabue, A., Vecchi, A., and Spreafico, F. (1976). *Eur. J. Cancer* **12**, 113.

Mathé, G., Pouillart, P., and Lapeyraque, F. (1969). *Br. J. Cancer* **23**, 814.

Mathé, G., Kamel, M., Dezfulian, M., Halle-Panenko, O., and Bourut, C. (1973). *Cancer Res.* **33**, 1987.

Mazurek, C., Chalvet, H., Stiffel, C., and Biozzi, G. (1976). *Int. J. Cancer* **17**, 511.

Migliore-Samour, D., Kovontzis, M., Jollès, P., Maral, R., Floc'h, F., and Werner, G. H. (1974). *Immunol. Commun.* **3**, 593.

Milas, L. (1975). *Lancet* **1**, 695.

Milas, L., and Mujagić, H. (1972). *Eur. J. Clin. Biol. Res.* **17**, 498.

Milas, L., and Withers, H. R. (1976). *Radiology* **118**, 211.

Milas, L., Gutterman, J. U., Bašić, I., Hunter, N., Mavligit, G. M., Hersh, E. M., and Withers, H. R. (1974a). *Int. J. Cancer* **14**, 493.

Milas, L., Hunter, N., Bašić, I., and Withers, H. R. (1974b). *J. Natl. Cancer Inst.* **52**, 1875.

Milas, L., Hunter, N., and Withers, R. H. (1974c). *Cancer Res.* **34**, 613.

Milas, L., Hunter, N., Bašić, I., and Withers, H. R. (1974d) *Cancer Res.* **34**, 2470.

Milas, L., Hunter, N., and Withers, H. R. (1975a). *Cancer Res.* **35**, 1274.

Milas, L., Hunter, N., Bašić, I., Mason, K., Grdina, D. J., and Withers, H. R. (1975b). *J. Natl. Cancer Inst.* **54**, 895.

Milas, L., Bašić, I., Kogelnik, H. D., and Withers, H. R. (1975c). *Cancer Res.* **35**, 2365.

Milas, L., Kogelnik, H. D., Bašić, I., Mason, K., Hunter, N., and Withers, H. R. (1975d). *Int. J. Cancer* **16**, 738.

Milas, L., Withers, H. R., and Hunter, N. (1975e). *Proc. Am. Assoc. Cancer Res.* **16**, 154.

Milas, L., Mason, K., and Withers, H. R. (1976). *Cancer Immunol. Immunother.* **1**, 233.

Minton, J. P., Rossio, J. L., Dixon, B., and Dodd, M. C. (1976). *Clin. Exp. Immunol.* **24**, 441.

Moore, A. R., and Hall, J. G. (1973). *Cell. Immunol.* **8**, 112.

Morahan, P. S., and Kaplan, A. M. (1976). *Int. J. Cancer* **17**, 82.

Morahan, P. S., Schuller, G. B., Snodgrass, M. J., and Kaplan, A. M. (1976). *J. Infect. Dis.* **133** (Suppl.), A 249.

Moroson, H., and Schechter, M. (1976). *Biomedicine.* **25**, 97.

Mosedale, B., and Smith, M. A. (1975). *Lancet* **1**, 1968.

Munder, P. G., and Modelell, M. (1974). *Recent Results Cancer Res.* **47**, 244.

Nathan, C. F., Karnovsky, M. L., and David, J. R. (1971). *J. Exp. Med.* **133**, 1356.

Neveu, T., Branellec, A., and Biozzi, G. (1964). *Ann. Inst. Pasteur, Paris* **106**, 771.

Nussenzweig, R. S. (1967). *Exp. Parasitol.* **21**, 224.

Ochoa, M., Jr., Wanebo, H. J., and Lewis, J. L., Jr. (1976). *Proc. Am. Assoc. Cancer Res.* **17**, 170.

Old, L. J., Clarke, D. A., Benacerraf, B., and Goldsmith, M. (1960). *Ann. N.Y. Acad. Sci.* **88**, 264.
Old, L. J., Benacerraf, B., Clarke, D. A., Carswell, E. A., and Stockert, E. (1961). *Cancer Res.* **21**, 1281.
Olivotto, M., and Bomford, R. (1974). *Int. J. Cancer* **13**, 478.
O'Neill, G. J., Henderson, D. C., and White, R. G. (1973). *Immunology* **24**, 977.
Ossorio, R. C., Fahey, J. L., Wilson, W., Platkin, D., Brossman, S., and Skinner, D. (1975). *Lancet* **2**, 1090.
Paslin, D., Dimitrov, N. V., and Heaton, C. (1974). *J. Natl. Cancer Inst.* **52**, 571.
Pearson, J. W., Pearson, G. R., Gibson, W. T., Chermann, J. C., and Chirigos, M. A. (1972). *Cancer Res.* **32**, 904.
Pearson, J. W., Chaparas, S. D., Torgersen, J. A., Perk, K., Chirigos, M. A., and Sher, N. A. (1974a). *Cancer Res.* **34**, 355.
Pearson, J. W., Chirigos, M. A., Charapas, S. D., and Sher, N. A. (1974b). *J. Natl. Cancer Inst.* **52**, 463.
Pearson, J. W., Perk, K., Chirigos, M. A., Pryor, J. W., and Fuhrman, F. S. (1975). *Int. J. Cancer* **16**, 142.
Peters, L. J., McBride, W. H., Mason, K. A., Hunter, N., Bašić, I., and Milas, L. (1977). Submitted for publication.
Philippon, A., Krazmierczak, A., and Nevot, P. (1972). *Ann. Inst. Pasteur, Paris* **123**, 349.
Pinckard, R. N., and Halonen, M. (1971). *J. Immunol.* **106**, 1602.
Pinckard, R. N., Weir, D. M., and McBride, W. H. (1967a). *Clin. Exp. Immunol.* **2**, 331.
Pinckard, R. N., Weir, D. M., and McBride, W. H. (1967b). *Clin. Exp. Immunol.* **2**, 343.
Pinckard, R. N., Weir, D. M., and McBride, W. H. (1968). *Clin. Exp. Immunol.* **3**, 413.
Presant, C. A., Smalley, R. V., and Vogler, W. R. (1976). *Proc. Am. Soc. Clin. Oncol.* **17**, 241.
Prévot, A. R., and Van Phi, J. T. (1964). *C. R. Hebd. Seances Acad. Sci.* **258**, 4619.
Proctor, J., Rudenstam, C. M., and Alexander, P. (1973). *Biomedicine* **19**, 248.
Puvion, F., Fray, A., and Halpern, B. (1975). *In* "Corynebacterium parvum: Applications in Experimental and Clinical Oncology" (B. Halpern, ed.), p. 137. Plenum, New York.
Puvion, F., Fray, A., and Halpern, B. (1976). *J. Ultrastruct. Res.* **54**, 95.
Rauchwerger, J. H., Gallagher, M. T., Monie, H. J., and Trentin, J. J. (1976). *Biomedicine.* **24**, 20.
Raynaud, M., Kouznetzova, B., Bizzini, B., and Cherman, J. C. (1972). *Ann. Inst. Pasteur, Paris* **122**, 695.
Reed, R. C., (1976). *Proc. Am. Assoc. Cancer Res.* **17**, 214.
Reed, R. C., Gutterman, J. U., Mavligit, G. M., and Hersh, E. M. (1975a). *Proc. Am. Soc. Clin. Oncol.* **16**, 228.
Reed, R. C., Gutterman, J. U., Mavligit, G. M., Burgess, A. A., and Hersh, E. M. (1975b). *In* "Corynebacterium parvum: Applications in Experimental and Clinical Oncology" (B. Halpern, ed.), p. 349. Plenum, New York.
Rees, R. C., and Potter, C. W. (1974). *J. Med. Microbiol.* **7**, 17.
Roberts, R. M., Walker, A., and Cetorelli, J. J. (1973). *Nature (London), New Biol.* **244**, 86.
Roth, S., and White, D. (1972). *Proc. Natl. Acad. Sci. U.S.A.* **69**, 485.
Roumiantzeff, M., Mynard, M. C., Coquet, B., Goldman, C., and Ayme, G. (1975a). *In* "Corynebacterium parvum: Applications in Experimental and Clinical Oncology" (B. Halpern, ed.), p. 11. Plenum, New York.
Roumiantzeff, M., Musetescu, M., Ayme, G., and Mynard, M. C. (1975b). *In Corynebac-*

terium parvum: "Applications in Experimental and Clinical Oncology" (B. Halpern, ed.), p. 202. Plenum, New York.

Ruitenberg, E. J., and Steerenberg, P. A. (1973). *Nature (London), New Biol.* **242**, 149.

Ruitenberg, E. J., and van Noorle Jansen, L. M. (1975). *Zentralbl. Bakteriol., Parasitenkd., Infeutionskr. Hyg., Abt. 1: Orig., Reine A* **231**, 197.

Russel, R. J., McInroy, R. J., Wilkinson, P. C., and White, R. G. (1976). *Immunology* **30**, 935.

Sadler, T. E., and Castro, J. E. (1975). *Br. J. Cancer* **31**, 359.

Sadler, T. E., and Castro, J. E. (1976). *Br. J. Surg.* **63**, 292.

Schorlemmer, H. U., Davies, P., and Allison, A. C. (1976). *Nature (London)* **261**, 48.

Schwarzenberg, L., and Mathé, G. (1975). *In* "*Corynebacterium parvum:* Applications in Experimental and Clinical Oncology" (B. Halpern, ed.), p. 372. Plenum, New York.

Scott, M. T. (1972a). *Cell. Immunol.* **5**, 459.

Scott, M. T. (1972b). *Cell. Immunol.* **5**, 469.

Scott, M. T. (1974a). *Cell. Immunol.* **13**, 251.

Scott, M. T. (1974b). *J. Natl. Cancer Inst.* **53**, 855.

Scott, M. T. (1974c). *J. Natl. Cancer Inst.* **53**, 861.

Scott, M. T. (1974d). *Semin. Oncol.* **1**, 367.

Scott, M. T. (1975a). *J. Natl. Cancer Inst.* **54**, 789.

Scott, M. T. (1975b). *J. Natl. Cancer Inst.* **55**, 65.

Scott, M. T. (1976). *J. Natl. Cancer Inst.* **56**, 675.

Scott, M. T., and Warner, S. L. (1976). *Cancer Res.* **36**, 1335.

Smith, S. E., and Scott, M. T. (1972). *Br. J. Cancer* **26**, 361.

Stiffel, C., Mouton, D., Bouthillier, Y., Decreusefond, C., and Biozzi, G. (1966). *RES, J. Reticuloendothel. Soc.* **3**, 439.

Stiffel, C., Mouton, D., Bouthillier, Y., Decreusefond, C., and Biozzi, G. (1970). *RES, J. Reticuloendothel. Soc.* **7**, 280.

Stiffel, C., Mouton, D., and Biozzi, G. (1971). *Ann. Inst. Pasteur, Paris* **120**, 412.

Stiffel, C., Mouton, D., and Biozzi, G. (1974). *Recent Results Cancer Res.* **47**, 239.

Stjernswärd, J., Jondal, M., Vánky, F., Wigzell, H., and Sealy, R. (1972). *Lancet* **1**, 1352.

Suit, H. D., Sedlacek, R., Wagner, M., and Orsi, L. (1975). *Nature (London)* **255**, 493.

Suit, H. D., Sedlacek, R., Silobrčić, V., and Lingood, R. M. (1976a). *Cancer (Philadelphia)* **37**, 2573.

Suit, H. D., Sedlacek, R., Wagner, M., Orsi, L., Silobrčić, V., and Rothman, J. (1976b). *Cancer Res.* **36**, 1305.

Swartzberg, J. E., Krahenbuhl, J. L., and Remington, J. S. (1975). *Infect. Immun.* **12**, 1037.

Takita, H., and Moayeri, H. (1976). *Proc. Am. Soc. Clin. Oncol.* **17**, 292.

Toujas, L., Dazord, L., Le Garrec, Y., and Sabolovic, D. (1972). *Experientia* **28**, 1223.

Toujas, L., Dazord, L., Houy, J. C., Guelfi, J., Fleury-Touzeau, F., and Pilet, C. (1974). *Rev. Pathol. Comp. Med. Exp.* **74**, 29.

Toujas, L., Dazord, L., and Guelfi, J. (1975). *In* "*Corynebacterium parvum:* Applications in Experimental and Clinical Oncology" (B. Halpern, ed.), p. 117. Plenum, New York.

Turner, R. J., Nguyen-Dang, T., and Manning, M. J. (1974). *RES, J. Reticuloendothel. Soc.* **16**, 232.

Tuttle, R. L., and North, R. J. (1975). *J. Natl. Cancer Inst.* **55**, 1403.

Tuttle, R. L., and North, R. J. (1976a). *RES, J. Reticuloendothel. Soc.* **20**, 197.

Tuttle, R. L., and North, R. J. (1976b). *RES, J. Reticuloendothel. Soc.* **20**, 209.

Valdivieso, M., Hersh, E. M., Rodriquez, V., Gutterman, J. U., and Freireich, E. J. (1976). *Proc. Am. Assoc. Cancer Res.* **17**, 170.

van Neil, C. B. (1928). "The Propionic Acid Bacteria." Boissevain, Harlem.

van Putten, L. M., Kram, L. K. J., van Dierendonck, H. H. C., Smink, T., and Füzy, M. (1975). *Int. J. Cancer* **15**, 588.

Warr, G. W., and Šljivić, V. S. (1974a). *Clin. Exp. Immunol.* **17**, 519.

Warr, G. W., and Šljivić, V. S. (1974b). *RES, J. Reticuloendothel. Soc.* **16**, 193.

Warr, G. W., and Šljivić, V. S. (1974c). *Tissue Cell Kinet.* **7**, 559.

Watson, S. R., and Šlijivić, V. S. (1976). *Clin. Exp. Immunol.* **23**, 149.

Weissmann, G., and Dingle, J. (1961). *Exp. Cell Res.* **25**, 207.

Wiener, E. (1975). *Cell. Immunol.* **19**, 1.

Wiener, E., and Bandieri, A. (1975). *Immunology* **29**, 265.

Wilkinson, P. C., O'Neill, G. J., McInroy, R. J., Cater, J. C., and Roberts, J. A. (1973a). *Immunopotentiation, Ciba Found. Symp., 1973* No. 18, p. 121.

Wilkinson, P. C., O'Neill, G. J., and Wapshaw, K. G. (1973b). *Immunology* **24**, 997.

Withers, H. R. (1974). *Adv. Radiat. Biol.* **4**, 241.

Wolmark, N., and Fisher, B. (1974). *Cancer Res.* **34**, 2869.

Wolmark, N., Levine, M., and Fisher, B. (1974). *RES, J. Reticuloendothel. Soc.* **16**, 252.

Woodruff, M. F. A., and Boak, J. L. (1966). *Br. J. Cancer* **20**, 345.

Woodruff, M. F. A., and Dunbar, N. (1973). *Immunopotentiation, Ciba Found. Symp., 1973* No. 18, p. 287.

Woodruff, M. F. A., and Dunbar, N. (1975). *Br. J. Cancer* **32**, 34.

Woodruff, M. F. A., and Inchley, M. P. (1971). *Br. J. Cancer* **25**, 584.

Woodruff, M. F. A., Inchley, M. P., and Dunbar, N. (1972). *Br. J. Cancer* **26**, 67.

Woodruff, M. F. A., Dunbar, N., and Ghaffar, A. (1973). *Proc. R. Soc. London, Ser. B* **184**, 97.

Woodruff, M. F. A., McBride, W. H., and Dunbar, N. (1974). *Clin. Exp. Immunol.* **17**, 509.

Woodruff, M. F. A., Clunie, G. J. A., McBride, W. H., McCormack, R. J. M., Walbaum, P. R., and James, K. (1975). *In* "Corynebacterium parvum: Applications in Experimental and Clinical Oncology" (B. Halpern, ed.), p. 383. Plenum, New York.

Yamamura, Y., Azuma, I., Sugimura, I., Kusumoto, S., and Shiba, T. (1976). *Proc. Jpn. Acad.* **52**, 58.

Yuhas, J. M., and Ullrich, R. L. (1976). *Cancer Res.* **36**, 161.

Yuhas, J. M., Toya, R. E., and Wagner, E. (1975). *Cancer Res.* **35**, 242.

Zola, H. (1975). *Clin. Exp. Immunol.* **22**, 514.

SUBJECT INDEX

A

2-Acetylaminofluorene, as intestinal
carcinogen, 120
cis-Aconitic acid, as carcinogenesis
inhibitor, 220
Adenomatous polyps
epidemiology of, 122–126, 130
large-bowel cancer and, 98–100, 108,
111–114
Age factors, in large-bowel cancer, 18–22
Alcohol, large-bowel cancer and use of,
76–78
Antioxidants, as carcinogenesis inhibitors,
203–215
Appendectomies, large-bowel cancer and,
91–92
Arteriosclerotic heart disease, large-bowel
cancer and, 80–82, 85–86
Azoxymethane, as carcinogen, 203

B

Bacteriodes, as fecal flora, 115–116
α-Benzene hexachloride, as
carcinogenesis inhibitor, 216
Benzo[a]pyrene, as carcinogen, 201
Benzyl isothiocyanate, as carcinogenesis
inhibitor, 204, 212–214
Bifidobacteria, as fecal flora, 115–116
Bis(ethylxanthogen), as carcinogenesis
inhibitor, 204
Bracken toxin, as intestinal carcinogen,
121
Breast cancer, large-bowel cancer and, 80,
83–84
Butylated hydroxyanisole, as
carcinogenesis inhibitor, 203–208
Butylated hydroxytoluene, as
carcinogenesis inhibitor, 203–208

C

C3Hf system, mammary tumors in
169–175
Carcinoembryonic antigens (CEA),
large-bowel cancer and, 90–91
Cell replication, in colorectal cancer,
119–120
Cellular immunity, C. parvum effects on,
262–264
Chemical carcinogenesis, inhibitors of,
197–226
Chemotherapy, C. parvum combined
with use of, 279–281
Chlordane, as carcinogenesis inhibitor,
216
Cholesterol, fecal conversion of, 116, 117
Clostridia, fecal, as possible cancer
indicator, 131
Clostridium paraputrificum, as fecal flora,
116
Colon-rectum ratios, of large-bowel
cancer, 10–13
Corynebacterium parvum
antitumor activity of, 257–306
of various fractions, 281–282
chemotherapy combined with use of,
279–281
clinical experience with, 290–296
effects on experimental neoplasia,
268–290
future prospects for, 296–299
hematopoietic influence of, 260–261
immune modulation by, 262–267
cellular immunity, 264–266
humoral immunity, 262–264
immunity to, 288–289
immunologic parameters following use
of, 295–296
immunoprophylaxis by, 269–272
immunotherapy by, 272–277
combination with active agent,
276–277

307

CONTENTS OF PREVIOUS VOLUMES

A
B   8
C   9
D   0
E   1
F   2
G   3
H   4
I   5
J   6